Robotic Approaches to Colorectal Surgery

Howard Ross • Sang W. Lee
Bradley J. Champagne
Alessio Pigazzi • David E. Rivadeneira
Editors

Robotic Approaches to Colorectal Surgery

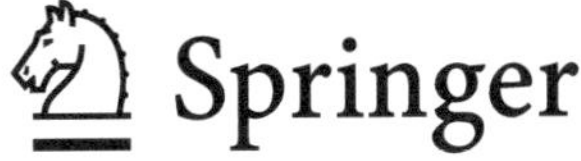

Editors
Howard Ross
Division of Colon and Rectal Surgery
  Department of Surgery
Temple University Health System
Philadelphia, PA, USA

Bradley J. Champagne
Division of Colorectal Surgery
University Hospitals Case Medical Center
Cleveland, USA

David E. Rivadeneira
North Shore-LIJ Health System
Huntington Hospital, Hofstra School
  of Medicine
Woodbury, NY, USA

Sang W. Lee
Chief of Colon & Rectal Surgery
Professor of Clinical Surgery
University of Southern California
Keck School of Medicine
Los Angels, CA

Alessio Pigazzi
University of California, Irvine
Orange, CA, USA

Videos can also be accessed at http://link.springer.com/
book/10.1007/978-3-319-09120-4

ISBN 978-3-319-35625-9   ISBN 978-3-319-09120-4   (eBook)
DOI 10.1007/978-3-319-09120-4

Springer International Publishing AG Switzerland is part of Springer Science+Business Media
(www.springer.com)

Foreword

The evolution of robotic surgery, from a platform initially developed to improve the surgical care of combat casualties to the most technically advanced surgical instrument ever introduced in many fields, has been nothing but extraordinary. After a lukewarm reception in cardiac surgery in the late 1990s, robotic systems have been embraced in urology and then in gynecology during the past decade, offering surgeons safe, precise, and reproducible approaches to complex pelvic surgery, and becoming the most widely utilized minimally invasive platforms in these specialties.

Although the adoption of robotics in general surgery has been somewhat slow, there is no doubt that the last few years have seen an exponential increase in the number of robotic procedures in this area. Moreover, no field in this specialty has been more promising for robotic applications than colorectal surgery. After the first robotic colectomy performed by Garth Ballantyne in 2002, the emphasis has mostly been on pelvic applications in subsequent years, with a number of centers from all over the world showing very promising results in terms of conversion rates and margin positivity with robotic total mesorectal excision (TME) compared to laparoscopic dissection. Indeed, in a recent analysis of the National Inpatient Sample (NIS), low anterior and abdomino-perineal resections were the most common robotic colorectal procedures with over 50 % of cases as opposed to just over 8 % with conventional laparoscopy [1]. Although robotic surgery accounted for less than 3 % of all NIS colorectal procedure in 2010, this figure has almost doubled in 2012 and is expected to continue to grow accordingly (Pigazzi et al. unpublished data).

One significant limitation of robotic surgery has been its poor applicability in multi-quadrant surgery. For this reason, many colorectal robotic procedures have been performed with hybrid laparoscopic-robotic approaches where reliance on a competent assistant is very important. However, new instrumentation such as the robotic stapler and vessel sealer, and improved arms design such as with the new Intuitive Surgical Xi system, are gradually rendering multi-quadrant robotic colorectal surgery a reproducible reality. By contrast, the problem of the added cost of robotic procedures still represents a significant obstacle to the spread of this technology, and this issue is likely to become more relevant as the current health care reform plan is rolled out.

In the absence of level I evidence showing the superiority of robotics over existing approaches, the burden will be increasingly on us to study and explain the potential benefits of this technology.

It is difficult to predict to what extent robotic surgery will replace laparoscopy in colon and rectal surgery. Personally, I think the role of laparoscopy will continue to be an important one for the foreseeable future—at least outside of the pelvis—in part because of the increased cost of and limited access to robotic surgical systems. But it is also a fairly widely accepted fact that the two fields are somewhat complementary: the best robotic colorectal surgeons have come from extensive laparoscopic experiences and many who have labored extensively with robotic surgery in the pelvis have later found themselves able to perform laparoscopic TME with greater confidence.

Given the current state of colorectal surgery and what lies ahead in the field, it is a great joy to see the attention dedicated to robotics in "Robotic Approaches to Colorectal Surgery." This textbook represents the most comprehensive and up-to-date reference for practitioners of the difficult art of minimal access colon and rectal surgery. The scope of procedures described in this book is unsurpassed in the literature and will be of great value to young and seasoned surgeons. To the editors of this important work goes my admiration and ever-lasting friendship.

Alessio Pigazzi, M.D., Ph.D.

Reference

1. Halabi WJ. World J Surg. 2013;37:2782–90.

Preface

Education is the most powerful weapon we can use to change the world

Nelson Mandela

When I was a medical student at the University of Rochester, James Adams, M.D., a beloved senior surgeon used to describe surgery as a dance, always moving and flowing steadily forward. The progression of open surgery, to laparoscopic surgery, to robotic surgery seems to illustrate that same directed progression to an end that seems almost at once ready to grasp yet at the same time transient and lost in the distance. We truly do not know where robotic surgery as applied to colon and rectal disease will end up. Certainly, the rapid evolution in robotic systems that are now better designed to facilitate operation in multiple quadrants is evidence that the reality of robotic colon and rectal surgery is here now. The promise of tables that tilt to allow better positioning of patients without undocking, surgical staplers that sense tissue properties and ensure staple height and formation, and tissue perfusion assessment devices all hint at the ability to more broadly apply robotics to more patients and with possibly better outcomes. The future likely holds haptic feedback, greater miniaturization, and an ability to better handle adhesions and inflamed tissues. Competition in the robotic marketplace and the ability to allow more surgeons exposure to robotic colon and rectal surgery will synergize improvements.

On behalf of all the editors of this text, we are truly excited to allow our work *Robotic Approaches to Colorectal Surgery* to instruct us in what is possible today, and illustrate the methods that will take us to the future. The state of the art is evolving so fast that each month seemingly new techniques and abilities arrive. We have been privileged to have contributions from surgeons who are pioneers, also dedicated to developing techniques and technologies to help our patients. The field of robotics requires the cooperation and collaboration of industry and caregivers. The contributors to this book have worked successfully with industry to develop technology that serves the needs of our patients. The world's patients with colon and rectal disease will now be better for it.

Robotic Approaches to Colorectal Surgery explores all facets of the application of robotics to colon and rectal disease. The text begins with a history of robotic surgery, describes particularly pertinent features of current systems, surgical anatomy, preoperative assessment, and troubleshooting with the aim of establishing a strong foundation for the performance of operations. Detailed instruction highlighting key features and multiple approaches to succeed with right, sigmoid, left, total, and proctocolectomy are offered. Low anterior resection, rectopexy, abdominal perineal resection, and transanal robotic resections are explored in-depth. The text also provides surgeons unique insight into preventing and treating complications, robotic surgery in the obese, training, the bedside assistant, and discussion of both the economics and realistic future of robotic colon and rectal surgery.

The textbook before you truly is a product of many, and for the tremendous efforts the authors and editorial team at Springer we are indebted and grateful. *Robotic Approaches to Colorectal Surgery* creates a written and visual foundation for the surgeon to depend upon in this rapidly developing field. The book was conceptualized to provide a centralized source of information by surgeons and for surgeons. The promise of improved care and outcomes for the patient with colon and rectal disease continues to drive refinements in technology and techniques and we are proud to add to the armamentarium of the surgeons of today and tomorrow.

I am forever indebted to my fellow coeditors, H.R., S.L., B.C., and A.P., for their friendship, guidance, and vision with this textbook. To my wife, Anabela, and daughters, Sophia and Gabriella, for their unwavering love and support. As far as my colleagues who believe there is no place for robotic surgery, "Once a new technology rolls over you if you're not part of the steamroller you're part of the road." Stewart Brand.

Internet Access to Video Clip

The owner of this text will be able to access these video clips through Springer with the following Internet link: http://link.springer.com/book/10.1007/978-3-319-09120-4.

Philadelphia, PA, USA   Howard Michael Ross

Acknowledgements

To my mentor, Dr. Edward Lee, who taught me the true art of minimally invasive colorectal surgery without a hand or a Robot! To my wife, Christina, for her unyielding support, spiritual guidance, and lifelong devotion to the most important job of all; raising our three precious gems. Lastly, to my late mother for her unconditional love and for instilling the importance of perspective.

Bradley J. Champagne, M.D., F.A.C.S., F.A.S.C.R.S.

I would like to acknowledge and thank my colleagues and friends for volunteering their precious time and expertise. To my coeditors, Howard, David, Brad, and Alessio, thank you for your hard work and friendship. Finally, and most importantly, I would like to thank my wife, Crystal, for her support, encouragement, and unwavering love; and my sons, Eric and Ryan, for making me a better person and making everything worthwhile.

Sang W. Lee, M.D., F.A.C.S., F.A.S.C.R.S.

Becoming a surgeon is the fulfillment of a dream that started when my father used to tell me as a child, "you can become anything you want, but if you are a physician you will always have a job, be able to feed your family, and do something good for society." Producing a textbook to apply robotics to colon and rectal surgery has been an honor and privilege. I owe so much to my teachers, colleagues, patients, and family who have been so generous with their time, support, insights, and patience. I am eternally grateful. To my wife Stacy, Molly, Leo, and Emily, I am so appreciative and thankful for all you have given me.

Howard M. Ross, M.D., F.A.C.S., F.A.S.C.R.S.

Contents

Contributors

Editors

Bradley J. Champagne, M.D., F.A.C.S., F.A.S.C.R.S. University Hospitals-Case Medical Center, Cleveland, OH, USA

Sang W. Lee, M.D., F.A.C.S., F.A.S.C.R.S. Division of Colorectal Surgery, New York-Presbyterian Hospital, Weill Cornell Medical Center, New York, NY, USA

Alessio Pigazzi, M.D., Ph.D. University of California, Irvine, Orange, CA, USA

David E. Rivadeneira, M.D., M.B.A., F.A.S.C.R.S. North Shore-LIJ Health System, Huntington Hospital, Hofstra School of Medicine, Woodbury, NY, USA

Howard Ross, M.D. Division of Colon and Rectal Surgery, Temple University School of Medicine, Philadelphia, PA, USA

Authors

Farrell Adkins, M.D. Department of Colorectal Surgery, Cleveland Clinic Florida, Weston, FL, USA

Matthew Albert, M.D., F.A.C.S., F.A.S.C.R.S. Department of Colorectal Surgery, Florida Hospital, Altamonte Springs, FL, USA

Doaa Alsaleh, M.D. Division of Colorectal Surgery, New York-Presbyterian Hospital, Weill Cornell Medical Center, New York, NY, USA

Sam Atallah, M.D., F.A.C.S., F.A.S.C.R.S. Department of Colorectal Surgery, Florida Hospital, Altamonte Springs, FL, USA

Emre Balık, M.D. Department of General Surgery, Koc University School of Medicine, Istanbul, Turkey

Amir Loucas Bastawrous, M.D., M.B.A. Department of Surgery, Swedish Cancer Institute, Seattle, WA, USA

Joshua I.S. Bleier, M.D., F.A.C.S., F.A.S.C.R.S. Pennsylvania Hospital/ Hospital of the University of Pennsylvania, Philadelphia, PA, USA

Sarah Boostrom, M.D., F.A.C.S. Department of Surgery, Baylor University Medical Center, Dallas, TX, USA

Luis Carlos Cajas-Monson, M.D., M.P.H. Department of General Surgery, UCSD Health System, San Diego, CA, USA

Gentry Caton, M.D. Department of Surgery, Baylor University Medical Center, Dallas, TX, USA

Robert K. Cleary, M.D. Department of Surgery, St Joseph Mercy Hospital Ann Arbor, Division of Colon & Rectal Surgery, Ann Arbor, MI, USA

Aneel Damle, M.D., M.B.A. Department of Surgery, University of Massachusetts Medical Center, Worcester, MA, USA

Jacob Eisdorfer, D.O., F.A.C.S North Shore-LIJ Health System, Huntington Hospital, Hofstra School of Medicine, Woodbury, NY, USA

Anthony Firilas, M.D. Roper St Francis Physicians Partners, Charleston, SC, USA

James W. Fleshman, M.D., F.A.C.S., F.A.S.C.R.S. Department of Surgery, Baylor University Medical Center, Dallas, TX, USA

Todd D. Francone, M.D., M.P.H. Department of Colon and Rectal Surgery, Lahey Hospital & Medical Center, Burlington, MA, USA

Julio Garcia-Aguilar, M.D., Ph.D. Department of Surgery, Memorial Sloan Kettering Cancer Center, New York, NY, USA

Maher Ghanem, M.D. Department of Surgery, Central Michigan University (CMU) College of Medicine, Saginaw, MI, USA

Cristina R. Harnsberger, M.D. Department of Surgery, University of California, San Diego, CA, USA

Raquel Gonzalez Heredia, M.D., Ph.D. Division of General, Minimally Invasive and Robotic Surgery, University of Illinois at Chicago, Chicago, IL, USA

Roel Hompes, M.D. Department of Colorectal Surgery, Oxford University Hospitals, Oxford, UK

Brian R. Kann, M.D., F.A.C.S., F.A.S.C.R.S. Penn Presbyterian Hospital, Philadelphia, PA, USA

Kevin R. Kasten, M.D. Division of Colon and Rectal Surgery, Brody School of Medicine at East Carolina University, Greenville, NC, USA

Seon Hahn Kim, M.D., Ph.D. Department of Surgery, Division of Colorectal Surgery, Korea University Anam Hospital, Seoul, South Korea

Jorge A. Lagares-Garcia, M.D., F.A.C.S., F.A.S.C.R.S. Division of Colon and Rectal Surgery, Department of Surgery, Charleston Colorectal Surgery, Roper Hospital, Charleston, SC, USA

David W. Larson, M.D., M.B.A. Division of Colon and Rectal Surgery, Mayo Clinic, Rochester, MN, USA

Mary Arnold Long, A.P.R.N. Department of Nursing, Roper Hospital, Charleston, SC, USA

Slawomir J. Marecik, M.D., F.A.C.S., F.A.S.C.R.S. Department of Colorectal Surgery, Advocate Lutheran General Hospital, University of Illinois at Chicago, Park Ridge, IL, USA

David J. Maron, M.D., M.B.A. Department of Colorectal Surgery, Cleveland Clinic Florida, Weston, FL, USA

Justin A. Maykel, M.D. Division of Colon and Rectal Surgery, Department of Surgery, University of Massachusetts Medical Center, Worcester, MA, USA

Elizabeth McKeown, M.D. Swedish Colon and Rectal Clinic, Seattle, WA, USA

Amit Merchea, M.D. Section of Colon and Rectal Surgery, Mayo Clinic, Jacksonville, FL, USA

Lee J. Milas, M.D. Department of General Surgery, The George Washington University School of Medicine, Yardley, PA, USA

W. Conan Mustain, M.D. University Hospitals—Case Medical Center, Cleveland, OH, USA

Govind Nandakumar, M.D. Division of Colorectal Surgery, New York-Presbyterian Hospital, Weill Cornell Medical Center, New York, NY, USA

Vincent Obias, M.D. Division of Colon and Rectal Surgery, George Washington University Hospital, Washington, DC, USA

Seung Yeop Oh, M.D. Department of Surgery, Ajou University School of Medicine, Suwon, South Korea

Kelly Olino, M.D. Department of Surgery, Memorial Sloan Kettering Cancer Center, New York, NY, USA

Ajit Pai, M.D., F.A.C.S. Department of Colon and Rectal Surgery, Advocate Lutheran General Hospital and University of Illinois at Chicago, Park Ridge, IL, USA

John J. Park, M.D., F.A.C.S., F.A.S.C.R.S. Department of Colon and Rectal Surgery, Chicago Medical School at Rosalind Franklin University of Medicine and Science, Advocate Lutheran General Hospital, Park Ridge, IL, USA

Carlos Martinez Parra, M.D. Division of General and Transplant Surgery, University of Illinois at Chicago, Chicago, IL, USA

Carrie Y. Peterson, M.D. Division of Colorectal Surgery, New York-Presbyterian Hospital, Weill Cornell Medical Center, New York, NY, USA

Matthew M. Philp, M.D. Division of Colon and Rectal Surgery, Department of Surgery, Temple University Hospital, Philadelphia, PA, USA

Leela M. Prasad, M.D., F.A.C.S., F.A.S.C.R.S. Department of Surgery, Advocate Lutheran General Hospital, Park Ridge, IL, USA
University of Illinois College of Medicine at Chicago, Park Ridge, IL, USA
Division of Colon and Rectal Surgery, Advocate Lutheran General Hospital, Park Ridge, IL, USA

Sonia Ramamoorthy, M.D., F.A.C.S., F.A.S.C.R.S. Department of General Surgery, UC San Diego Health System, San Diego, CA, USA

Elizabeth R. Raskin, M.D., F.A.C.S., F.A.S.C.R.S. Division of Colon and Rectal Surgery, Department of Surgery, University of Minnesota, St. Paul, MN, USA

Rebecca Rhee, M.D. Division of Colorectal Surgery, Maimonides Medical Center, Brooklyn, NY, USA

Tushar Samdani, M.D. Department of Surgery, Memorial Sloan Kettering Cancer Center, New York, NY, USA

Anthony J. Senagore, M.D., M.S., M.B.A. Department of Surgery, Central Michigan University (CMU) College of Medicine, Saginaw, MI, USA

Anna Serur, M.D., F.A.C.S., F.A.S.C.R.S. Division of Colon and Rectal Surgery, Maimonides Medical Center, Brooklyn, NY, USA

Samuel Shaheen, M.D. Department of Surgery, Central Michigan University (CMU) College of Medicine, Saginaw, MI, USA

Nak Song Sung, M.D. Department of Surgery, Division of Colorectal Surgery, Korea University Anam Hospital, Seoul, South Korea

Konstantin Umanskiy, M.D. Department of Surgery, University of Chicago, Chicago, IL, USA

Hsin-Hung Yeh, B.Med., F.R.A.C.S. Department of Colorectal Surgery, Korea University Anam Hospital, Seoul, Korea

Part I

Robotic Surgery

History of the Robotic Surgical System

1

Joshua I.S. Bleier and Brian R. Kann

Abstract

Robotics has its roots back to ancient human history. The current conception of the surgical robot began with NASA, as a government project in telepresence surgery for use in remote battlefield surgery. The concept then quickly evolved into what we use today in the operating room. The da Vinci robot, the most commonly used robotic platform, is now pervasively used for all types of surgery. This chapter serves to explore the origins of the surgical robot and provide a brief overview of its current and, perhaps, future applications.

Keywords

Telepresence • Surgical robot • da Vinci • History

The origin of the surgical robot has its roots deep in human history. Although the term "robot" evolved relatively recently in the twentieth century as detailed in the 1920s play "R.U.R. Rossum's Universal robots" by Czech author Karel Capek, in which these were automatons used for forced labor of dreary tasks, "robots" appeared in human history as far back as 1000 BC. In ancient China, Yan Shi, a mechanical engineer, presented his king with a life-sized mechanical humanoid. In ancient Greece, the mathematician Archytas was credited with designing a steam-powered mechanical pigeon in the fourth century BC. Later, early in the first century, Heron of Alexandria allegedly created a speaking automaton. Notably, Leonardo da Vinci, in sketches contained from recovered notebooks, clearly detailed a mechanical knight based on his research in the Vitruvian Man [1] (Fig. 1.1). The timeline of our interactions with "robots" started early in human history and continues to be redrawn until the present day.

The modern concept of the surgical robot had its origins in the development of virtual reality based on NASA's use of a head-mounted display

J.I.S. Bleier, M.D., F.A.C.S., F.A.S.C.R.S. (✉)
Pennsylvania Hospital/Hospital of the University of Pennsylvania, 800 Walnut St. 20th Floor, Philadelphia, PA 19106, USA
e-mail: Joshua.bleier@uphs.upenn.edu

B.R. Kann, M.D., F.A.C.S., F.A.S.C.R.S.
Penn Presbyterian Hospital, Philadelphia, PA, USA

H. Ross et al. (eds.), *Robotic Approaches to Colorectal Surgery*,
DOI 10.1007/978-3-319-09120-4_1

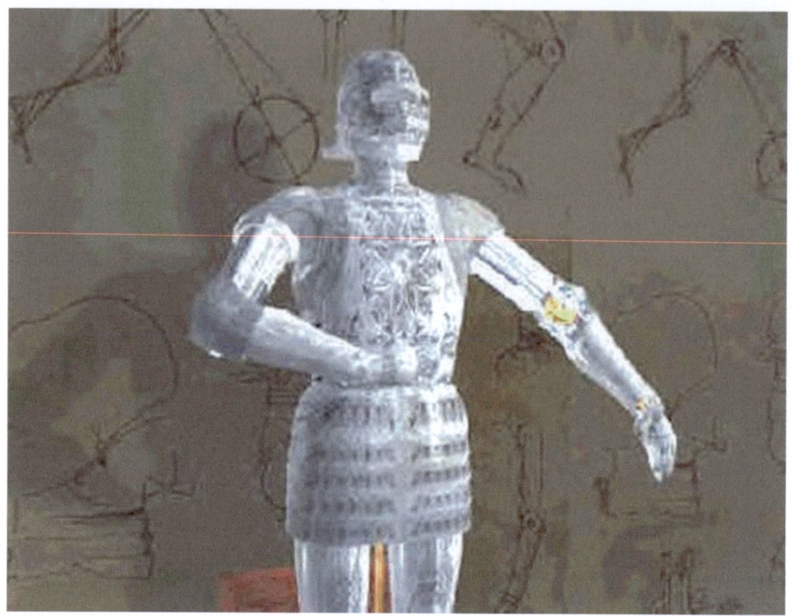

Fig. 1.1 Design drawings of the lost da Vinci writings (from Institute and Museum of the History of Science, Florence, Italy). *With permission from Ilya A. Volfson, Jeffrey A. Stock. History of Robotic Surgery. In: Jeffrey A. Stock MD, Michael P. Esposito MD, Vincent J. Lanteri MD, David M. Albala MD, edds. Current Clinical Urology: Urologic Robotic Surgery. Springer, New York 2008: pp 3–25. © Springer*

for visualizing the data being returned from Voyager's exploratory mission. Scott Fisher and Joe Rosen combined this with the use of robotic waldoes and coined the term "telepresence," founding Telepresence Research Inc., envisioning the use in telepresence surgery. Rosen and Fisher collaborated with Phil Green, a PhD at Stanford Research Institute, and, with other roboticists, worked to develop an interface allowing surgeons to operate virtually, with the sense that their robotic hands are directly in front of their eyes [2].

During this time, in the late 1980s, laparoscopy was also becoming mainstream, and the concept of a potential remote interface became a reality. It seemed that robotics could provide assistance to make up for the loss of three-dimensional visualization and impairment of dexterity that laparoscopy caused.

In 1985, Unimation's PUMA 560 system, the first non-laparoscopic robotic device, was used to perform the first documented robotic-assisted surgical procedure, when it was used for a percutaneous brain biopsy (Fig. 1.2) [3]. In the early 1990s, Hap Paul, a veterinary surgeon, and

William Barger, an orthopedic surgeon, began developing a surgical system based on IBM's Puma arm to develop a robot to be used in hip replacement surgery. The Puma system was an early robotic interface, which enabled more precise preoperative planning in order to best match a femur with a prosthesis. The collaboration yielded ROBODOC (Integrated Surgical Systems, Sacramento, CA), a device that improved the ability to core out the femoral shaft from 75 % (standard human accuracy) to 96 % (Fig. 1.3).

In London, surgeon John Wickham, MD, and Brian Davies, PhD, used a system similar to ROBODOC (PROBOT) in its coring abilities, to perform a transurethral resection of the prostate. This was aided by a mechanically constrained ring in order to enhance safety and ensure precise movements of the robotic arm (Fig. 1.4).

Research is continued by the US military to develop a medical application for the use of remote telepresence surgery. In 1992, Risk Satava and Don Jenkins, working with Defense Advanced Research Projects Agency (DARPA), developed the MEDFAST (medical forward

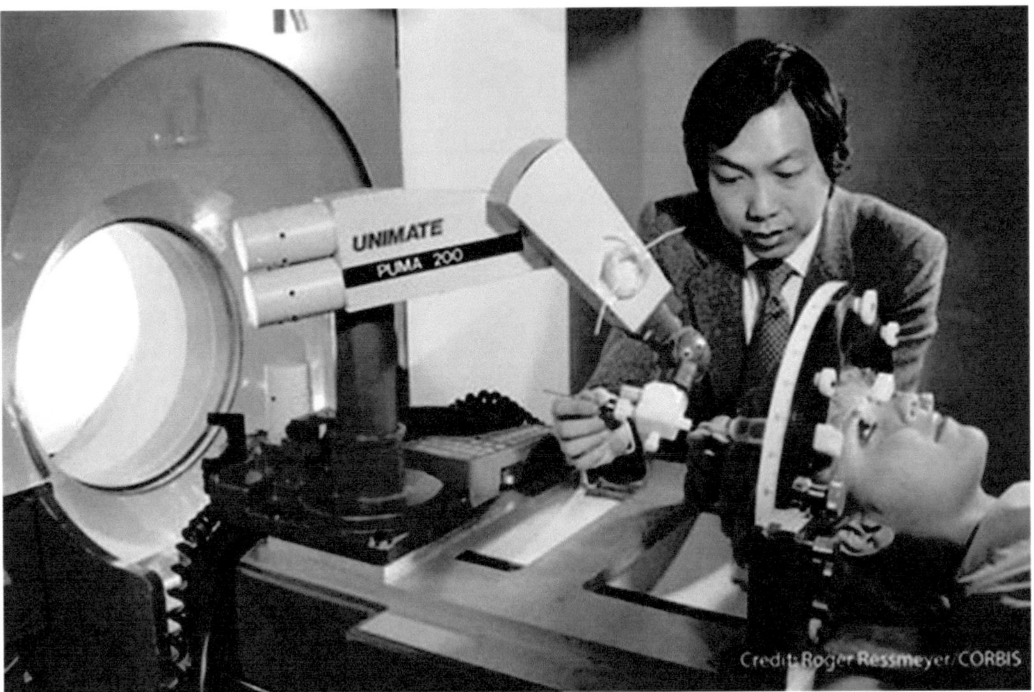

Fig. 1.2 Puma 200 robot. *With permission from M.L. Lorentziadis A Short History of the Invasion of Robots in Surgery. Hellenic Journal of Surgery (2014) 86:3, 117–121. © Springer*

advanced surgical treatment) application. The goal was to maneuver the vehicle, a Bradley Fighting Vehicle (Fig. 1.5), onto the battlefield where injured soldiers could be treated by a field medic and surgery could be performed using the robotic arms mounted inside, while surgeons were stationed at a MASH (Mobile Advanced Surgical Hospital) unit. In 1996, a successful demonstration over a 5 km distance provided a proof of principle, though ultimately this system never took hold, mostly due to a shift from open battlefield grounds to more urban environments in which this model was not feasible.

Despite the success of ROBODOC, because of a prolonged approval process through the FDA, the first true mainstream application of the surgical robot was in the use of laparoscopy. Yulun Wang, a PhD working with DARPA, developed the AESOP system (Automated Endoscopic System for Optimal Positioning) (Computer Motion Inc., Santa Barbara,

California). This was developed in order to provide a robotic first assist for the positioning and use of the laparoscopic camera (Fig. 1.6).

At the same time as AESOP was becoming more prevalent, Frederick Moll, MD, licensed Green's telepresence surgery device and formed Intuitive Surgical Inc. After some redesigning, the da Vinci system was born (Fig. 1.7). In April 1997, this system was used to perform the first true robotic surgery in Brussels by Drs. Himpens and Cardiere. In 1998, the da Vinci system was used to perform the first robotic valve surgery [4]. Soon after this, Computer Motion Inc. launched their system, ZEUS (Fig. 1.8). This system was similar to the da Vinci system in that robotic manipulator arms performed the surgery; however, the user interface was different in that it provided an ergonomically enhanced interface and an enhanced two-dimensional display. Initially the ZEUS system did not provide wristed instruments, although these were later introduced.

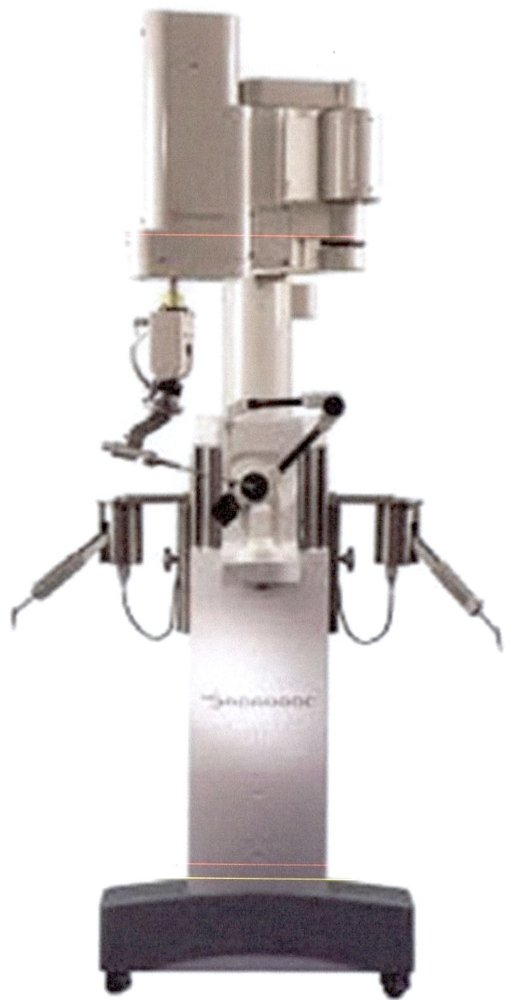

Fig. 1.3 ROBODOC surgical system. *With permission from M.L. Lorentziadis A Short History of the Invasion of Robots in Surgery. Hellenic Journal of Surgery (2014) 86:3, 117–121. © Springer*

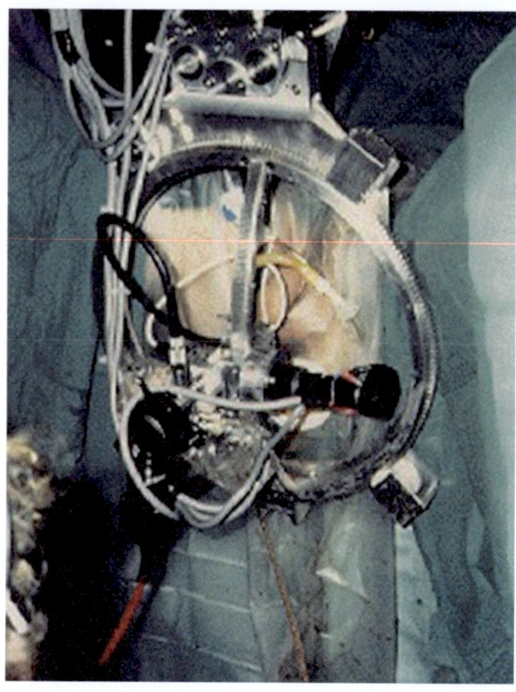

Fig. 1.4 PROBOT surgical robotic system (from http://www.imperial.ac.uk/ mechatronicsinmedicine/projects/probot/index.html). *With permission from Ilya A. Volfson, Jeffrey A. Stock. History of Robotic Surgery. In: Jeffrey A. Stock MD, Michael P. Esposito MD, Vincent J. Lanteri MD, David M. Albala MD, edds. Current Clinical Urology: Urologic Robotic Surgery. Springer, New York 2008: pp 3–25. © Springer*

This was used for the first full endoscopic robotic procedure, a fallopian tube reanastomosis.

Finally, in 2003, Intuitive Surgical Inc. bought Computer Motion Inc. and the rest, as they say, "is history." The da Vinci robotic surgical system was introduced to the market in 1999. At that time, it included a three-dimensional vision system, three arms, and the EndoWrist® technology. In 2003, its first major upgrade included the addition of a fourth arm to allow for enhanced manipulation and retraction. In 2006, the "S" system was released offering a high-definition vision and a multi-image display. In 2009, the "Si" system was released offering dual console capacity for enhanced training and collaboration as well as another enhancement of the visual system. Finally, this year (2014), Intuitive launched the "Xi" system which allowed for improved use and multi-quadrant surgery, upgrading the technology of its optics systems and using technology to improve the process of arm positioning and port placement. In addition, Intuitive Surgical Inc. introduced a fluorescence imaging system, Firefly™, to allow for direct visualization of tissue perfusion as well as the addition of energy and stapling tools married to the armature. The various da Vinci systems will be more fully discussed later in this chapter.

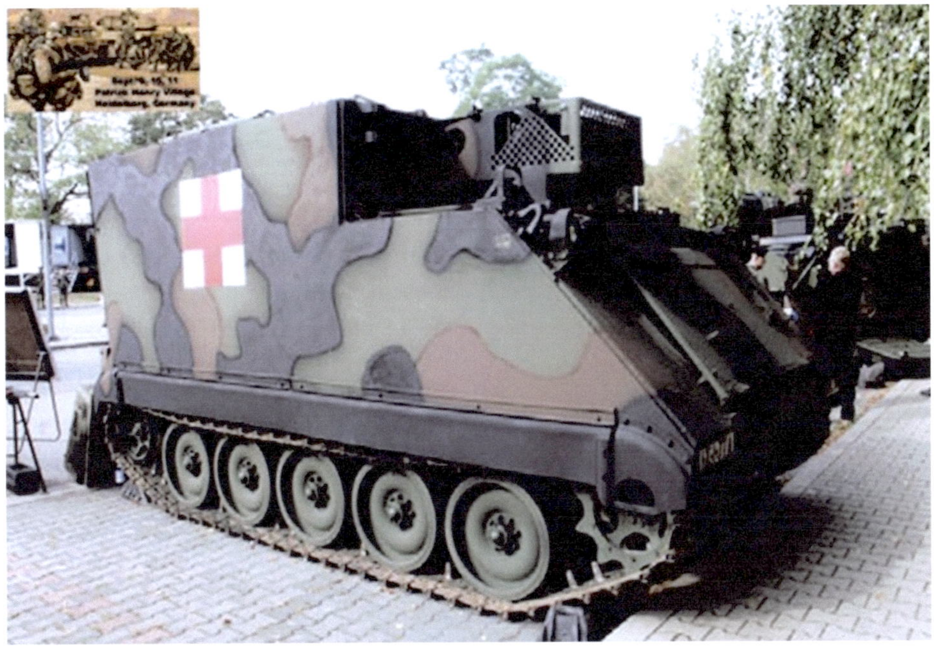

Fig. 1.5 Bradley Fighting Vehicle. *With permission from M.L. Lorentziadis A Short History of the Invasion of Robots in Surgery. Hellenic Journal of Surgery (2014) 86:3, 117–121. © Springer*

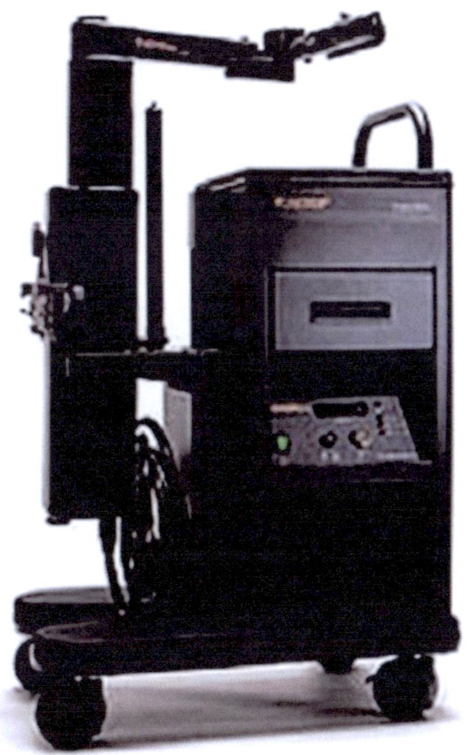

Fig. 1.6 AESOP (Automated Endoscopic System for Optimal Positioning). *With permission from M.L. Lorentziadis A Short History of the Invasion of Robots in Surgery. Hellenic Journal of Surgery (2014) 86:3, 117–121. © Springer*

1.1 Current Applications

Although the first robotic-assisted coronary artery bypass was performed in Germany in 1998 [5], the Food and Drug Administration (FDA) only granted approval for selected robotic-assisted laparoscopic procedures in the Unites States in 2000. Since then, applications for robotic-assisted surgery have expanded exponentially. This section reviews some of the current applications and surgical procedures for which robotic assistance has been utilized over the past decade and a half.

1.1.1 Urology

1.1.1.1 Robotic Radical Prostatectomy

Prostate cancer is the second leading cause of cancer in men in the USA and worldwide. Radical prostatectomy is the standard surgical management for patients with localized disease; however, it is associated with high morbidity rates. Laparoscopic radical prostatectomy was introduced in 1997 by Schuessler et al. with the goal of reducing the morbidity associated with the open operation [6]. However, the technical

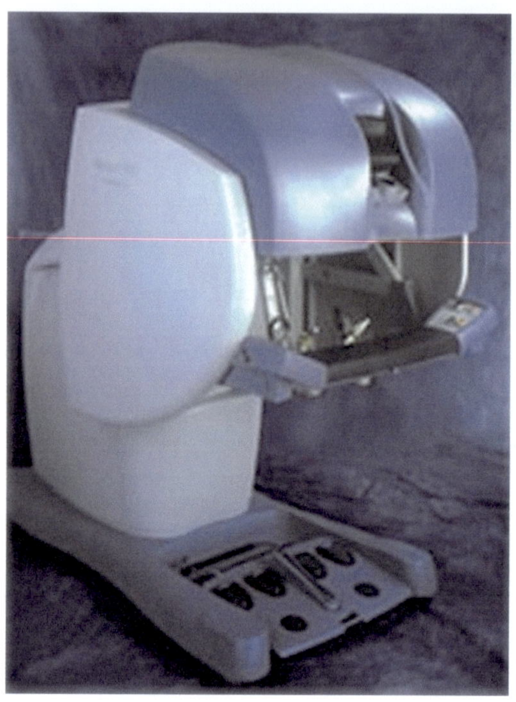

Fig. 1.7 da Vinci surgical system console. *With permission from Ilya A. Volfson, Jeffrey A. Stock. History of Robotic Surgery. In: Jeffrey A. Stock MD, Michael P. Esposito MD, Vincent J. Lanteri MD, David M. Albala MD, edds. Current Clinical Urology: Urologic Robotic Surgery. Springer, New York 2008: pp 3–25. © Springer*

challenges of laparoscopic radical prostatectomy proved to be difficult for the average urologist with limited laparoscopic experience and limited case volumes, and widespread adoption of the laparoscopic approach was not seen.

The introduction of the da Vinci® Surgical System paved the way for minimally invasive prostatectomy. Since the initial report by Menon et al. in 2002 [7] describing robotic prostatectomy utilizing the da Vinci® system, robotic prostatectomy has become the most widely performed robotic surgical procedure in the world. The robotic technique offers the advantages of improved ergonomics, easier laparoscopic suturing, and shorter learning curves. Following US FDA approval for the use of the da Vinci® system for radical prostatectomy in 2001, there was a 955 % increase in the number of robotic prostatectomies performed in the USA between 2003 and 2009 [8], with as many as 90 % of radical

prostatectomies in the USA being performed robotically [9].

Interestingly, widespread adoption of robotic radical prostatectomy occurred in the early 2000s despite the lack of any convincing evidence demonstrating a clear benefit. It was not until 2012 when Trinh et al. demonstrated improved perioperative outcomes for patients undergoing robotic prostatectomy compared with open or laparoscopic prostatectomy, with fewer intraoperative and postoperative complications, decreased likelihood of requiring blood transfusion, and shorter length of stay [10]. Interestingly, despite the robot's overwhelming prevalence, well-powered, randomized controlled trials demonstrating superior oncologic and functional (urinary continence and sexual potency) outcomes with the use of robotic-assisted prostatectomy are still lacking. Nevertheless, it is still considered by most to be the current gold standard in the surgical management of prostate cancer.

1.1.1.2 Robotic Partial Nephrectomy

In 2014, there will be an estimated 64,000 new cases of kidney cancer diagnosed and 13,860 deaths related to kidney cancer in the USA [11]. Given that radical nephrectomy has been shown to be an independent risk factor for new-onset chronic renal failure [12], there has been a trend in recent years toward performing partial nephrectomy when technically feasible. For small (<4 cm) early stage cancers, long-term cancer-free survival rates are comparable to those with radical nephrectomy; the incidence of local recurrence for partial nephrectomy is estimated at 0–10 % and is 0–3 % for tumors less than 4 cm [13].

While most would consider open partial nephrectomy the gold standard for nephron-sparing surgery, the procedure is associated with significant morbidity related to the muscle-cutting flank incision, namely, a high rate of hernia, pain, and paresthesia. In an effort to reduce the morbidity associated with open partial nephrectomy, laparoscopic partial nephrectomy was introduced and began to be more widely utilized in the late 1990s and early 2000s.

While laparoscopic partial nephrectomy is associated with shorter length of stay, decreased

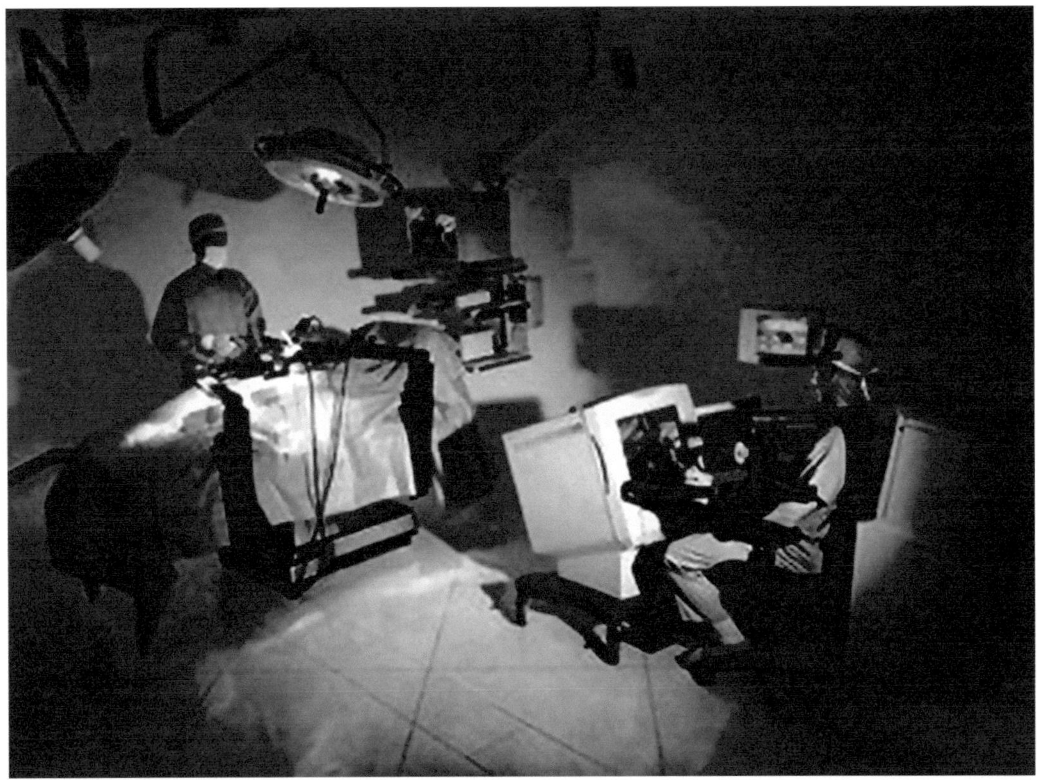

Fig. 1.8 ZEUS Robotic Surgical System. *With permission from Faust RA, Kant AJ, Lorincz A et al. Robotic endoscopic surgery in a porcine model of the infant neck. J Robotic Surg 2007;1:75–83*

operative blood loss, and fewer wound-related complications, it is also a very technically challenging procedure with prolonged learning curves and has not quite gained the widespread acceptance that some thought it would. In fact, an unintended consequence of the push for more minimally invasive procedures for renal cancer was the resurgence in the number of radical nephrectomies being performed, as many viewed laparoscopic radical nephrectomy as a less technically challenging procedure than partial nephrectomy that still imparted the benefits of minimally invasive surgery (MIS) [14].

Robot-assisted partial nephrectomy has now largely replaced the traditional laparoscopic approach to partial nephrectomy, as it preserves the advantages of MIS, while at the same time being more technically feasible than laparoscopic partial nephrectomy, with a shorter learning curve. A number of case series have demonstrated

equivalent early oncologic outcomes with robot-assisted partial nephrectomy compared with the traditional laparoscopic approach [15, 16]. A recent study utilizing data from the American College of Surgeons' National Surgical Quality Improvement Program (NSQIP) database demonstrated that, when compared with the open approach, minimally invasive (including both laparoscopic and robot-assisted) partial nephrectomy resulted in shorter length of stay, fewer blood transfusions, and fewer complications, including pneumonia, wound infection, sepsis, and acute kidney injury requiring dialysis [17].

1.1.1.3 Robotic Cystectomy

Radical cystectomy is the standard surgical procedure for node-positive or muscle-invasive bladder cancer, but it can be associated with morbidity rates of up to 50 % and mortality rates as high as 5 % [18]. Laparoscopic cystectomy was first introduced in 1992 with the primary goal of reducing the morbidity rates seen with the open procedure and decreasing length of stay. While laparoscopic cystectomy has been shown to be associated with less morbidity, fewer blood transfusions, less postoperative pain, and shorter length of stay when compared with open cystectomy [19], it suffers from the same drawbacks as laparoscopic partial nephrectomy, namely, extreme technical challenges and a long learning curve.

The first robotic-assisted radical cystectomy was performed in 2003 [20]. The robotic approach has since been seen as a means to potentially overcome the technical challenges of laparoscopic cystectomy. However, the procedure is still in its relative infancy, and there is a paucity of level I data comparing robotic-assisted cystectomy with open and laparoscopic cystectomy. A prospective, randomized controlled trial published by Bochner that randomized patients to open vs. robotic-assisted radical nephrectomy demonstrated similar perioperative complication rates and length of hospital stay. In this study, the robotic-assisted approach was associated with less intraoperative blood loss, but had an average operative time 127 min longer than the open technique; the authors concluded that this argued against the benefit of robotic-assisted cystectomy in terms of minimizing perioperative morbidity [21]. A recent non-randomized, retrospective study comparing open and robotic-assisted radical cystectomy showed no difference in surgical margin status and lymph node yield, though there were less need for transfusion and a 20 % reduction in length of stay in the robotic group [22].

While preliminary reports of robotic-assisted cystectomy are encouraging, long-term functional and oncologic results are still widely unknown. Certainly, the procedure seems to hold promise for the future, though further study is clearly needed before it gains the acceptance that robotic prostatectomy has seen.

1.1.2 Cardiothoracic Surgery

One of the earliest applications of robotic surgery was in cardiothoracic surgery, with a robotic-assisted mitral valve repair being performed by Carpentier in 1998 [23]. Robotic-assisted cardiac procedures currently being performed include mitral valve repair and replacement, coronary artery bypass grafting, closure of atrial septal defects, implantation of pacing leads, and resection of intracardiac tumors. Robotic mitral valve surgery is probably the most widely used application of robotic assistance in cardiac surgery and has been shown to be associated with decreased rates of postoperative atrial fibrillation and pulmonary effusion, as well as decreased length of stay, while maintaining similar perioperative complication rates to those seen with open procedures [24, 25]. The complexity of the procedure and longer operative times are felt by its proponents to be offset by the shorter length of stay and other potential benefits of the minimally invasive approach to mitral valve surgery.

Robotic-assisted thoracic surgical procedures currently being performed include pulmonary resection and mediastinal lymphadenectomy for lung cancer, thymectomy, and removal of mediastinal tumors. The adoption of robotic lobectomy has gained significant momentum in recent years, despite the majority of trials showing equivocal results. A recent national database review did demonstrate that robotic pulmonary resections were associated with significant reductions in mortality, length of stay, and overall complication rates compared with open thoracotomy [26]. Robotic-assisted esophagectomy has also been recently introduced, with early reports suggesting similar outcomes to those seen with laparoscopic and open esophagectomy [27].

Despite being one of the pioneering specialties in the development and implementation of robotic-assisted surgical technology, it is still somewhat unclear as to whether or not there is a distinct advantage afforded to patients undergoing robotic-assisted cardiothoracic procedures compared with those undergoing open procedures. Given prolonged operative times and the increased cost associated with the use of robotic technology, combined with largely equivocal results in the literature thus far, further evidence and results from well-powered, randomized controlled trials are needed before robotic-assisted cardiothoracic surgery becomes a standard of care.

1.1.3 Colon and Rectal Surgery

While laparoscopic colon and rectal resection for benign disease has been performed for some time now, laparoscopic resection for malignant disease did not become an accepted means of surgical treatment until the results of the Clinical Outcomes of Surgical Therapy (COST) trial were published in 2004, demonstrating equivalent oncologic outcomes between laparoscopic and open colectomy [28]. The use of laparoscopy for colorectal resection, however, is fraught with a number of difficulties, including the need to work in multiple quadrants, lack of fixation of the transverse and sigmoid colon, and difficult access to the pelvis. The addition of robotic technology to traditional laparoscopic techniques has sought to overcome the difficulty of operating in the pelvis but augments the challenge of operating in different quadrants and provides zero tactile feedback.

Colon and rectal surgical procedures that have been described using a robotic-assisted approach include segmental and total abdominal colectomy, low anterior resection, abdominoperineal resection, restorative proctocolectomy, and rectopexy (with and without sigmoid colectomy) for rectal prolapse. The number of publications describing techniques and outcomes for robotic-assisted colon and rectal surgery continues to grow exponentially, yet a great deal of controversy still remains regarding the exact role of robotics in colon and rectal surgery.

While a number of studies have shown robotic colon and rectal surgery to be safe and technically feasible [29–31], two of the major deterrents to its more widespread adoption, similar to that seen in other specialties, are longer operating times (including operating room setup and breakdown) and greater cost. In fact, a recent study comparing robotic-assisted and conventional laparoscopic right colectomy [32] found that while there were equivalent morbidity rates, lymph node retrieval, blood loss, and length of stay, the robotic group clearly had significantly longer operative times and increased cost, arguing that robotic surgery for right colectomy may only be disadvantageous.

An area where some feel that longer operative times and increased cost may be justified is the in the realm of rectal cancer surgery. Total mesorectal excision (TME) has become the gold standard in surgery for rectal cancer [33], but this can be a challenging procedure to perform laparoscopically, particularly in obese patients and those with a narrow pelvis. The quest for a complete, intact TME specimen, coupled with the desire to minimize pelvic autonomic nerve injury and postoperative genitourinary dysfunction, has raised the bar in terms of the need for surgical precision when operating in the pelvis. Proponents of robotic-assisted rectal resection argue that improved outcomes in terms of oncologic and functional outcome may be achievable due to more precise identification of anatomic planes and neurovascular structures, aided by the magnified, three-dimensional high-definition images provided by the robotic platform as well as improved tissue handling facilitated by wristed instruments.

A body of evidence is growing in the literature indicating that robotic surgery may be equivalent to open and conventional laparoscopy for rectal cancer. De Souza et al. published a comparative series of robotic vs. open TME that demonstrated similar perioperative morbidity, length of stay, and wound infection rates between the two groups, while the robotic group has less blood loss but longer operative times [34]. A number of other studies have demonstrated similar and, in some cases, better complication rates and short- to intermediate-term oncologic results for robotic-assisted rectal resection when compared to open and conventional laparoscopic rectal resection [35–37]. A recent meta-analysis comparing robotic-assisted and laparoscopic TME published by Xiong showed that robotic TME is safe and feasible and the short- and medium-term oncologic and functional outcomes are equivalent to laparoscopic TME [38].

As previously discussed, one of the proposed benefits of robotic-assisted surgery for rectal cancer is the potential for better visualization of the neurovascular bundles in the pelvis and reduced rates of genitourinary dysfunction. However, data supporting this fact had been lacking until recently, when Kim et al., in 2012, reported that robotic TME, in their experience, was associated with earlier recovery of normal voiding and sexual function compared to patients undergoing conventional laparoscopic TME [39]; others have since reported similar findings [40, 41].

The issues of increased cost and operative time have been major deterrents to the more widespread use of robotic TME. However, Byrn et al. have actually shown that the issues of longer operative time and increased cost may become offset with experience and increased surgical volume. They compared their first 43 robotic-assisted rectal resections with their next 42 robotic-assisted rectal resections and found that, despite the latter group having a higher body mass index, shorter operative times were seen; direct hospital costs were also lower in the latter group, though this did not reach statistical significance [42].

The future of robotic colon and rectal surgery remains somewhat unclear. Many continue to raise the question as to whether the potential benefits are offset by the increased cost and operative time. Additionally, data regarding improved functional outcome for robotic-assisted rectal surgery are just beginning to appear in the literature, and we are still awaiting long-term results with regard to oncologic outcomes. It has been proposed that with the further development and advancement of single-site robotic technology and techniques, there may be further increased interest in advancing robotic-assisted colon and rectal surgery in coming years [43].

1.1.4 General Surgery

Robotic applications in general surgery are widespread and include gynecology [44–51], cholecystectomy, bariatric surgery, anti-reflux surgery, hepatobiliary surgery, gastrectomy, and splenectomy. Conclusions regarding any clear benefit of the robotic-assisted approach for these procedures, as well as their safety and efficacy, are limited due to a lack of well-powered, prospective randomized clinical trials. Nonetheless, as robotic surgery becomes more accepted, newer applications for this technology continue to be explored within the realm of general surgery.

After the initial introduction of robotic-assisted surgical technology in urologic and cardiac surgery, robotic cholecystectomy was seen by many as a way for general surgeons to "practice" their robotic skills on a less complicated procedure before attempting to broaden the spectrum of applications to more complex tasks [52]. However, the issues of higher cost and prolonged operative times hampered the widespread adoption of robotic-assisted cholecystectomy. In fact, a review of data from the NIS Database found that robotic-assisted cholecystectomy was associated with a statistically *higher* complication rate than that seen with conventional laparoscopic cholecystectomy [53]. As single-site robotic technology continues to advance and more experience with the procedure is gained, robotic-assisted single-site cholecystectomy may become a more accepted option, as decreased operative times may lead to less of a cost differential when compared with conventional laparoscopic cholecystectomy [54, 55].

Obesity is a nationwide epidemic, and bariatric surgical procedures in appropriately selected patients can provide durable weight loss and reduce obesity-related comorbidities. The application of robotic technology to bariatric surgical procedures has seen a dramatic rise in recent years. A recent systematic review showed that perioperative complication rates and short-term outcomes are similar between robotic-assisted and conventional laparoscopic bariatric procedures and the learning curve may actually be shorter for the robotic approach [56]. However, prospective randomized trials and long-term outcomes are still needed to better define the role of robotics in bariatric surgery.

Robotic surgery has also been used with increased frequency for anti-reflux procedures, such as Nissen fundoplication. In a recent review of data from the University HealthSystem Consortium (UHC) of patients undergoing anti-reflux surgery, robotic procedures and conventional laparoscopic procedures had similar morbidity, mortality, and length of stay, though the robotic group demonstrated higher readmission rates and substantially higher cost [57]. However, operative times have actually been reported in more recent series to be lower with the robotic approach [58].

Recent studies have also demonstrated the feasibility and safety of robotic-assisted hepatectomy in terms of perioperative morbidity and mortality [59]. In a comparison of robotic-assisted and conventional laparoscopic hepatectomy, Tsung et al. demonstrated similar perioperative outcomes. While operative times were longer with the robotic approach, a higher percentage of cases performed with robotic assistance were able to be completed in a purely minimally invasive approach, without conversion to open surgery or the use of hand port or hybrid approach [60]. Lai et al. have reported 2-year overall and disease-free survival rates of 94 % and 74 %, respectively, utilizing robotic-assisted hepatectomy for resectable hepatocellular carcinoma [61]. However, data regarding long-term oncologic outcomes are still lacking.

As interest in minimally invasive pancreatic surgery has grown in recent years, the robotic approach has been seen as a means to attempt to overcome the technical difficulties and limitations of conventional laparoscopic pancreatectomy. A recent comparison of robotic-assisted and laparoscopic pancreaticoduodenectomy by Orti-Rodriguez and Rahman showed no differences in operative times, morbidity, and mortality; however, the laparoscopic approach was actually found to be superior to the robotic approach in terms of less blood loss, shorter length of stay, fewer postoperative fistulae, and fewer conversions to open procedures [62]. In contrast, a meta-analysis comparing open and robotic-assisted pancreaticoduodenectomy showed that complication rates, reoperation, and surgical margin positivity were significantly lower following robotic surgery [63]. Despite promising initial reports, more experience with the use of this technique and further data regarding long-term oncologic outcomes and cost-effectiveness are likely needed before robotic pancreatic surgery becomes more widely utilized.

Reports of safety and efficacy with the use of robotic surgery for other general surgical procedures, such as gastrectomy and splenectomy, are also being published with increasing frequency [64–77]. Robotic approaches to these procedures are still in their relative infancy, and prospective randomized trials showing clear advantages of the robotic approach over open and conventional laparoscopic approaches have yet to be reported.

1.1.5   Current Prototypes

The da Vinci® Surgical System (Intuitive Surgical Inc., Sunnyvale, CA), first introduced in 1999, is the sole robotic surgical system currently commercially available. The system is comprised of three main components: the surgeon's console, a patient-side robotic cart that has four robotic arms (one for the camera and three for surgical instruments) that are manipulated by the surgeon at the console, and a high-definition three-dimensional vision system. The da Vinci® Surgical System was first approved by the FDA for use in the USA in 2000. At that time, the patient-side robotic cart had only three arms; an upgraded version with a fourth arm was introduced in 2003. Since then, the da Vinci® Surgical System has gone through three generational upgrades: the da Vinci® S in 2006, the da Vinci® Si in 2009, and the latest generation, the da Vinci® Xi, which was introduced in 2014.

The da Vinci® Xi Surgical System has a number of advancements designed to make the system easier to use and broaden its potential applications. One of the major changes is that instead of the arms extending outward from the main body of the patient-side cart, they now extend downward from an overhead boom, which allows the arms to rotate as a group and frees up space inside the surgical field, allowing unobstructed access to the patient. The endoscope can now also be attached to any one of the four arms, instead of being limited to one arm. This allows for improved visualization and four-quadrant access to the abdomen without undocking, repositioning the patient-side cart, and redocking, which can be time-consuming.

The newly designed endoscope is smaller and more compact, providing better definition and clarity, while being less cumbersome. White balancing, calibration, and draping are not required, and the endoscope is easily interchangeable between any of the four arms on the patient-side cart at any point in the operation, allowing more flexibility and expanded visualization. Docking of the patient cart is now facilitated by a laser targeting system, which simplifies the process of positioning the cart appropriately in relation to the position of the patient. Once the endoscope is pointed at an intended surgical site, the system will configure itself into the optimal position for the procedure.

The robotic arms are now smaller and lighter, with an extended range of motion that, when coupled with longer instrument shafts, allow for greater reach within the abdomen and pelvis. The mechanism used to dock the robotic arms with the laparoscopic trocars in the patient's abdominal wall has also been greatly simplified, allowing for faster docking and undocking.

Lastly, the da Vinci® Xi Surgical System is compatible with all of the advanced da Vinci® technology, including the single-site surgery platform, intracorporeal stapler, vessel sealer, and Firefly Fluorescence Imaging System, which allows for real-time imaging of blood vessels, tissue perfusion, and bile ducts. All of the advances with the latest iteration of the da Vinci® Surgical System are intended to create a scalable platform that allows for the application of these advanced technologies, with the intent of broadening the scope of robotic-assisted surgery's clinical applications.

1.1.5.1 Future Developments

It is almost redundant to include a section on the future development of robotic surgery; since this is such an actively evolving technology, likely all of our speculation will be fact or confirmed history by the time this textbook is published; however, current research can certainly spark speculation. Even before the da Vinci Xi model was launched, robotic trailblazers have been pushing the envelope. The ENT surgeons have fully realized the use of the robot with natural orifice surgery, the TORS (trans-oral robotic surgery) platform. Active development of single-arm platforms with multiple robotically controlled manipulator tips will advance our capabilities with single-incision laparoscopic/robotic surgery (SILS). In vivo tests have already shown proof of principle [71]. Major advances have been made in urologic procedures with completely intracorporeal renal autotransplantation [72]. Currently, adaptations of this use are being adapted to use the robot for NOTES (natural orifice translumenal endoscopic surgery). NOSCAR, the Natural Orifice Surgery Consortium for Assessment and Research, was developed to explore the frontiers of this technology. Adaptation of this technology has been used to push the limits of transanal endoscopic microsurgery (TEM) using the robot [73, 74], as well as the use of the robot for completely transanal TME [75].

Perhaps the natural extension of NOTES surgery is true incisionless surgery, using miniaturized, robotically controlled manipulators. Zygomalas published an excellent review detailing the current status of the various prototypes of miniature robots that have been tried to test the paradigm of intracorporeal robot operating [76]. True miniaturization already exists, with the development of microelectromechanical systems (MEMS), but the primary issue regarding these systems has to do with the fact that with the radical reduction in scale comes an equal reduction in the force that can be generated by the robots, greatly limiting the scope of their usefulness. Similarly, nanotechnology is advancing at a fast rate, and such experimental "microbots" are already in existence and have been used for invasive intraocular surgery, demonstrating that such untethered microbots can be controlled effectively [77].

Technological advances grow almost as fast as human imagination. No longer are the limits to MIS dictated by patient characteristics as they were during the advent of MIS; rather, they are dictated now only by our ability to come up with new ideas. The future for robotic surgery and its extension are truly boundless, and it will be exciting to see how far we can go. Perhaps Star Trek's sick bay and tricorder are only around the corner.

1.1.5.2 Key Points

- Modern-day robotics has its roots in NASA's development of virtual reality.
- Its first practical application was developed as the Green Telepresence Surgery System for DARPA.
- Unimation's PUMA system was the first robotic system to be used clinically.
- The AESOP system and the da Vinci system were developed in parallel.
- Current clinical applications of the robotics are growing daily but include urology, gynecology, colorectal surgery, and cardiac surgery.

References

1. Yates DR, Vaessen C, Roupret M. From Leonardo to da Vinci: the history of robot-assisted surgery in urology. BJU Int. 2011;108(11):1708–13; discussion 1714.
2. Satava RM. Surgical robotics: the early chronicles: a personal historical perspective. Surg Laparosc Endosc Percutan Tech. 2002;12(1):6–16.
3. Kwoh YS, Hou J, Jonckheere EA, Hayati S. A robot with improved absolute positioning accuracy for CT guided stereotactic brain surgery. IEEE Trans Biomed Eng. 1988;35(2):153–60.
4. Falk V, Walther T, Autschbach R, Diegeler A, Battellini R, Mohr FW. Robot-assisted minimally invasive solo mitral valve operation. J Thorac Cardiovasc Surg. 1998;115(2):470–1.
5. Pugin F, Bucher P, Morel P. History of robotic surgery: from AESOP® and ZEUS® to da Vinci®. J Visc Surg. 2011;148(5 Suppl):e3–8.
6. Schuessler WW, Schulam PG, Clayman RV, Kavoussi LR. Laparoscopic radical prostatectomy: initial short-term experience. Urology. 1997;50(6):854–7.
7. Menon M, Tewari A, Baize B, Guillonneau B, Vallancien G. Prospective comparison of radical retropubic prostatectomy and robot-assisted anatomic prostatectomy: the Vattikuti Urology Institute experience. Urology. 2002;60(5):864–8.
8. Lowrance WT, Eastham JA, Savage C, Maschino AC, Laudone VP, Dechet CB, et al. Contemporary open and robotic radical prostatectomy practice patterns among urologists in the United States. J Urol. 2012;187(6):2087–92.
9. Tsui C, Klein R, Garabrant M. Minimally invasive surgery: national trends in adoption and future directions for hospital strategy. Surg Endosc. 2013;27(7): 2253–7.
10. Trinh QD, Sammon J, Sun M, Ravi P, Ghani KR, Bianchi M, et al. Perioperative outcomes of robot-assisted radical prostatectomy compared with open radical prostatectomy: results from the nationwide inpatient sample. Eur Urol. 2012;61(4):679–85.
11. American Cancer Society. What are the key statistics about kidney cancer. 2014. http://www.cancer.org/cancer/kidneycancer/detailedguide/kidney-cancer-adult-key-statistics. Accessed 25 Aug 2014.
12. Huang WC, Levey AS, Serio AM, Snyder M, Vickers AJ, Raj GV, et al. Chronic kidney disease after nephrectomy in patients with renal cortical tumours: a retrospective cohort study. Lancet Oncol. 2006;7(9): 735–40.
13. Uzzo RG, Novick AC. Nephron sparing surgery for renal tumors: indications, techniques and outcomes. J Urol. 2001;166(1):6–18.
14. Abouassaly R, Alibhai SM, Tomlinson G, Timilshina N, Finelli A. Unintended consequences of laparoscopic surgery on partial nephrectomy for kidney cancer. J Urol. 2010;183(2):467–72.
15. Benway BM, Bhayani SB, Rogers CG, Dulabon LM, Patel MN, Lipkin M, et al. Robot assisted partial nephrectomy versus laparoscopic partial nephrectomy for renal tumors: a multi-institutional analysis of perioperative outcomes. J Urol. 2009;182(3):866–72.
16. Khalifeh A, Autorino R, Hillyer SP, Laydner H, Eyraud R, Panumatrassamee K, et al. Comparative outcomes and assessment of trifecta in 500 robotic and laparoscopic partial nephrectomy cases: a single surgeon experience. J Urol. 2013;189(4):1236–42.
17. Liu JJ, Leppert JT, Maxwell BG, Panousis P, Chung BI. Trends and perioperative outcomes for laparoscopic and robotic nephrectomy using the National Surgical Quality Improvement Program (NSQIP) database. Urol Oncol. 2014;32(4):473–9.
18. Stein JP, Lieskovsky G, Cote R, Groshen S, Feng AC, Boyd S, et al. Radical cystectomy in the treatment of invasive bladder cancer: long-term results in 1,054 patients. J Clin Oncol. 2001;19(3):666–75.
19. Guillotreau J, Game X, Mouzin M, Doumerc N, Mallet R, Sallusto F, et al. Radical cystectomy for bladder cancer: morbidity of laparoscopic versus open surgery. J Urol. 2009;181(2):554–9. discussion 559.
20. Beecken WD, Wolfram M, Engl T, Bentas W, Probst M, Blaheta R, et al. Robotic-assisted laparoscopic radical cystectomy and intra-abdominal formation of an orthotopic ileal neobladder. Eur Urol. 2003;44(3): 337–9.
21. Bochner BH, Sjoberg DD, Laudone VP, Group MSKCCBCST. A randomized trial of robot-assisted laparoscopic radical cystectomy. N Engl J Med. 2014;371(4):389–90.
22. Niegisch G, Albers P, Rabenalt R. Perioperative complications and oncological safety of robot-assisted (RARC) vs. open radical cystectomy (ORC). Urol Oncol. 2014;32(7):966–74.
23. Carpentier A, Loulmet D, Aupecle B, Kieffer JP, Tournay D, Guibourt P, et al. Computer assisted open heart surgery. First case operated on with success. C R Acad Sci III. 1998;321(5):437–42.
24. Mihaljevic T, Jarrett CM, Gillinov AM, Williams SJ, DeVilliers PA, Stewart WJ, et al. Robotic repair of posterior mitral valve prolapse versus conventional approaches: potential realized. J Thorac Cardiovasc Surg. 2011;141(1):72–80. e1–4.
25. Seco M, Cao C, Modi P, Bannon PG, Wilson MK, Vallely MP, et al. Systematic review of robotic minimally invasive mitral valve surgery. Ann Cardiothorac Surg. 2013;2(6):704–16.
26. Kent M, Wang T, Whyte R, Curran T, Flores R, Gangadharan S. Open, video-assisted thoracic surgery, and robotic lobectomy: review of a national database. Ann Thorac Surg. 2014;97(1):236–42. discussion 242-4.
27. Sarkaria IS, Rizk NP. Robotic-assisted minimally invasive esophagectomy: the Ivor Lewis approach. Thorac Surg Clin. 2014;24(2):211–22. 2.
28. Clinical Outcomes of Surgical Therapy Study Group. A comparison of laparoscopically assisted and open colectomy for colon cancer. N Engl J Med. 2004;350(20):2050–9.
29. Casillas Jr MA, Leichtle SW, Wahl WL, Lampman RM, Welch KB, Wellock T, et al. Improved perioperative and short-term outcomes of robotic versus

conventional laparoscopic colorectal operations. Am J Surg. 2014;208(1):33–40.

30. Delaney CP, Lynch AC, Senagore AJ, Fazio VW. Comparison of robotically performed and traditional laparoscopic colorectal surgery. Dis Colon Rectum. 2003;46(12):1633–9.

31. Deutsch GB, Sathyanarayana SA, Gunabushanam V, Mishra N, Rubach E, Zemon H, et al. Robotic vs. Laparoscopic colorectal surgery: an institutional experience. Surg Endosc. 2012;26(4):956–63.

32. deSouza AL, Prasad LM, Park JJ, Marecik SJ, Blumetti J, Abcarian H. Robotic assistance in right hemicolectomy: is there a role? Dis Colon Rectum. 2010;53(7):1000–6.

33. Heald RJ, Moran BJ, Ryall RD, Sexton R, MacFarlane JK. Rectal cancer: the Basingstoke experience of total mesorectal excision, 1978–1997. Arch Surg. 1998; 133(8):894–9.

34. deSouza AL, Prasad LM, Ricci J, Park JJ, Marecik SJ, Zimmern A, et al. A comparison of open and robotic total mesorectal excision for rectal adenocarcinoma. Dis Colon Rectum. 2011;54(3):275–82.

35. Baek JH, McKenzie S, Garcia-Aguilar J, Pigazzi A. Oncologic outcomes of robotic-assisted total mesorectal excision for the treatment of rectal cancer. Ann Surg. 2010;251(5):882–6.

36. Hara M, Sng K, Yoo BE, Shin JW, Lee DW, Kim SH. Robotic-assisted surgery for rectal adenocarcinoma: short-term and midterm outcomes from 200 consecutive cases at a single institution. Dis Colon Rectum. 2014;57(5):570–7.

37. Saklani AP, Lim DR, Hur H, Min BS, Baik SH, Lee KY, et al. Robotic versus laparoscopic surgery for mid-low rectal cancer after neoadjuvant chemoradiation therapy: comparison of oncologic outcomes. Int J Colorectal Dis. 2013;28(12):1689–98.

38. Xiong B, Ma L, Zhang C, Cheng Y. Robotic versus laparoscopic total mesorectal excision for rectal cancer: a meta-analysis. J Surg Res. 2014;188(2):404–14.

39. Kim JY, Kim NK, Lee KY, Hur H, Min BS, Kim JH. A comparative study of voiding and sexual function after total mesorectal excision with autonomic nerve preservation for rectal cancer: laparoscopic versus robotic surgery. Ann Surg Oncol. 2012;19(8): 2485–93.

40. Luca F, Valvo M, Ghezzi TL, Zuccaro M, Cenciarelli S, Trovato C, et al. Impact of robotic surgery on sexual and urinary functions after fully robotic nerve-sparing total mesorectal excision for rectal cancer. Ann Surg. 2013;257(4):672–8.

41. D'Annibale A, Pernazza G, Monsellato I, Pende V, Lucandri G, Mazzocchi P, et al. Total mesorectal excision: a comparison of oncological and functional outcomes between robotic and laparoscopic surgery for rectal cancer. Surg Endosc. 2013;27(6):1887–95.

42. Byrn JC, Hrabe JE, Charlton ME. An initial experience with 85 consecutive robotic-assisted rectal dissections: improved operating times and lower costs with experience. Surg Endosc. 2014;28(11):3101–7.

43. Ostrowitz MB, Eschete D, Zemon H, DeNoto G. Robotic-assisted single-incision right colectomy: early experience. Int J Med Robot. 2009;5(4):465–70.

44. ACOG Committee Opinion No. 444: choosing the route of hysterectomy for benign disease. Obstet Gynecol. 2009;14(5):1156–1158.

45. Rosero EB, Kho KA, Joshi GP, Giesecke M, Schaffer JI. Comparison of robotic and laparoscopic hysterectomy for benign gynecologic disease. Obstet Gynecol. 2013;122(4):778–86.

46. Liu H, Lu D, Wang L, Shi G, Song H, Clarke J. Robotic surgery for benign gynaecological disease. Cochrane Database Syst Rev. 2012;2, CD008978.

47. Wright JD, Ananth CV, Lewin SN, Burke WM, Lu YS, Neugut AI, et al. Robotically assisted vs laparoscopic hysterectomy among women with benign gynecologic disease. JAMA. 2013;309(7):689–98.

48. Weinberg L, Rao S, Escobar PF. Robotic surgery in gynecology: an updated systematic review. Obstet Gynecol Int. 2011;2011:852061.

49. Gaia G, Holloway RW, Santoro L, Ahmad S, Di Silverio E, Spinillo A. Robotic-assisted hysterectomy for endometrial cancer compared with traditional laparoscopic and laparotomy approaches: a systematic review. Obstet Gynecol. 2010;116(6):1422–31.

50. Backes FJ, Brudie LA, Farrell MR, Ahmad S, Finkler NJ, Bigsby GE, et al. Short- and long-term morbidity and outcomes after robotic surgery for comprehensive endometrial cancer staging. Gynecol Oncol. 2012; 125(3):546–51.

51. Cardenas-Goicoechea J, Shepherd A, Momeni M, Mandeli J, Chuang L, Gretz H, et al. Survival analysis of robotic versus traditional laparoscopic surgical staging for endometrial cancer. Am J Obstet Gynecol. 2014;210(2):160.e1–e11.

52. Jayaraman S, Davies W, Schlachta CM. Getting started with robotics in general surgery with cholecystectomy: the Canadian experience. Can J Surg. 2009;52(5):374–8.

53. Salman M, Bell T, Martin J, Bhuva K, Grim R, Ahuja V. Use, cost, complications, and mortality of robotic versus nonrobotic general surgery procedures based on a nationwide database. Am Surg. 2013;79(6):553–60.

54. Vidovszky TJ, Carr AD, Farinholt GN, Ho HS, Smith WH, Ali MR. Single-site robotic cholecystectomy in a broadly inclusive patient population: a prospective study. Ann Surg. 2014;260(1):134–41.

55. Konstantinidis KM, Hirides P, Hirides S, Chrysocheris P, Georgiou M. Cholecystectomy using a novel Single-Site(®) robotic platform: early experience from 45 consecutive cases. Surg Endosc. 2012;26(9):2687–94.

56. Fourman MM, Saber AA. Robotic bariatric surgery: a systematic review. Surg Obes Relat Dis. 2012;8(4): 483–8.

57. Owen B, Simorov A, Siref A, Shostrom V, Oleynikov D. How does robotic anti-reflux surgery compare with traditional open and laparoscopic techniques: a cost and outcomes analysis. Surg Endosc. 2014;28(5):1686–90.

58. Muller-Stich BP, Reiter MA, Wente MN, Bintintan VV, Koninger J, Buchler MW, et al. Robot-assisted versus conventional laparoscopic fundoplication: short-term outcome of a pilot randomized controlled trial. Surg Endosc. 2007;21(10):1800–5.
59. Boggi U, Caniglia F, Amorese G. Laparoscopic robot-assisted major hepatectomy. J Hepatobiliary Pancreat Sci. 2014;21(1):3–10.
60. Tsung A, Geller DA, Sukato DC, Sabbaghian S, Tohme S, Steel J, et al. Robotic versus laparoscopic hepatectomy: a matched comparison. Ann Surg. 2014;259(3):549–55.
61. Lai EC, Yang GP, Tang CN. Robot-assisted laparoscopic liver resection for hepatocellular carcinoma: short-term outcome. Am J Surg. 2013;205(6):697–702.
62. Orti-Rodriguez RJ, Rahman SH. A comparative review between laparoscopic and robotic pancreaticoduodenectomies. Surg Laparosc Endosc Percutan Tech. 2014;24(2):103–8.
63. Zhang J, Wu WM, You L, Zhao YP. Robotic versus open pancreatectomy: a systematic review and meta-analysis. Ann Surg Oncol. 2013;20(6):1774–80.
64. Park JY, Kim YW, Ryu KW, Eom BW, Yoon HM, Reim D. Emerging role of robot-assisted gastrectomy: analysis of consecutive 200 cases. J Gastric Cancer. 2013;13(4):255–62.
65. Vasilescu C, Stanciulea O, Tudor S. Laparoscopic versus robotic subtotal splenectomy in hereditary spherocytosis. Potential advantages and limits of an expensive approach. Surg Endosc. 2012;26(10):2802–9.
66. Sun GH, Peress L, Pynnonen MA. Systematic review and meta-analysis of robotic vs conventional thyroidectomy approaches for thyroid disease. Otolaryngol Head Neck Surg. 2014;150(4):520–32.
67. Abdelgadir Adam M, Speicher P, Pura J, Dinan MA, Reed SD, Roman SA, et al. Robotic thyroidectomy for cancer in the US: patterns of Use and short-term outcomes. Ann Surg Oncol. 2014;21(12):3859–64.
68. O'Malley Jr BW, Weinstein GS, Snyder W, Hockstein NG. Transoral robotic surgery (TORS) for base of tongue neoplasms. Laryngoscope. 2006;116(8):1465–72.
69. Hans S, Delas B, Gorphe P, Menard M, Brasnu D. Transoral robotic surgery in head and neck cancer. Eur Ann Otorhinolaryngol Head Neck Dis. 2012;129(1):32–7.
70. Van Abel KM, Moore EJ. The rise of transoral robotic surgery in the head and neck: emerging applications. Expert Rev Anticancer Ther. 2012;12(3):373–80.
71. Wortman TD, Mondry JM, Farritor SM, Oleynikov D. Single-site colectomy with miniature in vivo robotic platform. IEEE Trans Biomed Eng. 2013;60(4):926–9.
72. Gordon ZN, Angell J, Abaza R. Completely intracorporeal robotic renal autotransplantation. J Urol. 2014;192(5):1516–22.
73. Hompes R, Rauh SM, Ris F, Tuynman JB, Mortensen NJ. Robotic transanal minimally invasive surgery for local excision of rectal neoplasms. Br J Surg. 2014;101(5):578–81.
74. Bardakcioglu O. Robotic transanal access surgery. Surg Endosc. 2013;27(4):1407–9.
75. Gomez Ruiz M, Palazuelos CM, Martin Parra JI, Alonso Martin J, Cagigas Fernandez C, del Castillo DJ, et al. New technique of transanal proctectomy with completely robotic total mesorrectal excision for rectal cancer. Cir Esp. 2014;92(5):356–61.
76. Zygomalas A, Kehagias I, Giokas K, Koutsouris D. Miniature surgical robots in the Era of NOTES and LESS: dream or reality? Surg Innov. 2015;22(1):97–107.
77. Ullrich F, Bergeles C, Pokki J, Ergeneman O, Erni S, Chatzipirpiridis G, et al. Mobility experiments with microrobots for minimally invasive intraocular surgery. Invest Ophthalmol Vis Sci. 2013;54(4):2853–63.

Evolution of Robotic Approaches for Colorectal Surgery

Elizabeth R. Raskin

Abstract

The evolution of robotic surgery is not unlike the process described by Charles Darwin (Fig. 2.1) in his seminal treatise, *On the Origin of Species*. His premise of natural selection is based on the concept that certain genetic traits of an organism encode for enhanced robustness and fecundity. Organisms capable of adapting to their environments reproduced, passed on their genetic material, and survived. The development of minimally invasive surgery (MIS) is analogous in that techniques which have translated into improved outcomes and perceived advantages have established themselves in surgical culture and continue to develop.

Keywords

Evolution • History • Robotic surgery • Colorectal surgery • Minimally invasive surgery

> In the long history of humankind (and animal kind, too) those who learned to collaborate and improvise most effectively have prevailed. —Charles Darwin

The evolution of robotic surgery is not unlike the process described by Charles Darwin (Fig. 2.1) in his seminal treatise, *On the Origin of Species*. His premise of natural selection is based on the concept that certain genetic traits of an organism encode for enhanced robustness and fecundity. Organisms capable of adapting to their environments reproduced, passed on their genetic material, and survived. The development of minimally invasive surgery (MIS) is analogous in that techniques that have translated into improved outcomes and perceived advantages have established themselves in surgical culture and continue to develop.

Technologic advancement has lent itself to the development of innovative surgical technique and has changed the surgical standard of care in several areas. Laparoscopic cholecystectomy is a technique that has demonstrated clear-cut advantages over its open surgery predecessor. From decreased postoperative pain to shorter length of stay, the superiority of this approach from a short-term outcome standpoint catapulted it to

E.R. Raskin, M.D., F.A.C.S., F.A.S.C.R.S. (✉)
Division of Colon and Rectal Surgery,
Department of Surgery, University of Minnesota,
St. Paul, MN, USA
e-mail: eraskin@crsal.org

© Springer International Publishing Switzerland 2015
H. Ross et al. (eds.), *Robotic Approaches to Colorectal Surgery*,
DOI 10.1007/978-3-319-09120-4_2

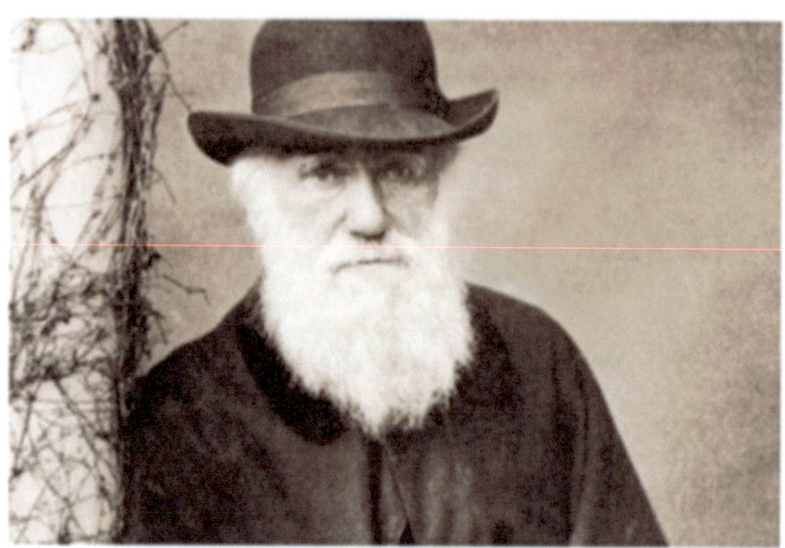

Fig. 2.1 Charles Darwin

the standard of care for surgical treatment of routine gallbladder disease [1–4]. Although not extinct, open cholecystectomy represents less than 10 % of gallbladder resections performed annually. Similarly, routine tubal ligation is almost exclusively performed in a laparoscopic manner, avoiding the unnecessary morbidity of a laparotomy.

While shown to be oncologically sound and to significantly reduce postoperative pain and length of stay [5–8], laparoscopic colectomy (LC) has experienced a flatter trajectory in its evolution with less than a 50 % implementation for colorectal resections. Attributed to the technical challenges of the approach and significant learning curve [9, 10], the lack of significant adoption of the laparoscopic approach may signify the establishment of an intermediate surgical technique. To clarify, the outcome advantages and technical feasibility may not demonstrate enough robustness to supplant the standard open approach [11]. Some of the technical obstacles of laparoscopic colectomy include inadequate optics with poor resolution of 2D images, incongruous eye–hand coordination, decreased dexterity of laparoscopic instruments, and reduced sensory information with a loss of accurate haptic feedback.

Evolution is a concept that relies upon constant, random mutation. Although not random, but rather the result of conscious innovation, the introduction of robotic technology to the field of surgery can be viewed as one such mutation. From rudimentary instruments such as the PUMA 560, designed to perform more precise biopsying of the brain and prostate, to the more sophisticated platforms of the ZEUS and da Vinci® systems which enable surgeons to perform complex minimally invasive resections, robotic technology has emerged as a variant of MIS aimed at addressing the technical limitations of laparoscopy and expanding the benefits to patients. With its origin in cardiothoracic surgery, robotic surgery has metastasized to such specialties as urology, gynecology, ENT, and colorectal surgery. Within the field of colorectal surgery, surgeons have reported on the expansion of their capabilities and technique in regards to the optics, dexterity of instruments, and stability of the current robotic platform. The goal of this chapter is to address the evolution of robotic technology and robotic surgical technique.

2.1 The Dawn of Laparoscopic Surgery

Interest in evaluating the occult spaces of the human body using tube instruments and rudimentary light sources was first noted in artifacts from ancient Mesopotamian and Greek civilizations.

However, the development of modern endoscopic technology truly found its beginnings in the early nineteenth century when several European physicians contrived the first cystoscope which was used to look into the vagina, urethra, and bladder. The term "celiacoscopy" was coined by the German surgeon Georg Kelling (1866–1945) in 1901 after inserting a cystoscope into the abdomen of a laboratory dog followed by cadaveric and live humans [12]. Kelling had experimented with high-pressure insufflation of air into the abdominal cavity (Lufftamponade) as a means to halt intra-abdominal bleeding. To evaluate the effect of the air tamponade on the intra-abdominal contents, he began inserting a cystoscope.

While Kelling never published his results, Hans Christian Jacobaeus (1879–1937), a Swedish internist, did report on the first use of "laparothoracoscopy" in 1910 during his investigation of pneumoperitoneum as a treatment for tubercular peritonitis. He chronicled the use of this novel endoscopic technique in 97 patients, using the large volume of ascites created in the condition as a means of inflating the abdomen and protecting from intestinal injury.

Slow progress ensued over the next 50 years in the field of laparoscopy, but culminated in a publication by American surgeon, Raoul Palmer, in the early 1950s describing the first diagnostic laparoscopy. German gynecologist, Kurt Semm, led the charge for pelviscopic and laparoscopic surgery in the mid-1950s, developing techniques such as minimally invasive adnexectomy, hysterectomy, and appendectomy. As an instrument maker, he invented many sophisticated laparoscopic instruments such as a CO_2-pneumatic insufflator, a thermocoagulator, and several intracorporeal knot-tying devices. Unfortunately, Semm was harshly ridiculed by his gynecologic colleagues and many international societies, with opponents demanding that he undergo a "brain scan" for "only a person with brain damage would perform laparoscopic surgery" [13]. With passion and perseverance, Semm continued his work and began to influence open-minded surgeons in both Europe and the USA.

The late twentieth century ushered in an era of laparoscopic implementation and diversification.

The first descriptions of laparoscopic cholecystectomy were reported by Erich Mühe (Germany, 1985), Philippe Mouret (France, 1987), Francois Dubois (France, 1988), and McKernan/Saye (USA, 1988). After presenting a paper describing the first laparoscopic cholecystectomy at the German Surgical Society (GSS) meeting in 1986, his paper was rejected, much like the work of Semm some 30 years before. Mühe was later given the highest honor by the GSS in 1992, recognizing the substantial contribution he had made toward the development of laparoscopic surgery. The use of trocars, specialized instruments such as graspers and scissors, and vessel clips was introduced in these early procedures. Interestingly, Mühe had developed his own "galloscope" through which he performed the first laparoscopic cholecystectomies (Fig. 2.2). The galloscope consisted of side-viewing optics, a light source, a duct for insufflation, and instrumentation chan-

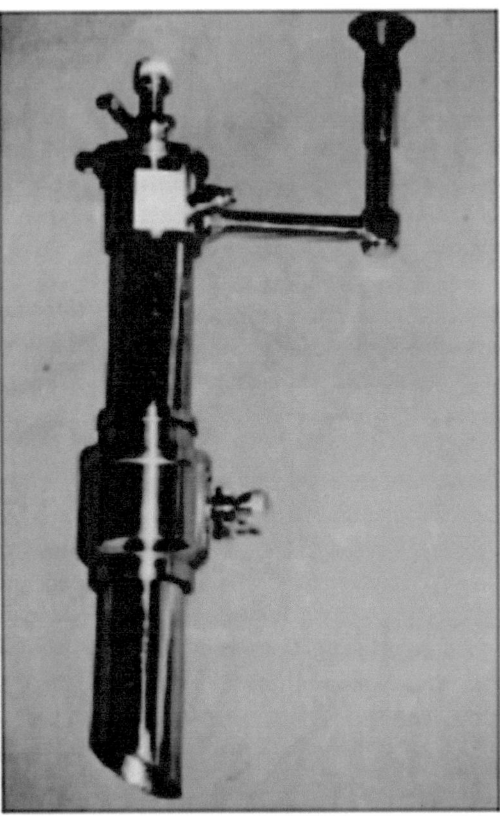

Fig. 2.2 The Mühe "galloscope" through which was used to perform the first laparoscopic cholecystectomy

nels with valves. He adopted early on a single-incision approach, described as an "open tube laparoscopic cholecystectomy," which necessitated a single 2.5 cm incision created directly above the gallbladder for his galloscope and required no insufflation [14, 15]. This technique was not adopted universally, as the multi-port approach with insufflation demonstrated the advantages of enhanced visualization and range of motion for instruments.

As laparoscopic cholecystectomy gained momentum, surgeons began to expand the use of laparoscopic technology to include such procedures as appendectomy, adrenalectomy, gastrectomy, and colectomy. Large series and randomized controlled trials emerged in the literature demonstrating the feasibility, safety, and oncologic soundness of laparoscopic colectomy for both benign and malignant colorectal disease [16–18].

2.2 Robotic Technology

While early surgical robotic technology was originally created to enhance precision in biopsying, the development of more complex robotic surgery platforms was first driven by the National Aeronautics and Space Administration (NASA) and the US military in hopes of achieving telepresence surgery. Telepresence surgery refers to the concept of performing surgery from a remote location outside of the operating room, such as the battlefield or space station. When physicians became exposed to this new research, they recognized a very imminent application of robotic technology in the current operating room. The collaboration between surgeons and roboticists culminated in a variety of telepresence devices such as AESOP, PROBOT, and ROBODOC which provided very specific, but limited surgical activities (i.e., voice-activated, "third-arm" camera assistance, more precise prostate biopsying, and femur manipulation in hip replacements) [19]. AESOP's voice-activated technology was incorporated into the ZEUS Robotic Surgical System (ZRSS) by Computer Motion, an early master–slave platform that consisted of three robotic arms controlled by the surgeon sitting at a remote console. ZRSS was cleared by the FDA in 2001, but was discontinued when a merger between Computer Motion and Intuitive Surgical occurred in 2003.

In 2000, Intuitive Surgical launched their first FDA-approved robotic surgery platform, the da Vinci® Surgical System, and has been the most widely used surgical platform to date. The da Vinci® Surgical System is comprised of a patient-side cart with four interactive arms controlled by the surgeon at the console using his forefingers and thumbs to manipulate the master controls.

2.3 Optics

From the primitive light-sensitive "eyespot" of simple unicellular organisms to the more complex optical systems of vertebrates, the evolution of modern optics has relied upon 540 million years of gradual mutation. Luckily, surgical optics have developed over a much shorter period of time. Building upon the early developments of such visionaries as Austrian Philipp Bozzini who created the *Lichtleiter* (Fig. 2.3) in 1805, the first illuminated scope which consisted of a rudimentary viewing tube, a series of mirrors, and a candle as a light source, and German dentist Julius Bruck who first linked a medical scope to an electric light source (1867), physicists have been pushing the boundaries of medical optics with the hope of enhancing surgical capabilities. The development of fiber-optic technology in the 1950s allowed for improved illumination but exposed the deficits of lens design. A series of small lenses were required to propagate the light through the shaft of the early scopes, but high-quality lenses were exceptionally difficult to manufacture. British physicist Harold Hopkins unveiled his "rod lens" design, which eliminated the need for lenses by using glass rods to transduce the light and allowed for the development of smaller scope diameter.

Until analog medical cameras were made available in the 1970s to attach to the scopes, the surgeon was required to utilize the eyepiece for

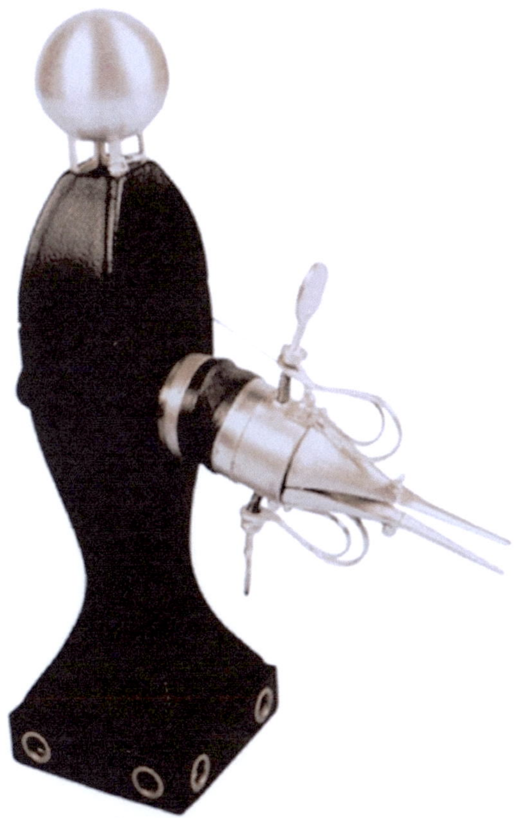

Fig. 2.3 The *Lichtleiter* created by Austrian Philipp Bozzini in 1805, the first illuminated scope which consisted of a rudimentary viewing tube, a series of mirrors, and a candle as a light source

visualization of the surgical field. The development of medical cameras utilizing silicon chip technology or charge-coupled devices (CCD) in 1982 was considered a groundbreaking technologic advancement in that it allowed for the storage of a digital image of the surgical scene that could be transmitted more efficiently and with greater resolution than its analog predecessor. These higher-quality images could be projected onto monitors that could be viewed by the entire surgical team. Standard laparoscopic images are 2-D and result in the loss of binocular cues, limited depth perception, and increased motion parallax [20].

Robotic surgery optical technology has revolutionized MIS optics in that it has allowed for 3-D visualization of the surgical field at the remote console. 3-D technology is centered around the concept of stereopsis or creation of depth perception. The robotic system creates depth of field using two cameras and two different lenses, projecting images that are slightly different in each eye. A 3-D image is the result of the ocular disparity registered by the brain. Enhanced depth perception has been associated with a shorter learning curve in particular MIS skills such as intracorporeal knot tying and suturing [21, 22].

2.4 The Surgical Hand

The acquisition of human stereoscopic vision accompanied the evolution of the prehensile hand. With the densest concentration of nerve endings of the entire body centered at its fingertips, the hand is the organ that is most intimately associated with the sense of touch. Haptic feedback generated by the hand is responsible for spatial recognition and interpretation of density and texture of objects, cognitive skills essential to surgical performance. As MIS became a prominent surgical technique, a reduction of sensory information resulted as direct contact of the hand with the surgical field was replaced with crude feedback from rigid laparoscopic instruments. Decreased dexterity and range of motion are often cited as drawbacks of laparoscopy and contribute to the steep learning curve of complex MIS procedures. The robotic "hands" of the current system attempt to regain some of these lost functions by providing wristed instruments with 90 degrees of articulation and 7 degrees of freedom. While little to no haptic feedback exists with this platform, the concept of *surgical synesthesia* has been suggested, referring to the development of a sense of "touch" from the visual cues gained as an object is touched [20, 23, 24].

In addition to the specialized hands, the stability of the robotic platform allows for more precise fine motor activities, such as dissection, tissue manipulation, and suturing. The significant tremor reduction of the robotic platform is considered an advantage over both laparoscopic and open surgery.

2.5   Ergonomics of the Robotic Surgeon

Chronic musculoskeletal and vertebral disk injuries have been associated with the prolonged ergonomic stress of traditional laparoscopy [25–27]. Many of the chronic back, neck, and shoulder injuries described are attributed to the incongruous technical maneuvers required with straight-stick laparoscopic instruments, awkward body positioning, and non-ergonomic positioning of the operating table and video console [28]. Surgeon laparoscopic case volume and workload over time have been specifically linked to chronic musculoskeletal pain and discomfort [29]. It has been suggested that less surgeon fatigue occurs during robotic surgery as the operator sits in a more comfortable position at the console, manipulating lightweight master controls.

In a quantitative comparison study evaluating muscle activation during traditional laparoscopic surgery (TLS) versus robotic-assisted surgery (RAS), surface electromyography measurements were recorded from the surgeon's biceps, triceps, deltoid, and trapezius muscle groups [30]. Significantly elevated muscle activation was noted in the biceps, triceps, and deltoid muscles during TLS, compared to RAS. Similar levels of muscle activation were noted in the trapezius muscles in both TLS and RAS. These findings suggest that the more ergonomic design of the robotic surgery platform may minimize surgeon muscular fatigue over time and perhaps improve overall productivity and longevity of practice.

2.6   Evolution of Robotic Surgical Technique

Robotic surgical technique for numerous procedures has developed after many painstaking hours in the laboratory and operating room. From the number of trocars utilized to the positioning of instruments, current surgical instrument configuration has largely been established through a trial-and-error process. Some of the first robotic surgical experiences describe techniques used for cardiac and gynecologic procedures. In 2000,

Kappert et al. [31] reported on their "three-point stab incision" trocar arrangement for closed-chest coronary artery bypass while Lapietra et al. [32] described a three-port approach for the thoracoscope and two needle holders, with the use of a fourth "service entrance" incision in the seventh interspace for suture passing, retractor blade placement, and introduction of the valve prosthesis for mitral valve surgery. In the first reported series of hysterectomy with bilateral salpingo-oophorectomy, a four- to five-port approach was detailed by Diaz-Arrastia et al., utilizing a camera port, two robotic arm ports, and 1–2 laparoscopic assistant ports [33].

Trocar placement is typically based on the laparoscopic concept of triangulation of instruments around the target organ; however, the robotic ports require unique spacing to avoid arm collision once docked. Body habitus can complicate trocar placement by either limiting the spacing in the thin or petite patient or obscuring the abdominal landmarks in the obese patient. It is recommended that the spacing between trocars be at least 8 cm with approximately 18–20 cm between the camera port and the target organ. With respect to the iliac crests, at least 2–3 cm clearance should be allowed for the laterally placed ports. These earliest reports employed the three-armed da Vinci® Standard Surgery System. A fourth-arm upgrade to this system became available several years later, as well as a four-arm model, the da Vinci® S System.

Esposito et al. described their approach to radical prostatectomy using a four-arm model, noting the advantages of the fourth arm for retraction and rotation of the prostate during key events: dissection of the bladder neck and seminal vesicles, mobilization of the prostate off of the rectum, and dissection of vascular pedicles and neurovascular bundles [34]. By locking the fourth arm into place, more efficient dissection and exposure was made possible by the primary working arms. Similar findings were reported by Newlin et al. regarding foregut surgery, but the authors cautioned that the fixed retractor arm could pose a potential risk for tearing and avulsing structures if tissues are moved in relation to its fixed position [35].

Technical reports of colorectal procedures began surfacing in the early 2000s with authors touting the benefits of "single-surgeon surgery" [36]. The majority of these publications described a "hybrid" approach involving standard laparoscopy for portions of the operation [37–39]. Unlike the fields of urology and gynecology, colorectal surgery typically requires dissection and mobilization in multiple abdominal quadrants. A hybrid robotic-assisted sigmoid and anterior resections involved a laparoscopic-assisted takedown of the splenic flexure, transection of the bowel with a laparoscopic stapler, and division of vascular pedicles with laparoscopic energy devices, while the robot was utilized for the pelvic dissection. Technique for non-hybrid totally robotic colorectal resections evolved which entailed a "double-docking" approach [40–43]. Koh et al. described their approach for left-sided colon and rectal resections utilizing two phases of robotic application [40]. "Phase 1" involved docking the robot with the target anatomy toward the left colon allowing for the takedown of the splenic flexure, colonic mobilization, and ligation of the vascular pedicle. A second docking was then performed to allow for the pelvic dissection.

Single-stage totally robotic resections developed as surgeons discovered optimal placement of trocars with some of the newer generations of robotic systems (i.e., S, Si, and Xi) which have increased range of motion and less spacing requirements for arms [44–46]. A "one-step" approach for total mesorectal excision (TME) (Fig. 2.4) has been described with the first step involving a three-arm setup through which the initial exposure, primary vascular control, and medial-to-lateral mobilization of descending and splenic flexure are accomplished [44]. The second step employs the fourth arm for the TME dissection.

2.7 Conclusion

From rudimentary optical devices involving candles and mirrors to the modern and sophisticated robotic surgical systems currently employed in hospitals around the world, surgical innovation has evolved steadily over the past 150 years. The field of MIS has proven to offer advantages to patients in both short- and long-term outcomes. The lack of complete adoption of MIS for colorectal surgery and other surgical fields illuminates some of the limitations posed by laparoscopy. Although initially developed to realize the possibility of telepresence surgery, robotic surgical technology emerged as a response to some of the technical challenges of standard laparoscopy. Technique has coevolved with instrumentation

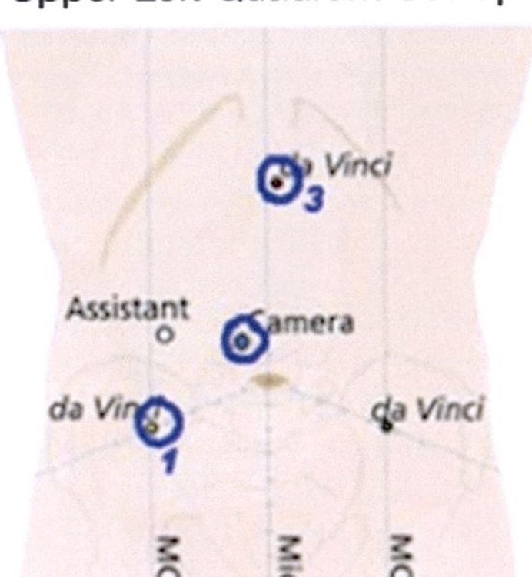

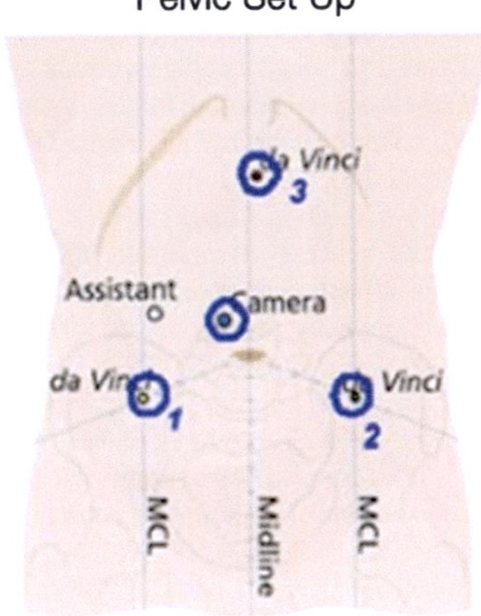

Fig. 2.4 A "one-step" approach for total mesorectal excision (TME)

and advanced robotic surgical systems. Robotic experience from other surgical fields has lent itself toward strategies regarding port placement and use of the fourth arm. The field of colorectal surgery has seen the rise of multiple robotic approaches, including hybrid and non-hybrid operations with different docking strategies, designed to improve mobilization and dissection. As surgeons continue to collaborate with physicists and innovators to advance surgical technology, it seems evident that the boundaries of robotic surgical capabilities will be limited by the extent of our imaginations.

References

1. Neugebauer E, Troidi H, Spangenberger W, Dietrich A, Lefering R. Conventional versus laparoscopic cholecystectomy and the randomized controlled trial: Cholecystectomy Study Group. Br J Surg. 1991;78(2):150–4.
2. Kunz R, Ortu K, Vogel J, Steinacker JM, Meitinger A, Bruckner U, Beger HG. Laparoscopic cholecystectomy versus mini-laparoscopic cholecystectomy: results of a prospective, randomized study. Chirurg. 1992;63(4):291–5.
3. Trondsen E, Reiertsen O, Anderson OK, Kjaersgaard P. Laparoscopic and open cholecystectomy. A prospective, randomized study. Eur J Surg. 1993; 159(4):217–21.
4. Barkun JS, Barkun AN, Meakins JL. Laparoscopic versus open cholecystectomy: the Canadian experience. The McGill Gallstone Treatment Group. Am J Surg. 1993;165(4):455–8.
5. Jacobs M, Verdeja JC, Goldstein HS. Minimally invasive colon resection (laparoscopic colectomy). Surg Laparosc Endosc. 1991;1(3):144–50.
6. Lacy AM, Garcia-Valdecasas JC, Delgado S, Castells A, Taura P, Pique JM, Visa J. Laparoscopy-assisted colectomy versus open colectomy for treatment of non-metastatic colon cancer: a randomised trial. Lancet. 2002;359(9325):2224–9.
7. Kuntz C, Wunsch A, Rosch R, Autschbach F, Windeler J, Herfarth C. Short- and long-term results after laparoscopic vs conventional colon resection in a tumor-bearing small animal model. Surg Endosc. 2000;14(6):561–7.
8. Biondi A, Grosso G, Mistretta A, Marventano S, Toscano C, Gruttadauria S, Basile F. Laparoscopic-assisted versus open surgery for colorectal cancer: short- and long-term outcomes comparison. J Laparoendosc Adv Surg Tech A. 2013;23(1):1–7.
9. Tekkis PP, Senagore AJ, Delany CP, et al. Evaluation of the learning curve in laparoscopic colorectal surgery: comparison of right-sided and left-sided resections. Ann Surg. 2005;242:83–91.
10. Reichenbach DJ, Tackett AD, Harris J, et al. Laparoscopic colon resection early in the learning curve: what is the appropriate setting? Ann Surg. 2006;243:730–5.
11. Biondi A, Grosso G, Mistretta A, Marventano S, Toscano C, Drago F, Gangi S, Basile F. Laparoscopic vs. open approach for colorectal cancer: evolution over time of minimal invasive surgery. BMC Surg. 2013;13 Suppl 2:S12.
12. Litzynski GS. Laparoscopy—the early attempts: spotlighting Georg Kelling and Hans Christian Jacobaeus. JSLS. 1997;1(1):83–5.
13. Bhattacharya K. Kurt Semm: a laparoscopic crusader. J Minim Access Surg. 2007;3(1):35–6.
14. Reynolds W. The first laparoscopic cholecystectomy. JSLS. 2001;5(1):89–94.
15. Dobbins TA, Young JM, Solomon MJ. Uptake and outcomes of laparoscopically assisted resection for colon and rectal cancer in Australia: a population-based study. Dis Colon Rectum. 2014;57(4):415–22.
16. Fleshman J, et al. Laparoscopic colectomy for cancer is not inferior to open surgery based on 5-year data from the COST Study Group trial. Ann Surg. 2007;246(4):655–62.
17. Jayne DG, et al. Randomized trial of laparoscopic-assisted resection of colorectal carcinoma: 3-year results of the UK MRC CLASICC Trial Group. J Clin Oncol. 2007;25(21):3061–8.
18. Guillou PJ, et al. Short-term endpoints of conventional versus laparoscopic-assisted surgery in patients with colorectal cancer (MRC CLASICC trial): multi-centre, randomised controlled trial. Lancet. 2005; 365(9472):1718–26.
19. Lafranco A, Castellanos A, Desai J, Meyers W. Robotic surgery: a current perspective. Ann Surg. 2004;239(1):14–21.
20. Healey A. Speculation on the neuropsychology of teleoperation: implications for presence research and minimally invasive surgery. Presence. 2008;17(2):199–211.
21. Buckley CE, et al. The impact of aptitude on the learning curve for laparoscopic suturing. Am J Surg. 2014;207(2):263–70.
22. Mistry M, Roach VA, Wilson TD. Application of stereoscopic visualization on surgical skill acquisition in novices. J Surg Educ. 2013;70(5):563–70.
23. Tewari AK, et al. Visual cues as a surrogate for tactile feedback during robotic-assisted laparoscopic prostatectomy: posterolateral margin rates in 1340 consecutive patients. BJU Int. 2010;106(4):528–36.
24. Lécuyer A. Simulating haptic feedback using vision: a survey of research and applications of pseudo-haptic feedback. Presence. 2009;18:139–53.
25. Cass GK, Vyas S, Akande V. Prolonged laparoscopic surgery is associated with an increased risk of vertebral disc prolapse. J Obstet Gynaecol. 2014;34(1): 74–8.
26. Tiiam IM, Goossens RH, Schout BM, Koldewijn EL, Hendrikx AJ, Muijtjens AM, Scherpbier AJ, Witjes

JA. Ergonomics in endourology and laparoscopy: an overview of musculoskeletal problems in urology. J Endourol. 2014;28(5):605–11.

27. Zihni AM, Ohu I, Cavallo JA, Cho S, Awad MM. Ergonomic analysis of robot-assisted and traditional laparoscopic procedures. Surg Endosc. 2014;28(12):3379–84.

28. Zihni AM, Ohu I, Cavallo JA, Ousley J, Cho S, Awad MM. FLS tasks can be used as an ergonomic discriminator between laparoscopic and robotic surgery. Surg Endosc. 2014;28(8):2459–65.

29. Stomberg MW, Tronstad SE, Hedberg K, Bengtsson J, Jonsson P, Johansen L, Lindvall B. Work-related musculoskeletal disorders when performing laparoscopic surgery. Surg Laparosc Endosc Percutan Tech. 2010;20(1):49–53.

30. Lee GI, Lee MR, Clanton T, Sutton E, Park AE, Marohn MR. Comparative assessment of physical and cognitive ergonomics associated with robotic and traditional laparoscopic surgeries. Surg Endosc. 2014;28(2):456–65.

31. Kappert U, et al. Robotic coronary artery surgery: the evolution of a new minimally-invasive approach in coronary artery surgery. Thorac Cardiovasc Surg. 2000;48(4):193–7.

32. Lapietra A, et al. Robotic-assisted instruments enhance minimally-invasive mitral valve surgery. Ann Thorac Surg. 2000;70(3):835–8.

33. Diaz-Arrastia C, Jurnalov C, Gomez G, Townsend C. Laparoscopic hysterectomy using a computer-enhanced surgical robot. Surg Endosc. 2002;16(9):1271–3.

34. Esposito MP, Ilbeigi P, Ahmed M, Lanteri V. Use of fourth arm in da Vinci® robot-assisted extraperitoneal laparoscopic prostatectomy: novel technique. Urology. 2005;66(3):649–52.

35. Newlin ME, Melvin SW. Initial experience with the four-arm computer-enhanced telesurgery device in foregut surgery. J Laparoendosc Adv Surg Tech A. 2004;14(3):121–4.

36. Hildebrandt U, Plusczyk T, Kessler K, Menger MD. Single-surgeon surgery in laparoscopic colonic resection. Dis Colon Rectum. 2003;46(12):1640–5.

37. Zimmern A, Prasad L, Desouza A, Marecik S, Park J, Abcarian H. Robotic colon and rectal surgery: a series of 131 cases. World J Surg. 2010;34(8):1954–8.

38. Baik SH, et al. Robotic tumor-specific mesorectal excision of rectal cancer: short-term outcomes of a pilot randomized trial. Surg Endosc. 2008;22:1601–8.

39. Hellan M, Anderson C, Ellenhorn JD, Paz B, Pigazzi A. Short-term outcomes after robotic-assisted total mesorectal excision for rectal cancer. Ann Surg Oncol. 2007;14:3168–73.

40. Koh DC, Tsang CB, Kim SH. A new application of the four-arm standard da Vinci® surgical system: totally robotic-assisted left-sided colon or rectal resection. Surg Endosc. 2011;25(6):1945–52.

41. Baik SH, et al. Robotic total mesorectal excision for rectal cancer using four robotic arms. Surg Endosc. 2008;22(3):792–7.

42. D'Annibale A, Morpurgo E, Fiscon V, Trevisan P, Sovernigo G, Orsini C, Guidolin D. Robotic and laparoscopic surgery for treatment of colorectal diseases. Dis Colon Rectum. 2004;47(12):2162–8.

43. Denoto G, Rubach E, Ravikumar TS. A standardized technique for robotically performed sigmoid colectomy. J Laparoendosc Adv Surg Tech A. 2006;16(6):551–6.

44. Hellan M, Stein H, Pigazzi A. Totally robotic low anterior resection with total mesorectal excision and splenic flexure mobilization. Surg Endosc. 2009;23:447–51.

45. Choi DJ, Kim SH, Lee PJ, Kim J, Woo SU. Single-stage totally robotic dissection for rectal cancer surgery: technique and short-term outcome in 50 consecutive patients. Dis Colon Rectum. 2009;52(11):1824–30.

46. Luca F, et al. Full robotic left colon and rectal cancer resection: technique and early outcome. Ann Surg Oncol. 2009;16(5):1274–8.

The Robot

3

Jacob Eisdorfer and David E. Rivadeneira

Abstract

There has been an increase in the use of minimally invasive approaches for many colorectal procedures during the past three decades. Many colorectal surgeons have embraced laparoscopic surgery as their technique of choice for most of the procedures that they perform. It is well known that laparoscopic surgery results in smaller incisions, less postoperative pain, and shorter lengths of stay. Robotic Surgery is an alternative method of performing laparoscopic colon and rectal surgery. Many have suggested that it is the optimal method by which to perform these procedures. This technology has expanded greatly since it was first used for colon and rectal surgery in 2001. Worldwide, the number of robot-assisted procedures that are performed nearly tripled in 2007–2011, from 80,000 to 205,000. We will discuss the most commonly used robotic platform, the advantages and disadvantages of robotic surgery, and the considerations that impact on a successful robotic program at an institution.

Keywords

Robot • Robotic surgery • Minimally invasive surgery • Robotic system • da Vinci • Colorectal surgery • Robotic platform • Vision card • Patient cart

There has been an increase in the use of minimally invasive approaches for many colorectal procedures during the past three decades. Many colorectal surgeons have embraced laparoscopic surgery as their technique of choice for most of the procedures that they perform. It is well known that laparoscopic surgery results in smaller incisions, less postoperative pain, and shorter lengths of stay. Robotic Surgery is an alternative method of performing laparoscopic colon and rectal surgery. Many have suggested that it is the optimal method by which to perform these procedures. This technology has expanded greatly since it was first used for colon and rectal surgery in 2001 [1]. Worldwide, the number of robot-assisted procedures that are performed nearly tripled in 2007–2011, from 80,000 to 205,000 [2].

J. Eisdorfer, D.O., F.A.C.S. • D.E. Rivadeneira, M.D., M.B.A., F.A.S.C.R.S. (✉)
North Shore-LIJ Health System, Huntington Hospital, Hofstra School of Medicine,
321 B Crossways Pk. Dr., Woodbury, NY 11797, USA
e-mail: drivadeneira@nshs.edu

© Springer International Publishing Switzerland 2015
H. Ross et al. (eds.), *Robotic Approaches to Colorectal Surgery*,
DOI 10.1007/978-3-319-09120-4_3

We will discuss the most commonly used robotic platform, the advantages and disadvantages of robotic surgery, and the considerations that impact on a successful robotic program at an institution.

3.1 A Guide to the Currently Used Robotic System and Robotic Components

The most frequently used robotic system today is the da Vinci Si (Intuitive Surgical, Inc., Sunnyvale, CA). It consists of a vision cart, a patient cart, and a surgeon console. Firstly, the vision cart (Fig. 3.1) consists of a touch screen monitor; this provides interactive control of video and audio at the patient side and also allows for the ability to draw directly on the screen's endoscopic view, known as telestration. This is particularly useful when trying to point out anatomy to the operating surgeon. The system's core, which is the system's central processing point, is housed in the vision cart. The camera assembly, which provides the three-dimensional, high-definition view, is also part of the vision cart, as is the illuminator, which is the light source for the endoscope. A 0° and 30° endoscope is available; the 30° endoscope can be positioned up or down; this is determined when attaching it to the camera assembly. The three-dimensional image is created by capturing two independent views from 2- to 5-mm endoscopes fitted into the endoscope and then displaying them into two channels which is viewed at the surgeon console's stereo viewer (Fig. 3.2). This provides a three-dimensional, high-definition, bright, and stable image.

The patient cart (Fig. 3.3) is the robotic component that interfaces with the patient directly. It consists of setup joints, which are used to position the arms. There are three instrument arms and one camera arm. The setup joints are connected to the camera and instrument arms, the camera arm holds and manipulates the camera, and the instrument arms do the same for the instruments. The camera arm is what provides the perfectly stable image. Each arm has its own clutch buttons that allow for movements of the arms during docking. Positioning the joints properly is essential to a procedure with the most intra-abdominal reach and the least arm collisions. In general the camera port, target anatomy, and center column of the patient cart should be placed in a straight line, such that the robotic arms are working toward the patient cart. The camera arm joints should be positioned such that the second camera arm joint is opposite arm number three. Also, the camera arm joints should be set up so that it is in its "sweet spot"; the sweet spot is indicated by a thick blue line on joint number two. The blue arrow should be within the boundaries of the thick blue line. This helps to insure that the patient cart is at an appropriate distance from the patient, which will improve arm mobility. Lastly, the camera port, target anat-omy, camera port clutch button, third camera arm joint, and patient cart center column should be in a straight line. Exceptions to this exist when side docking; in this case, all other alignment remains true with the exception of the target anatomy which will be 30°–45° from the line created by the other points previously mentioned. The instrument arms should be placed at 45° angles to each other. If care is taken to establish ideal joint position, this will greatly impact on the seamlessness of the procedure. The movement of the patient cart is controlled with the shift switches and the motor drive control. The use of these components must be understood well by the surgeon and the nursing staff because it is essential to docking the robot properly. The patient cart is moved to the patient side using motor drive. This is accomplished by moving the shift switch into the drive position, indicated by the "D." It is recommended that two people be used to move the cart, one to move it and one to direct that person. The throttle-enable switch is held in, and then the throttle is rotated away from you to move forward and toward you to move back. The cart can also be moved in neutral when the shift switch is in the neutral position indicated by the "N" and physically pushing the cart. The shift switch must be on "D" when docking is complete in order to set the breaks. Putting any port in a cannula mount will disable the motor drive and prevent the cart from moving in drive mode.

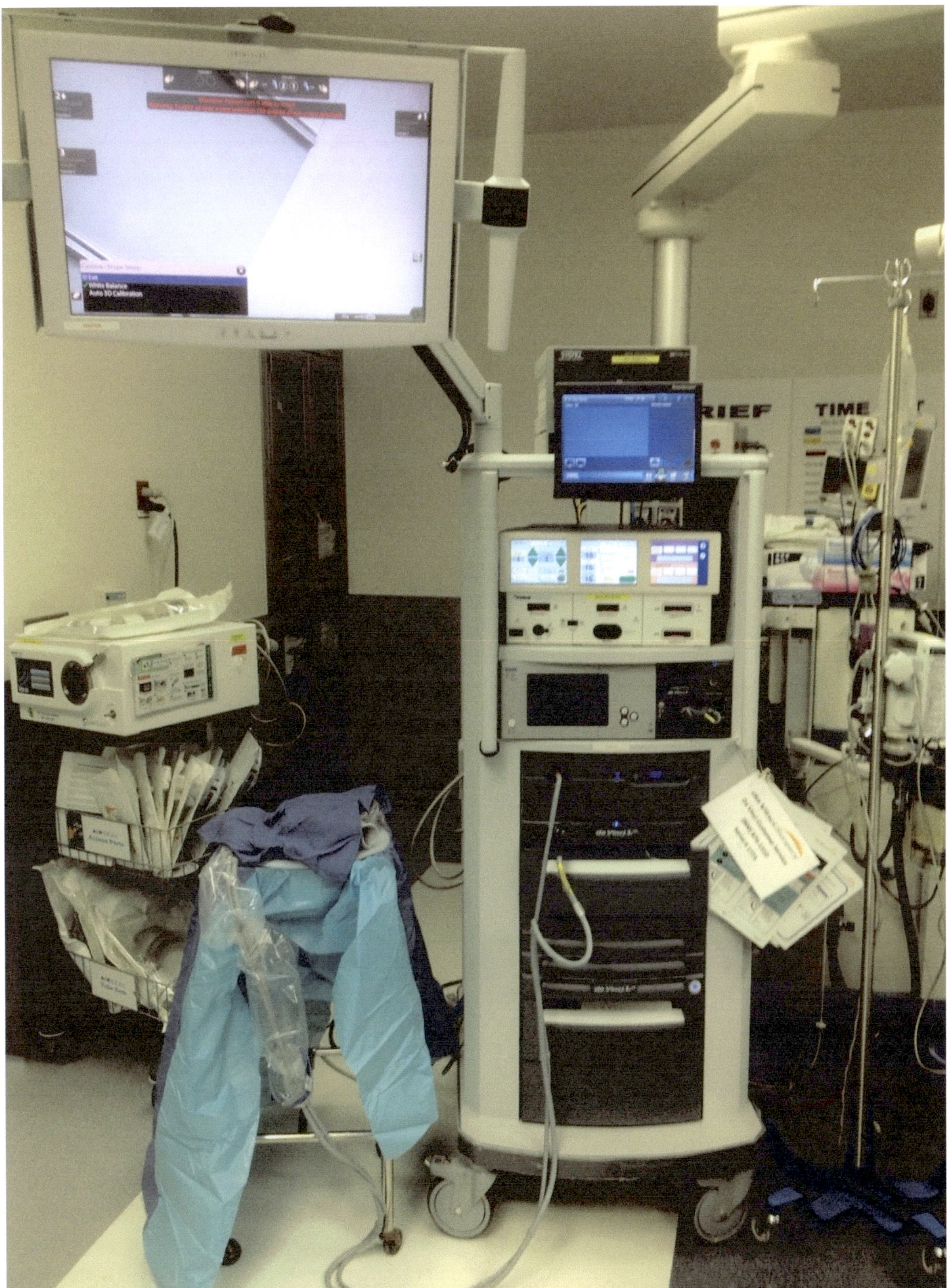

Fig. 3.1 Vision cart

Fig. 3.2 Stereo viewer

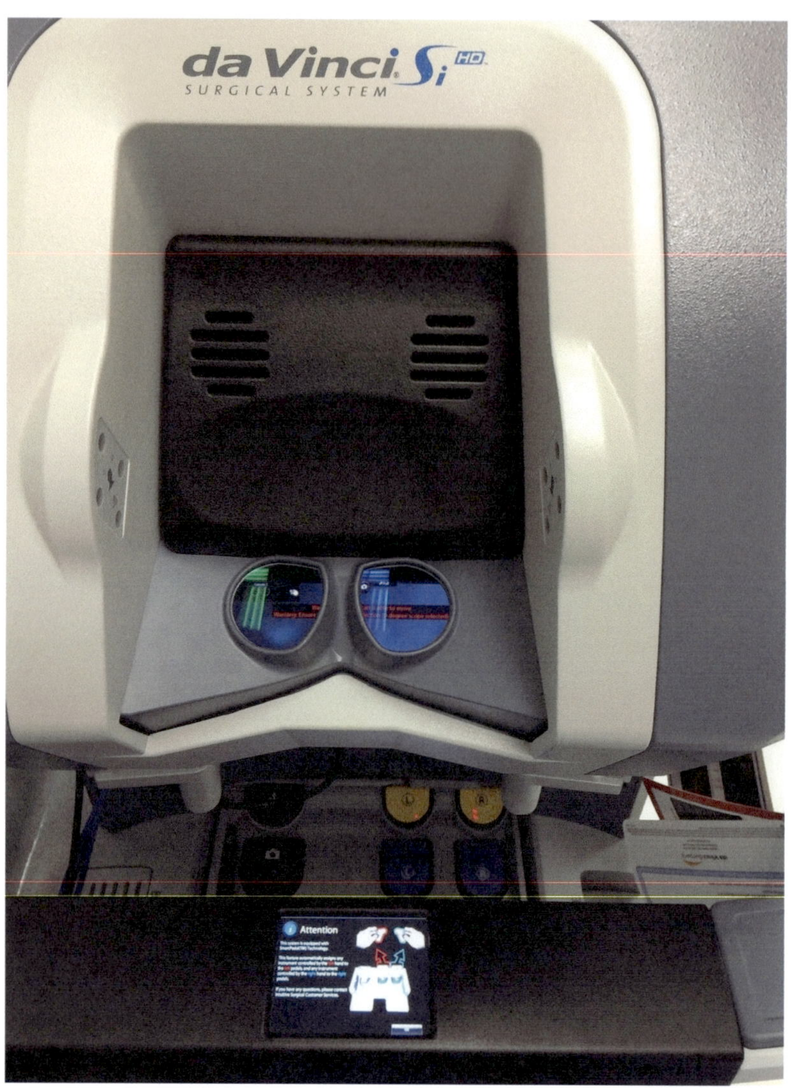

The surgeon console is the surgeon's interface with the da Vinci system; it also consists of many components. The stereo viewer provides the three-dimensional, high-definition video feed of the surgical field in real time. It also has a head and neck support for added ergonomic comfort. The stereo viewer also displays detailed messaging and icons that convey system settings for the surgeon during the procedure. These are displayed in specific locations throughout the procedure. The messages alert the surgeon to any changes or errors with the system. Next to the stereo viewer are infrared sensors that activate the surgeon console and robotic instruments when the surgeon's head is against the stereo viewer; the instruments do not move when the head is removed. This prevents inadvertent movement of the instruments. The master controllers (Fig. 3.4) are where the surgeon places his fingers (Fig. 3.5) in order to control the instruments and the endoscope. The master controllers are the surgeon's interface to the EndoWrist instruments, which afford 7 degrees of freedom, 180 degrees of articulation, and 540 degrees of rotation. The master controllers also provide ergonomic comfort and tremor filtration. Movements are simultaneously and seamlessly replicated at the patient cart. The master controllers also have a finger

Fig. 3.3 Patient cart

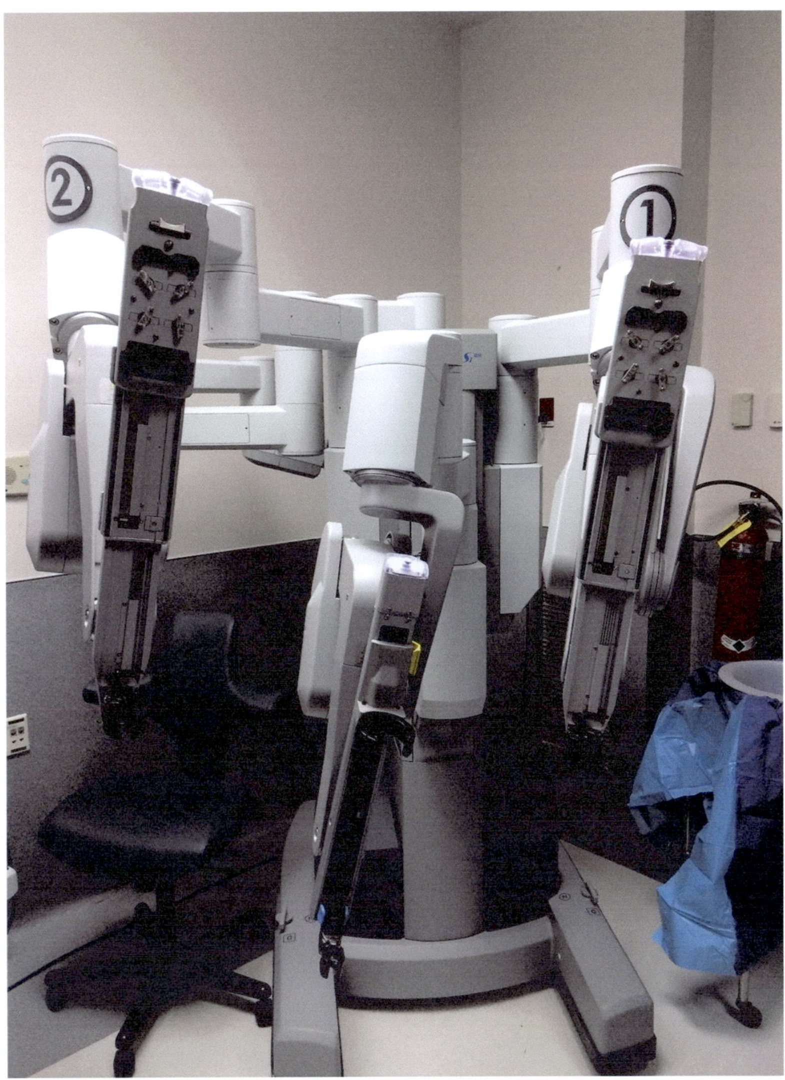

clutch option, which some surgeons prefer to the foot pedal master clutch. The finger clutch allows for clutching a single master controller without the other, unlike the master clutch foot pedal, which will allow for clutching of both master controllers. The da Vinci Si has 1.5 cubic feet of working space for the master controllers; the surgeon should use the master and finger clutches to establish a comfortable working environment and avoid collisions between the master controllers; this must be constantly adjusted throughout the procedure. The surgeon must also "match grips" by grasping the master controllers to match the position and grip of the EndoWrist instrument tips in the patient's body. This prevents unwanted activation of the instruments and therefore tissue damage. It is advantageous to frequently clutch and keep the master controllers close, to avoid reaching for tissues and avoid surgeon strain. The left-side pod houses the ergonomic control lever; this allows one to adjust the height and tilt of the stereo viewer, move the arm rest up and down, and move the foot switch panel (Fig. 3.6) in and out; these are important for optimal comfort during the procedure. The right-side pod contains the power button and the emergency stop button. The power button will power on the surgeon console (Fig. 3.7) in standalone mode or when

Fig. 3.4 Master controllers

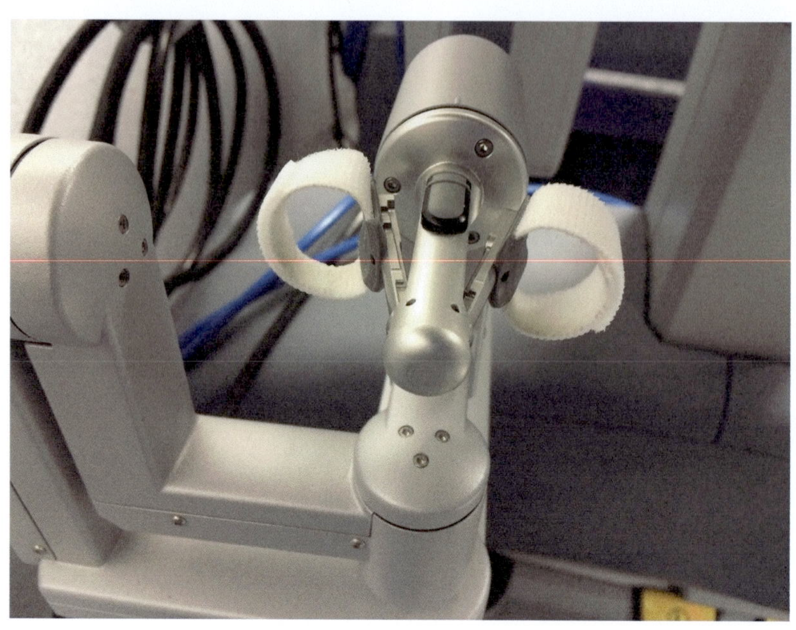

Fig. 3.5 Master controller
with surgeon

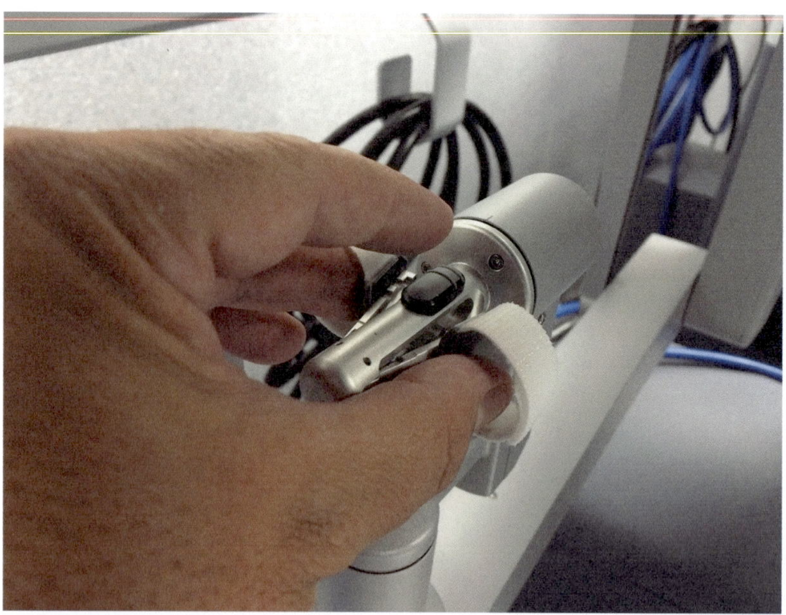

Fig. 3.6 Foot switch panel

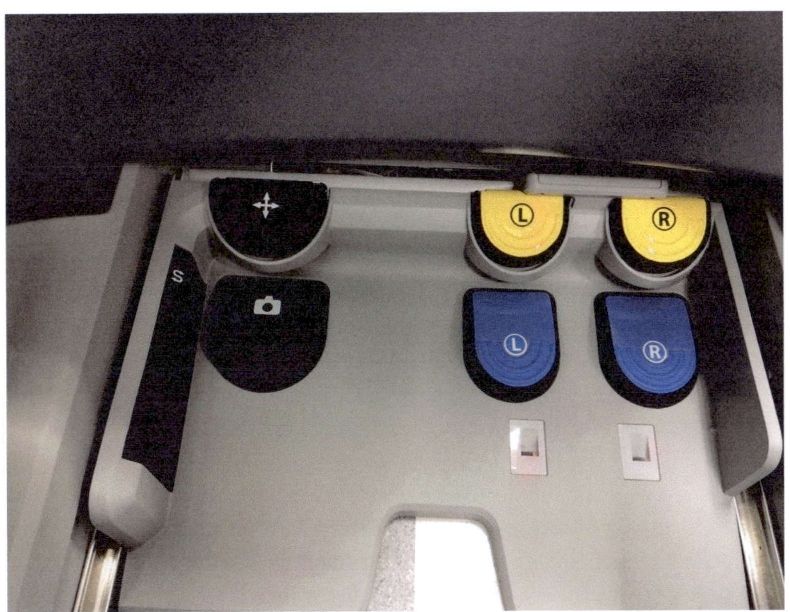

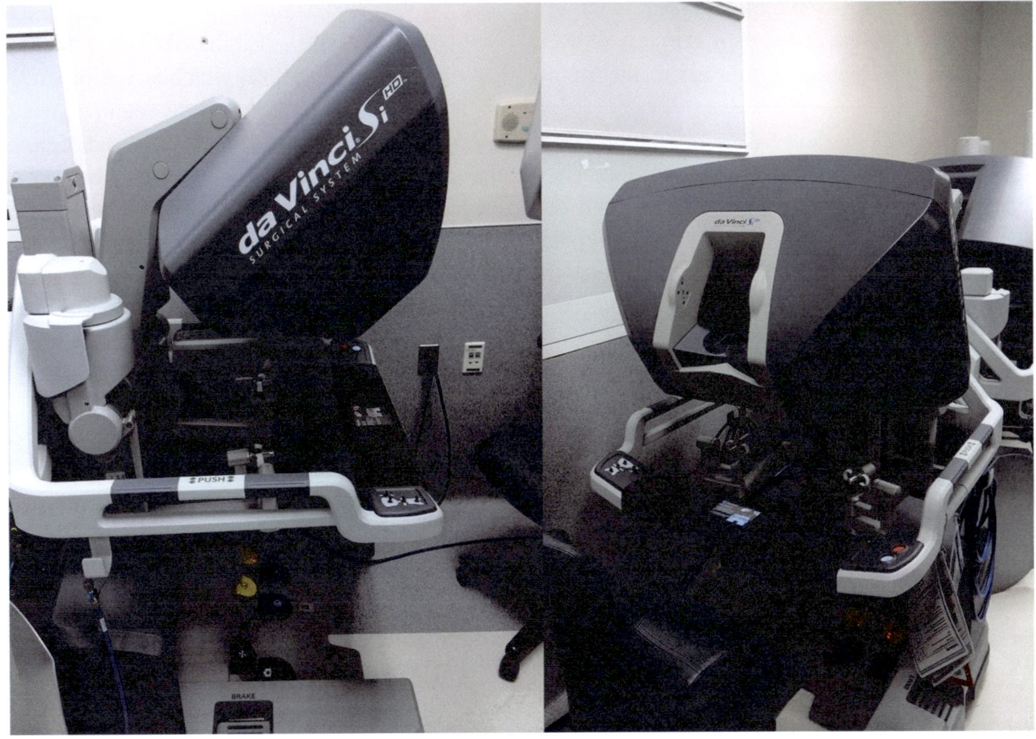

Fig. 3.7 Surgeon console

attached to the other system components can be used to power on the entire system. Pressing the emergency stop button will automatically stop system operation. The touch pad controls the system's audio and video. It acts as the interface for the surgeon to adjust and save personal preferences. The foot switch panel houses the foot pedals. The pedals allow for arm swapping, master clutching, camera control, and integrated instrument activation control. The foot switches are where the actions of many instruments are executed; examples are the energy for monopolar instruments, bipolar instruments, vessel-sealing devices, and the stapler. The Si has two tiers of pedals and a pedal on the side of the panel. On the right side, there are two sets of cut and coagulation pedals, which can control two instruments. The pedal on the side of the panel is for arm switching, and the left-side pedals are for the camera and for master clutching.

There are many EndoWrist instruments available for the da Vinci; we will discuss those most commonly used in colorectal surgery. All instruments have a fixed number of uses; the system automatically tracks the number of uses and will not work if it has exceeded its maximum allowed uses. This information is relayed in the stereo viewer.

The monopolar curved scissors or "Hot Shears" can provide monopolar current. They function like laparoscopic endoshears with the added benefit of being wristed with the typical degrees of freedom described earlier. There are multiple graspers, scissors, and monopolar cautery devices; these are the most commonly used in colon and rectal surgery. The Hot Shears open to 38° and the jaws are 1.3-cm long. The permanent cautery hook is similar to the laparoscopic hook cautery, its hook is 1.6-cm long, and the permanent cautery spatula is 1.7-cm long. The Cadiere forceps are nontraumatic fenestrated graspers; they open 30°, and the jaws are 2.0-cm long; these are appropriate for handling bowel. The Double Fenestrated Grasper opens 60° and is 3.3-cm long; they have a very low closing force and can be used for bowel. The Fenestrated Bipolar Forceps open 45° and are 2.1-cm long

and have a medium closing force, but allow for bipolar cautery; they are considered to be the bipolar equivalent to the Cadiere forceps. There are also Maryland Bipolar Forceps; they are curved and fenestrated, open 45° and are 2.1-cm long, and have a medium closing force.

With regard to needle drivers, there are five to choose from; two provide scissors at the base of the jaw. The Large Needle Driver and Large SutureCut are for midsize needles. The Mega Needle Driver and Mega SutureCut are for large needles. And the Black Diamond Micro Forceps are for small needles. All of the instruments mentioned thus far can be used up to ten times. There are also small, medium, and large EndoWrist clip appliers; they can each be used for up to 100 closures.

There are two energy devices available (Fig. 3.8a–p), the HARMONIC ACE Curved Shears and the da Vinci Vessel Sealer, which is similar to the LigaSure in that it is a bipolar energy device. The HARMONIC can be used up to 30 times, and the Vessel Sealer can be used once. There is also a suction/irrigator which can be used once. da Vinci now has an EndoWrist Stapler, which is available in 45-mm length and two staple heights—a blue reload, which is 3.5 mm, and green reload which is 4.3 mm.

The new da Vinci Xi has many features, which are meant to overcome some of the limitations of the previous systems. It is available, but not in broad use as of yet. Many procedures, which require access to multiple quadrants of the abdomen, could not be performed with the da Vinci alone in a single dock. The Xi has thinner arms and instruments with longer reach; also the camera can be placed on any of the arms—these features are meant to make multi-quadrant surgery possible with the da Vinci. The Xi also has voice-guided instructions which makes setup more efficient. There is a laser guidance system that will position a boom, in the appropriate location over the patient to make docking more precise. Lastly, the camera is smaller and lighter (Fig. 3.9a), which is why it can be placed in any arm (Fig. 3.9b), but also allows for better definition and eliminating the need for draping, focusing, white balancing, and calibrating.

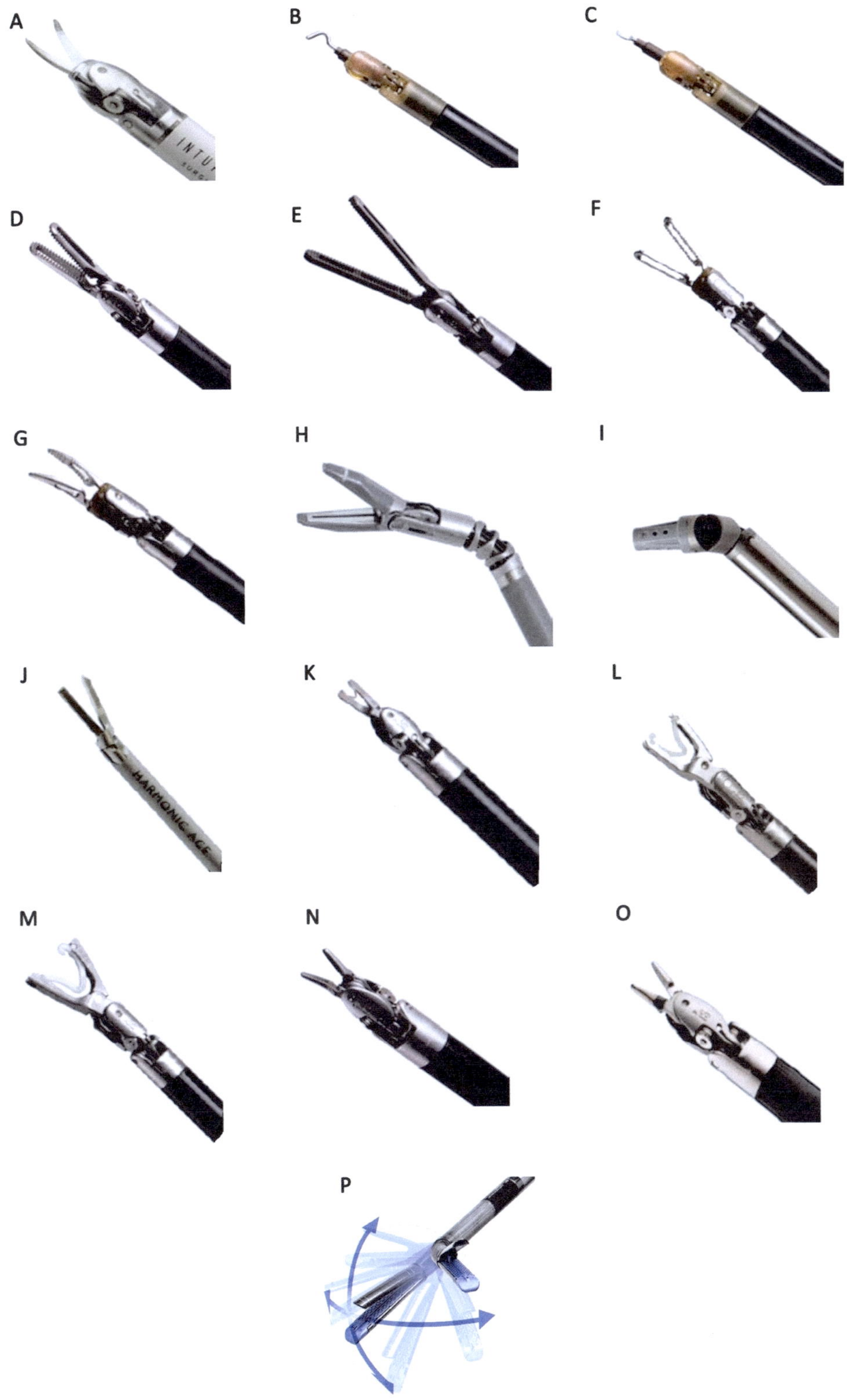

Fig. 3.8 Energy devices. (**a**) Hot Shears. (**b**) Permanent cautery hook. (**c**) Permanent cautery spatula. (**d**) Cadiere forceps. (**e**) Double Fenestrated Grasper. (**f**) Fenestrated Bipolar Forceps. (**g**) Maryland Bipolar Forceps. (**h**) Vessel Sealer. (**i**) Suction/irrigator. (**j**) HARMONIC ACE Curved Shears. (**k**) Small clip applier. (**l**) Medium-large clip applier. (**m**) Large clip applier. (**n**) Large Needle Driver. (**o**) Large SutureCut needle driver. (**p**) Stapler

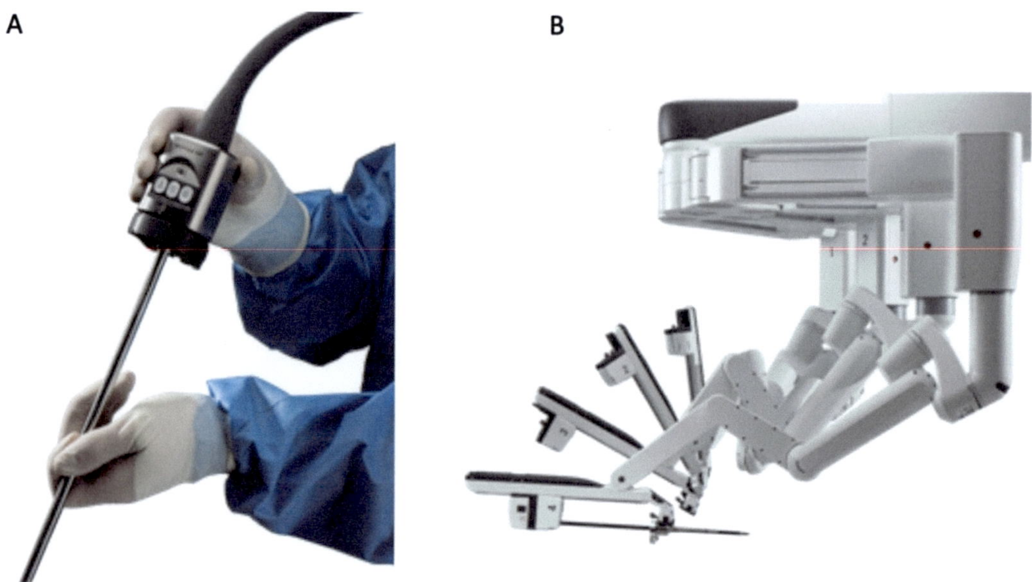

Fig. 3.9 (**a**) da Vinci smaller, lighter camera. (**b**) da Vinci Xi—thinner arms

3.2 Advantages and Disadvantages

One advantage of robotic surgery is the ergonomic position that the surgeon is able to be in during the procedure. This allows for less physical strain and fatigue during the procedure [3]. Also, the improved dexterity of the wristed robotic instruments is a clear advantage. Robotic interface can also downscale movements (5:1–2:1); this combined with the tremor filtering technology makes for a distinct benefit while operating. As discussed, the instruments of a robotic arm have an EndoWrist, which has functions of 7 degrees of freedom, 180 degrees of articulation, and 540 degrees of rotation. Its function is a technological advantage for dissection, especially in small spaces, and intracorporeal suturing. With regard to rectal surgery in particular, there are clear advantages. Robotic approach has particular advantage during pelvic dissection. The surgeon gets equal access to both sides of the pelvis, and the presence of the EndoWrist instruments permits a range of angles to approach the rectum from different directions, thus allowing sharp dissection around the lower part of the rectum and mesorectum [4]. Additionally, the three-dimensional, high-definition, completely stable optics produces superb visualization. Also, the ability for the surgeon to seamlessly control camera position and angle is a definite advantage (Fig. 3.10).

A disadvantage of robotic surgery is the limitation to a single quadrant of the abdomen, which is a significant shortcoming, certainly in colon and rectal surgery [4]. This is one of the reasons that this technique was initially thought of as most beneficial for work in the pelvis. However, many pelvic procedures that are performed require attention to the left upper quadrant as well. This is a concern that is supposedly addressed with the new Xi system. Also the patient cannot be repositioned during the procedure without undocking the robot [4]. For instance, if one would like steeper Trendelenberg or changing to reverse Trendelenberg position, this cannot be accomplished without manipulation of the patient cart and therefore undocking and redocking. Initially, robotic surgery was universally considered to take much longer than traditional laparoscopic surgery; this is no longer thought to be true [5]. In fact, a recent meta-analysis showed that the operative times were not significantly different between the two techniques. Another disadvantage is the lack of haptic feedback. Moreover, suture material can be torn

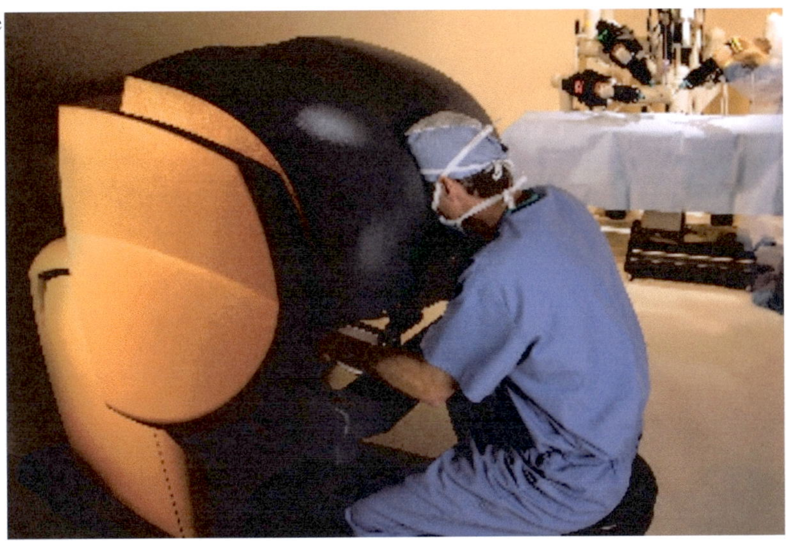

Fig. 3.10 Surgeon at console

frequently because of no tensile feedback during suturing using the robotic instrument. Also, tissue can be damaged due to lack of tactile feedback. These technological disadvantages can be overcome by learned visual sense, which many robotic surgeons attest to. However, experience is necessary [4]. This learning curve for performing safe and efficient robotic surgery also involves the assistant and the nursing staff. And finally, cost is a major concern. The initial capital investment is substantial, $1–2.5 million [6]. There is also an annual service agreement of which is priced at anywhere from $100,000 to $170,000 [7]. Finally and most significantly, the cost per procedure is also affected by the number of instruments and accessories that have a limited number of uses; this cost is anywhere from $1300–$2200 per procedure. During the first 9 months of 2013, sales of instruments and accessories increased by 18 % and represented 45 % of the company's total revenue [8]. One study showed an increase in operating room costs of approximately $2,000 per procedure [9].

3.3 The Importance of Having a Dedicated Team

It is essential and advantageous to have a dedicated team for robotic colon and rectal surgery. This consists of several components. The nursing staff in the operating room is essential to the success of any surgical procedure; this is especially true in robotic surgery, where there is more instrumentation and need for proper coordination. During a robotic procedure, the surgeon is not operating at the patient's side, but in fact is at a distance from the patient at the surgeon console. Therefore, the surgeon cannot observe the patient or his team members during the procedure. Also, much of the issues with the increased cost of robotic surgery revolve around efficiency and length of the procedure. For both these reasons, having a highly qualified dedicated nursing team is essential for the success of a robotic operation and therefore a robotic program. It has been suggested that a robotic team consist of an experienced, dedicated surgical technician and circulator. It is important that they are familiar with colon and rectal procedures and not simply robotic surgery in general. It is also important to have a managing nurse for the robotic program to oversee the training of new staff and update experienced staff as the program evolves [10]. There should be an ongoing dialogue about the progress of the robotic program at the institution. Initially, monthly meetings are recommended. All meetings regarding the robotic program at the institution should involve the surgeons, the nurse manager, and all members of the team. This is also an essential way to bring up issues as they arise and discuss change as the program grows; these are all aspects that are

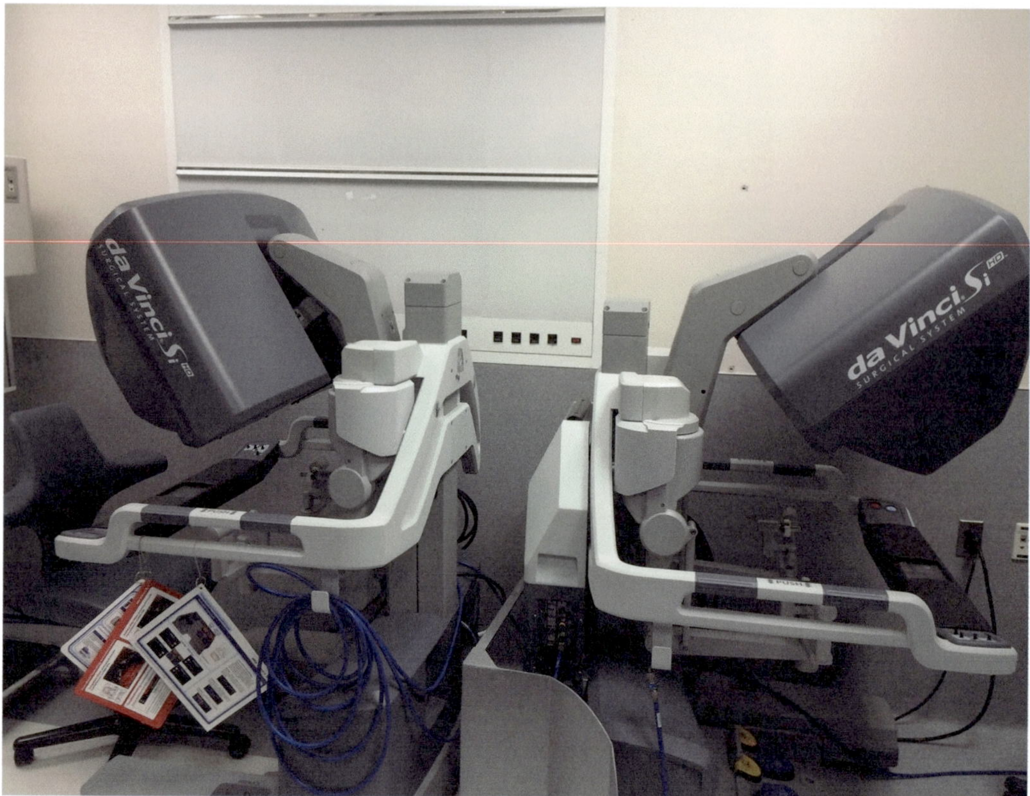

Fig. 3.11 Dual console

included in having a dedicated team. Dedicated surgical physician assistants are an asset to any robotic team. Again, due to the remote position of the operating surgeon, an appropriately trained physician assistant can effectively and efficiently accomplish all of the necessary patient side tasks during the procedure. Other options for assistants are less advantageous for many reasons. Having a second surgeon at the bedside in the long run will be costly. Utilizing trainees of any level as the lone assistant is not recommended; she will not be an effective assistant, and the experience will not truly benefit her education either. Training the resident or fellow at the bedside along with a physician assistant present and then also training them at the second console of a dual console (Fig. 3.11) robotic system are a far superior method.

3.4 Partnership with the Hospital Health System in Understanding Program Goals and Financial Support of the Program, Including Dedicated Teams

Likely, the most important element for the success of any new robotic program is the unity of vision between the surgery team and the hospital or health system administration. Of course the goal should always be to provide a better procedure for the patient with better outcomes. However, the path should be agreed upon as well to have the most effective program. Understanding each other's goals, needs, and expectations is necessary from the outset. Because success breeds more success, harnessing the achievements as they come and building upon them are also essential.

There must be a program coordinator; this person can be a healthcare professional such as a nurse, physician assistant, or physician or a non-healthcare professional with the skill and desire to perform all of the necessary tasks. This person will be a link between the administration and the operating room team. She is also responsible for the coordination of the program overall. She should have access to the administrative staff responsible for marketing, patient education, and other avenues of growth for the program [10].

Marketing is certainly part of the success of any new surgical program. In order to offer a new procedure on a large scale, the institution needs to draw patients who require this procedure; this is often patient driven, and therefore, direct patient marketing is necessary; however, marketing to referring physicians is also essential. The marketing team should consist of people who understand the geographical area, referral patterns, and the most effective methods to disseminate information about the new program.

Financial support is essential to the success of the program. Prior to going down the path of establishing a robotic program, the hospital or health system must have a realistic financial plan in place. The capital investment for the purchase of the robotic components and instruments and maintenance is one cost. Also, there is facility renovation to provide an appropriate operating room to perform the procedures. As discussed earlier, a dedicated team is essential; this involves staff retraining and often recruitment of new staff. The administration must often balance this against local payer mix and likely reimbursement for the procedures with the notion that providing a new and desired procedure will increase patient draw, with the appropriate marketing, of course. Additionally, an institution that provides the most up-to-date techniques with good outcomes will likely grow in all of its departments simply due to improved reputation and being considered "cutting edge." However, without the establishment of a realistic financial plan up front, a program is unlikely to flourish.

Ongoing reevaluation of the program's progress is essential. The program coordinator should be constantly evaluating the metrics that make the program successful. These include case volume, docking time, procedure time, conversion rate, complications, and outcomes. It is recommended that a meeting be held monthly that includes the coordinator, the entire robotic team, and all of the robotic surgeons. The data regarding the metrics that are being evaluated should be presented. There should be a discussion regarding the overall health of the program, the obstacles to its development, and new ideas for its growth. There should also be dialogue about the use of resources and the possible need for more resources. Lastly, is the program meeting its goals, should there be an expansion, and are their new applications for robotics that should be evaluated? This periodic assessment will identify any concerns and guarantee that the program continues to provide the best outcomes for our patients.

References

1. Baik SH. Robotic colorectal surgery. Yonsei Med J. 2008;49(6):891–6.
2. Hottenrott C. Robotic versus laparoscopic surgery for rectal cancer and cost-effectiveness analysis. Surg Endosc. 2011;25:3954–6.
3. Hellan M, Anderson C, Ellenhorn JDI, Paz B, Pigazzi A. Short-term outcomes after robotic-assisted total mesorectal excision for rectal cancer. Ann Surg Oncol. 2007;14(11):3168–73.
4. Aly EH. Robotic colorectal surgery: summary of the current evidence. Int J Colorectal Dis. 2014;29(1):1–8.
5. Liao G, Zhao Z, Lin S, Li R, Yuan Y, Du S, Chen J, Deng H. Robotic-assisted versus laparoscopic colorectal surgery: a meta-analysis of four randomized controlled trials. World J Surg Oncol. 2014;12(122):1–11.
6. Wormer BA, Dacey KT, Williams KB, Bradley III JF, Walters AL, Augenstein VA, Stefanidis D, Heniford BT. The first nationwide evaluation of robotic general surgery: a regionalized, small but safe start. Surg Endosc. 2014;28(3):767–76.
7. Intuitive Surgical, Inc. Investor presentation [internet]. http://investor.intuitivesurgical.com
8. Reynders, Mcveigh Capital Management, LLC. Intuitive Surgical (ISRG) [internet]. http://www.reyndersmcveigh.com/research/pdfdocs/Intuitive%20Surgical%202013-10-30-updt.pdf
9. Park JS, Choi GS, Park SY, Kim HJ, Ryuk JP. Randomized clinical trial of robot-assisted versus standard laparoscopic right colectomy. Br J Surg. 2012;99(9):1219–26.
10. Patel VR. Essential elements to the establishment and design of a successful robotic surgery programme. Int J Med Robot. 2006;2(1):28–35.

Part II

Preoperative

Aneel Damle and Justin A. Maykel

Abstract

Perioperative assessment in robotic colorectal surgery involves consideration of the patient, surgeon, and circumstances unique to robotics. Surgeons experience a learning curve so proper surgeon education is critical for optimizing outcomes. Patient selection is also essential to maximizing the benefits of the robotic surgery. This requires careful evaluation of robotic surgical indications and an understanding of the physiological effects of pneumoperitoneum. Finally, practitioners must understand the special considerations of robotics including docking, the lack of tactile feedback, the potential for peripheral nerve damage due to patient positioning and prolonged operative times, and the high operating and maintenance costs.

Keywords

Robotics • Laparoscopy • Colorectal surgery • Minimally invasive surgery • Learning curve • Patient selection • Pneumoperitoneum

Robotic-assisted surgery (RAS) requires special considerations both preoperatively and intraoperatively. Successful outcomes require the right surgeon, the right patient, the right team, and the right equipment. This chapter will demonstrate the importance of each of these factors.

A. Damle, M.D., M.B.A.
Department of Surgery, University of Massachusetts Medical Center, 67 Belmont Street, Worcester, MA 01605, USA

J.A. Maykel, M.D. (✉)
Division of Colon and Rectal Surgery, Department of Surgery, University of Massachusetts Medical Center, 67 Belmont Street, Worcester, MA 01605, USA
e-mail: Justin.Maykel@umassmemorial.org

4.1 Surgeon Skill and Training

4.1.1 The Learning Curve

The adoption of any novel surgical technique involves a learning curve to obtain proficiency and mastery. Following the introduction of laparoscopy in the 1990s, concerns were raised regarding the learning curve needed to master this new technique. Retrospective studies demonstrated 90 % of common bile duct injuries occurred during a surgeon's first 30 laparoscopic cholecystectomies, highlighting the danger of the learning curve [1]. However, compared to

© Springer International Publishing Switzerland 2015
H. Ross et al. (eds.), *Robotic Approaches to Colorectal Surgery*,
DOI 10.1007/978-3-319-09120-4_4

open cholecystectomy, numerous studies have since demonstrated that laparoscopic cholecystectomy is the superior operation in terms of cost and outcomes [2]. Similarly, RAS must address this concern through appropriate policies and procedures that can help surgeons overcome the learning curve while avoiding potential harm to patients.

Currently, it is unknown exactly how long the robotic learning curve is and which surgeons should embark upon it. Additionally, it is not clear which outcomes should be measured or how to define "proficiency." Multiple studies have attempted to evaluate these issues using operative time as a surrogate market for competence [3]. However, as surgeons take on increasingly complex cases, operative times tend to increase. Accordingly, this review will focus on studies using a multidimensional assessment such as the cumulative sum model.

Regarding the in vitro acquisition of robotic skills, early studies demonstrated a short learning curve of 4–6 h for experienced laparoscopists to successfully perform robotic intracorporeal knot tying at a level comparable to standard laparoscopy [4]. However, it has been a greater challenge to demonstrate how this learning curve applies more broadly to colon and rectal surgery.

A recent systematic review of laparoscopic and robotic colorectal surgical cases demonstrated a range of 5–310 cases to achieve proficiency in laparoscopy and 15–30 cases for robotics [3]. However, it should be noted that all six studies that evaluated the learning curve in RAS observed rectal resections only and did not include colon resections. In comparison, laparoscopic rectal resections have a learning curve of 60–80 cases. Measures of surgical competency included both patient outcomes and/or surgical efficiency. The only study to use multiple surgeons and both of these proficiency measurements cited a tighter learning curve in robotic rectal surgery of 21–23 cases [5].

This learning curve has been demonstrated to evolve along three distinct phases, as reported by Bokhari et al. when examining a single-surgeon experience with robotic rectosigmoid resections.

Each phase of the learning curve corresponded with the surgeon's ability to adapt to the changes of RAS [6]. The first phase deals with overcoming the lack of tactile feedback and recognizing visual cues for tissue tension and traction. The second phase involves understanding the spatial relationships of the robotic instruments outside the direct field of view and the ability to reposition them without direct visualization. The third phase develops the surgeon's ability to operate the robotic console without directly visualizing it or the patient. This final phase demonstrates an understanding of not only where the multiple robotic arms are within the patient but also their relationship to how the robotic system is docked. Of note, this study similarly reported that 15–25 cases were required to achieve competence.

Phase 1 of the learning curve included the first 15 cases and was associated with a steady decrease in surgeon console and docking time [6]. Phase 2 represented a plateau over the next ten cases. These 15–25 cases represent the learning curve required for competency. This number is similar to the learning curves reported for robotic cholecystectomy and Nissen fundoplication [7]. Phase 3 (>25 cases) represents the postlearning period where the surgeon is able to take on increasingly complex patients and procedures, which often leads to increased operative times. Similar findings regarding the three-phase model have been duplicated in other studies of robotic rectal resections [5].

Unlike rectal surgery, there are no studies to support the number of procedures required to achieve proficiency with robotic colon resections. However, proponents suggest that since right colectomies are straightforward procedures for colorectal surgeons and can be done with only two robotic arms, they can be undertaken in the early part of the learning curve [8]. A series of 40 robotic right colectomies demonstrated a mean operative time of 159 min. Although 41 min longer than the mean operative for laparoscopic colectomies at the same institution, the robotic colectomy times were similar to those reported in the literature for laparoscopic right colectomy (76–214 min) [8–10].

It is difficult and possibly misleading to describe an overall learning curve for the use of RAS as each procedure requires a different skill set. However, there is insufficient data to provide this information for each specific procedure. Therefore, surgeons must participate in clinical trials to collect this data. A systematic review of the literature recommended that surgeons complete 20–30 cases in addition to participating in a structured training course and have adequate mentorship before participating in robotic clinical trials [3]. Due to limited case volume utilizing this evolving technology, the number of surgeons able to accrue patients for such studies remains limited.

4.1.2 Is Laparoscopic Experience Required?

A proposed benefit of RAS is the reduced learning curve compared to laparoscopy [11]. It has been suggested that the controls of robotic surgery are more intuitive and similar to open surgery. This would allow open or even inexperienced laparoscopic surgeons to make the transition to RAS [12]. This has been demonstrated within the field of urology focusing on laparoscopic radical prostatectomy (LRP). Typically, for a skilled laparoscopist, the learning curve for an LRP is 40–60 cases. For a surgeon without prior laparoscopic experience, this number jumps to 80–100 cases [13]. However, Ahlering et al. demonstrated that after completing a 1-day robotic training course and two cadaveric robotic LRPs, the learning curve for experienced open surgeons who were laparoscopically naïve dropped to 8–12 cases.

Many authors caution inexperienced laparoscopic surgeons from proceeding directly into robotics [6, 7]. Although robotic surgery provides advantages over laparoscopy in three-dimensional vs. two-dimensional viewing, the field of view for both minimally invasive techniques is smaller. Expertise in all minimally invasive surgery (MIS) requires not only an understanding of what is directly in the field of view but an awareness of what is outside of it. The complexity required for this understanding is even higher with robotics due to the capability of the operator to use multiple arms that may not be visualized at all times. Further, surgeons without laparoscopic experience must convert a failed attempt at RAS to an open technique rather than laparoscopic which may lead to increased postoperative pain and length of stay (LOS). In addition, opponents state that even if the learning curve for robotic surgery is slightly lower than it is for laparoscopy, it is not substantial enough to justify the cost implications of learning robotic surgery rather than laparoscopy [14].

4.1.3 Training Surgeons

In order to perform RAS in a safe and effective manner, surgeons must have the proper training. In general surgery, completion of the fundamentals of laparoscopic surgery (FLS) program is required to be board eligible [15]. Currently, no such standardized and validated program exists for RAS [16]. Training is largely based on single-day courses followed by the implementation of skills into clinical practice [16]. However, as surgeons have recognized, this algorithm is not ideal, and multiple strategies for enhanced robotic training have been developed and implemented.

Many authors advocate for a stepwise approach to implement RAS into clinical practice. These steps include a didactic overview of the technology; mastery of skills in inanimate, animal, and cadaveric labs; and supervised live operating room procedures [17]. Although this intensive stepwise training allows surgeons to graduate up the latter, it does have its drawbacks. In particular, the capital investment required to operate multiple wet and dry labs in addition to owning a robotic operating system may be cost prohibitive for many medical centers.

Therefore, many programs divide training into acquisition of technical skills and mastery of intraoperative technique. Beginning with technical skills, Dulan et al. have been attempting to create a proficiency-based curriculum

Table 4.1 Robotic skills list [18]

1. Console setting	9. Clutching	17. Atraumatic handling
2. Docking	10. Instrument names	18. Blunt dissection
3. Robotic trocars	11. Instrument exchange	19. Fine dissection
4. Robotic positioning	12. Fourth arm control	20. Retraction
5. Communication	13. Basic eye-hand coordination	21. Cutting
6. Energy sources	14. Wrist articulation	22. Suturing interrupted
7. Robot component names	15. Depth perception	23. Suturing running
8. Camera	16. Instrument to instrument transfer	

similar to FLS [18]. Robotic surgical experts at an academic medical center identified 23 essential skills for robotic surgery ranging from learning console settings to suture running (Table 4.1). These skills are taught and tested via an online tutorial, a half-day interactive session, and nine inanimate exercises. This allows trainees to apply previously learned laparoscopic skills like peg transfer and pattern cutting to robotics while learning new techniques that are unique to robotics such as docking and operating the foot clutch.

Other simulators attempt to create more specialty-specific training. For example, Marecik et al. created a pelvic model to partner with a robotic simulator for colorectal surgery [19]. This allows surgeons to gain experience with robotic setup and use of the console in the context of their practice. Colorectal surgeons can experience proper docking and positioning, use of multiple robotic arms, and dissection between the pelvic sidewall and mesorectum in a simulated total mesorectal excision (TME). The materials to create this simulator (other than the robotic system) are inexpensive and easily obtainable. This provides significant advantages over virtual reality trainers, which are more expensive but have not been shown to offer any advantage in skill acquisition [20].

Other programs focus more heavily on operative technique. An academic MIS fellowship program required a fellow to first demonstrate proficiency in laparoscopy as well as completing 10 h of robotic training sessions before being allowed to operate with the robotic system [21].

The trainee then moved on to the operative portion with robotic-assisted Roux-en-Y gastric bypasses under the guidance of an expert robotic surgeon. Three specific subtasks of increasing difficulty were identified in the procedures. Task A, performing the posterior outer layer of the gastrojejunostomy (GJ) anastomosis, was performed during all 30 procedures. Operative times for this task decreased steadily through all 30 cases. Task B added the anterior outer layer of the GJ anastomosis, and operative times of the 20 cases did not differ significantly from the time of the faculty surgeon. Task C, enterotomy closure of the GIA-stapled inner layer, was performed by the fellow in the final ten cases. Trainee operative times were similar to what faculty times had been during the first ten cases. No patients in this series had any intraoperative complications such as anastomotic leak.

A similar methodology could easily be applied to colorectal surgery. For example, a robotic-assisted laparoscopic low anterior resection (LAR) could be divided into high ligation of the inferior mesenteric artery and mobilization of the descending colon, pelvic dissection and rectal mobilization, and colorectal anastomosis. This would allow colorectal trainees to receive graded responsibility under direct mentorship and ensure patients get the best outcomes.

Concerns for patient safety and surgeon accountability are of the highest importance. The current literature suggests that robotic surgery can be performed safely and effectively if surgeons train properly. Although no standardized and validated program exists, surgeons must be educated on robotic technology and become familiar with its use in a laboratory setting before operating on patients. While in the early portion of the learning curve, operating in increments of graded responsibility or with a mentor ensures the highest chance of success. Like other authors, we believe that patients and surgeons alike would benefit from a formal credentialing process addressing both the preclinical and clinical aspects of robotic surgical training [22].

4.2 Patient Selection

When adopting a new technology, appropriate patient selection is as important as selecting the best surgeons (Table 4.2). While there are no specific indications for robotic colorectal surgery over traditional approaches, the best applications of this technology are those that leverage the advantages that robotics has over laparoscopic or open surgery. These advantages include superior three-dimensional viewing, stabilization of instruments and camera, improved surgeon ergonomics, and mechanical advantages including instruments with 7 degrees of freedom and 90 degrees of articulation [23].

4.2.1 Robotic Colon Surgery

While the first robotic-assisted colectomy was reported in the literature in 2002, there are no consensus guidelines for indications for robotic colon resection that do not apply to the open or laparoscopic techniques [24]. Indications previously described in the literature for robotic colectomy include colonic adenoma, polyps, carcinoid, and diverticulitis [14]. Reported robotic resec-

tions include left, right, and subtotal colectomies. Operative techniques included both intracorporeal and extracorporeal, stapled, and robotic-assisted hand-sewn anastomoses [25]. While multiple studies have demonstrated robotic colectomy to be safe and feasible for both benign and malignant disease, none have demonstrated any objective benefit to justify the increased cost or increased operative time associated with robotics [8, 25, 26].

One reason for the lack of improvement with robotic colectomy may be that the advantages of robotics cannot be fully utilized for this operation. The advantages of robotic surgery apply best to operating in confined spaces, whereas colonic resection requires dissection in multiple abdominal quadrants and it can be difficult to retract the redundant colon in order to provide adequate countertraction [26]. However, some authors do report advantages with splenic flexure takedown and dissection of the inferior mesenteric vessels [26]. In addition, creation of an intracorporeal hand-sewn anastomosis is easier, allowing placement of the minilaparotomy extraction incision in the most convenient site for the patient [27].

Additional considerations in patient selection are the effects of prolonged anesthesia and pneumoperitoneum due to increased operative times. While the specific physiological effects of pneumoperitoneum will be discussed in the next section, comorbidities including severe chronic obstructive pulmonary disease (COPD), sepsis, chronic renal insufficiency, and heart failure must be taken into account when selecting patients for robotic surgery.

4.2.2 Robotic Rectal Surgery

In contrast to colon surgery, robotic-assisted rectal surgery may provide distinct improvements over open and laparoscopic approaches. While standard laparoscopy is widely accepted for colonic resections, it still faces significant limitations in rectal cancer, particularly in those requiring a complete TME [28]. The advantage of laparoscopy is that it provides unobstructed views

Table 4.2 Ideal patient for colorectal robotic surgery [28]

Sex	Male
Body habitus	Obese
Preoperative radiotherapy	Yes
Pathology	Malignancy
Tumor location	Lower two thirds of the rectum

of the rectal tissue planes and allows a more precise dissection due to the magnified view, and the pneumoperitoneum assists in opening tissue planes in the mesorectal dissection [29].

However, due to the confined space of the pelvis, fixed instrument tips with limited dexterity, and poor surgeon ergonomics, the distal dissection is technically challenging [29]. It often results in clashing of instruments and a crowded operative field, restricting view and requiring the involvement of an experienced assistant. The use of electrocautery introduces smoke into the surgical field, further disrupting visualization. In addition, localization of the exact distal margin of the tumor, particularly when in the low rectum, can be challenging without direct tactile sensation. Finally, limited maneuverability and articulation of staplers often lead to multiple angulated staple lines, increasing the risk of anastomotic leak [29]. Each of these factors contributes to the high learning curve for laparoscopic rectal procedures described above.

RAS may provide solutions to many of these problems. First, because the surgeon is the camera operator and the three-dimensional view is stabilized, visualization and depth perception are improved [28]. Second, the robotic endowrists allow for improved dexterity, decreasing the difficulty of intracorporeal suturing as well as giving the surgeon the ability to approach the mesorectum from multiple angles. Third, robotic suturing may allow surgeons to create a single-stapled, double-purse-string anastomosis that could potentially reduce leak rates [30]. Finally, robotics allows for improved ergonomics, allowing the surgeon to sit, and decreases the awkward hand and arm positioning encountered in laparoscopic rectal resections.

4.3 Physiology of Pneumoperitoneum

Similar to laparoscopy, intra-abdominal robotic procedures require the establishment of pneumoperitoneum, and special consideration of the physiological effects of sustained pneumoperitoneum

Table 4.3 Organ-specific physiological effects of pneumoperitoneum

Organ system	Mechanical effect		Biochemical effect
Pulmonary	↑	Functional residual capacity	↑ End-tidal CO_2
	↑	Dead space	
	↑	Atelectasis	
Cardiovascular	↓	Venous return	Metabolic acidosis
	↓	Cardiac output	
Renal	↓	Renal perfusion	↑ Renin
			↑ Antidiuretic hormone
			↑ Aldosterone

must be considered. Particularly due to the learning curve and increased operative times, these physiological effects may play an even larger role with RAS than they do with laparoscopy. An understanding of this topic plays an important role in patient selection and management. These physiological effects will be discussed in a system-based manner (Table 4.3).

Pneumoperitoneum is typically created with the insufflation of carbon dioxide (CO_2) gas. CO_2 is noncombustible, rapidly soluble in the blood, and relatively inexpensive [31]. There is no single ideal pressure to achieve pneumoperitoneum. Rather, the lowest intra-abdominal pressure that allows adequate exposure of the operative field should be used [32].

4.3.1 Pulmonary

When the peritoneal cavity is insufflated with CO_2 gas, a small portion is absorbed in the blood, but the majority combines with water in red blood cells to form carbonic acid and dissociates into hydrogen and bicarbonate [33]. CO_2 absorbed through the peritoneum is metabolized in a similar fashion.

This leads to an increase in end-tidal CO_2 as high as 50 % requiring an increase in minute ventilation to achieve eucapnia [33]. Regardless of whether or not the patient achieves this, most healthy patients can easily adapt using intracellular and plasma buffering systems. However, patients with diminished buffering capacity such as those with severe COPD or sepsis may be unable to tolerate the increased CO_2 load, resulting in acidosis and its sequelae.

In addition to the biochemical effects of CO_2, increased intra-abdominal pressure disrupts typical pulmonary mechanics [33]. Diaphragmatic movement is impaired resulting in a decreased functional residual capacity and increased dead space. Controlled ventilation with large tidal volumes can offset pulmonary problems by decreasing atelectasis. This can also be offset by increased positive end-expiratory pressure (PEEP); however, this must be balanced with the resulting cardiovascular effects, which will be described next. However, despite these changes, studies have demonstrated that laparoscopy results in smaller postoperative changes in pulmonary function tests compared to open surgery [33]. Overall, in healthy patients, changes to pulmonary mechanics are of minimal clinical significance.

Due to the resulting hypercapnia and respiratory acidosis, the monitoring of end-tidal CO_2 is mandatory during laparoscopy, whether traditional or robotic assisted. In patients with limited pulmonary reserves, capnoperitoneum carries an increased risk of CO_2 retention, increasing the difficulty of extubation. In patients with severe cardiopulmonary disease, arterial blood gas monitoring and continuous capnography are recommended [34].

4.3.2 Cardiovascular

The primary changes to the cardiovascular system due to CO_2 insufflation also result from hypercarbia and mechanical compression. These physiological effects occur most often during the early stages of insufflation [34].

The increase in end-tidal CO_2 may result in a mild hypercapnia (pCO_2 45–50 mmHg), which has little effect on hemodynamics. However, severe hypercapnia (pCO_2 55–70 mmHg) and the resulting acidosis may result in hemodynamic changes.

CO_2 has a direct effect of myocardial depression and vasodilation [33]. These effects trigger a compensatory sympathetic reaction resulting in a reflex tachycardia and vasoconstriction.

However, the primary effect of pneumoperitoneum on the cardiovascular system is due to mechanical compression of the venous system which lowers venous return. This compression, seen with intra-abdominal pressures from 12 to 15 mmHg, results in a decreased cardiac preload and cardiac output and a corresponding increase in heart rate, mean arterial pressure, and systemic and pulmonary vascular resistance [34].

Changes in patient positioning are often essential to gain proper visualization of the operative field. However, these changes can also affect hemodynamics. Reverse Trendelenburg position intensifies the physiological effects of pneumoperitoneum, while Trendelenburg position increases venous return [34]. Additionally, the use of PEEP of 10 cm H_2O during pneumoperitoneum to decrease atelectasis decreases preload and cardiac output [34].

It should be noted that the European Association of Endoscopic Surgery (EAES) in their 2001 clinical practice guidelines on pneumoperitoneum stated the effects of a 12–14 mmHg CO_2 pneumoperitoneum are not clinically relevant in healthy patients (ASA I or II) [34]. However, special consideration must be given to patients with underlying cardiac disease or other significant morbidities. Invasive blood pressure or circulating volume status measurements should be considered, and all of these patients should receive adequate preoperative beta-blockade, volume loading, and pneumatic compression of the lower limbs [34].

4.3.3 Renal

A systematic review on the effects of pneumoperitoneum on the renal system demonstrated a reduction in both renal perfusion and renal function [35]. This impairment is primarily mediated by direct compression of the renal parenchyma, arteries, and veins [34]. There is also an increase in the release of antidiuretic hormone, plasma renin activity, and serum aldosterone, which may further contribute to the decrease in urine output [36]. The level of depression is dependent upon multiple factors including preoperative renal function, volume status, intra-abdominal pressure, patient position, and duration of pneumoperitoneum. These changes appear to be temporary with function returning to normal after pneumoperitoneum is released. Although the decreases in renal perfusion and function are documented in the literature, it is unclear if they are of any clinical significance. The EAES guidelines state that while an intra-abdominal pressure of 12–14 mmHg in healthy patients is likely clinically insignificant, in patients with impaired renal function, intra-abdominal pressure should be kept as low as possible, and these patients should be volume loaded before and during times of increased intra-abdominal pressure [34].

4.4 Special Considerations for Robotic Surgery

Robotic surgery warrants several special considerations that do not apply to open or laparoscopic surgery (Table 4.4). These include robotic docking, the lack of tactile feedback, the potential for peripheral nerve damage, and the high cost.

4.4.1 Robotic Docking

In order to maximize the effectiveness of robotic systems, they must be precisely positioned [37]. Malpositioning can lead to clashing of surgical instruments or the need to re-dock the robot. Often, multiple dockings are required during a single procedure [28]. Both docking

Table 4.4 Special considerations for robotic surgery

• Robotic docking
• Lack of tactile and tensile feedback
• Capital and maintenance expenditures

and separation of the robot are time consuming, and the process varies considerably among institutions. For example, of the two recent case series evaluating the average docking time for robotic rectal procedures, one institution averaged 14 min per case, while the other averaged nearly 63 min per case [6, 7]. Finally, there is a concern that in the event of acute hemorrhage and the rapid need for open conversion, the time needed for robotic separation could affect patient safety [38].

This fundamental issue underscores the necessity for a dedicated robotics team. It is not just surgeons who graduate up the learning curve. In the previously mentioned studies evaluating docking time, there was a 48 and 49 % reduction in docking time between the first third and the last third of patients [6, 7]. As the team continues to gain experience with docking, positioning, and changing robotic instruments, total operative time will decrease.

4.4.2 Lack of Tactile and Tensile Feedback

Compared to open surgery, the haptic feedback from laparoscopic instruments has been demonstrated to provide surgeons with the ability to interpret the texture, shape, and consistency of objects [39]. However, a major limitation of the current robotic surgical systems is the lack of tactile or tensile feedback [23]. This may lead to breaking of suture during knot tying or tissue damage while creating traction [40]. In order to account for these factors, surgeons must learn to determine tissue strain by visualization [6]. While the ability to tie knots adequately without breaking suture can be mastered in a dry lab, the issue of iatrogenic injury is more complicated. For example, in colonic resection, redundant colon must be retracted to provide adequate counter tension. However, there have been reports of iatrogenic bowel injuries caused by robotic graspers [12]. There also exists a risk of iatrogenic injury that goes unrecognized at the time of surgery, particularly if the retracted tissue is out of the surgeon's field of view.

4.4.3 Potential Peripheral Nerve Damage

Injuries of the brachial plexus and common peroneal nerve have been documented after laparoscopic colorectal surgery [40]. This is often due to steep Trendelenburg positioning used to retract the small intestine out of the pelvis. Also, patients are often tilted down to the left or right or kept in lithotomy position. A systematic review found that prolonged operative time is the factor common to most peripheral nerve injuries in laparoscopy [42]. In addition, obesity was found to be a significant patient risk factor [41]. The Closed Claims Project, an analysis of 4000 anesthesia-related insurance claims, found 16 % of malpractice claims to be related to postoperative neuropathy [42].

Robotic surgery often requires steeper Trendelenburg positioning and generally has longer operative times [43]. Surgeons sitting at the console may not have a clear view to immediately recognize changes in patient position. A case series evaluating positioning injuries after urological surgery identified operative time, in-room time, ASA class, and quantity of IV fluids administered (which directly correlated with operative time) to be statistically significant [43]. Currently, there is insufficient evidence to determine if robotic colorectal surgery is associated with a higher risk of peripheral nerve injury. However, surgeons must be vigilant in minimizing risk factors including minimizing operative time and in-room time, judicious use of steep Trendelenburg position, and the creation of a positioning checklist. In addition, surgeons must perform and document a preoperative neurological exam to evaluate any preexisting nerve damage.

4.4.4 Large Capital Investment and High Operating Costs

Perhaps the biggest stumbling block for the implementation of robotic surgical systems is their cost. Robotic systems require financing of both the initial capital investment and ongoing operating costs. The 2013 average sale price for a *da Vinci* Surgical System was $1.53 million dollars (ranging from $1.0 to $2.3 million), and annual service agreements ranged from $100 to $170 thousand dollars per year [44]. In addition, robotic surgery requires single-use consumable products, further increasing the price [45]. However, despite the increased costs, robotic surgery does not result in additional reimbursement beyond the primary procedure code [46]. Therefore, centers that cannot make up for lower profit margins with increased volume will have difficulty providing robotic surgical services. This topic will be discussed in greater detail in Chap. 24.

4.5 Summary

Surgeons demonstrate a procedure-dependent learning curve when adopting robotic surgery. We recommend a stepwise approach to training beginning with didactics and a complete understanding of the technology, followed by robotic skills lab training to master skills such as intracorporeal suturing and knot tying, and finally operating room experience. This early experience should be with a mentor who is proficient in RAS. We also recommend that surgeons are experienced with laparoscopy before beginning robotics.

Data regarding patient selection is still in its early stages; however, there may be a benefit in short-term outcomes in obese male patients with low-lying rectal cancers who have completed neoadjuvant chemoradiation. Further study is warranted to determine if these benefits are widely generalizable. In addition, patients must be able to tolerate the physiological effects of prolonged pneumoperitoneum. Patients with heart failure, COPD, sepsis, and renal failure should be carefully evaluated to ensure they can tolerate the increased operative time associated with robotics.

Finally, there are a number of unique considerations that apply to robotic surgery. Docking and separation of the robot also have a learning curve, and an experienced team is required to maximize efficiency. Also, in contrast to open or laparoscopic surgery, robotic systems do not provide tactile or tensile feedback. This means that cues of tissue tension must be visual and acquisition of this skill is part of the learning curve. Due to prolonged operative times and the increased use of steep Trendelenburg positioning, patients may be at a higher risk for peripheral nerve injuries. Surgeons must remain cognizant of and attempt to minimize the factors associated with injury. Finally, the issue of cost must be considered. Robotic surgical systems are expensive to purchase, maintain, and operate. However, as reimbursement is not increased, centers that do not have sufficient volume may find robotic surgery to be prohibitively expensive.

References

1. Moore MJ, Bennett CL. The learning curve for laparoscopic cholecystectomy. Am J Surg. 1995;170(1): 55–9.
2. Glavic Z, Begic L, Simlesa D, Rukavina A. Treatment of acute cholecystitis. A comparison of open vs laparoscopic cholecystectomy. Surg Endosc. 2001;15(4): 398–401.
3. Barrie J, Jayne DG, Wright J, Czoski Murray CJ, Collinson FJ, Pavitt SH. Attaining surgical competency and its implications in surgical clinical trial design: a systematic review of the learning curve in laparoscopic and robot-assisted laparoscopic colorectal cancer surgery. Ann Surg Oncol. 2014;21(3):829–40.
4. Chang L, Satava RM, Pellegrini CA, Sinanan MN. Robotic surgery: identifying the learning curve through objective measurement of skill. Surg Endosc. 2003;17:1744–8.
5. Jiménez-Rodríguez RM, Díaz-Pavón JM, de la Portilla de Juan F, Prendes-Sillero D, Dussort HC, Padillo J. Learning curve for robotic-assisted laparoscopic rectal cancer surgery. Int J Colorectal Dis. 2013;28:815–21.
6. Bokhari MB, Patel CB, Ramos-Valadez DI, Ragupathi M, Haas EM. Learning curve for robotic-assisted laparoscopic colorectal surgery. Surg Endosc. 2011;25:855–60.
7. Guilianotti PC, Coratti A, Angelini M, Sbrana F, Cecconi S, Balestracci T. Robotics in general surgery: personal experience in a large community hospital. Arch Surg. 2003;138:777–84.
8. deSouza AL, Prasad LM, Park JJ, Marecik SJ, Blumetti J, Abcarian H. Robotic assistance in right hemicolectomy: is there a role? Dis Colon Rectum. 2010;53:1000–6.
9. Fabozzi M, Allieta R, Grimaldi L, Reggio S, Amato B, Danzi M. Open vs totally laparoscopic right colectomy: technique and results. BMC Surg. 2013;13 Suppl 1:A20.
10. Salloum RM, Butler DC, Schwartz SI. Economic evaluation of minimally invasive colectomy. J Am Coll Surg. 2006;202(2):269–74.
11. Peterson CY, Weiser MR. Robotic colorectal surgery. J Gastrointest Surg. 2014;18:398–403.
12. Mirnezami AH, Mirnezami R, Venkatasubramaniam AK, Chandrakumaran K, Cecil TD, Moran BJ. Robotic colorectal surgery: hype or new hope? A systematic review of robotics in colorectal surgery. Colorectal Dis. 2009;12:1084–93.
13. Ahlering TE, Skarecky D, Lee D, Clayman RV. Successful transfer of open surgical skills to a laparoscopic environment using a robotic interface: initial experience with laparoscopic radical prostatectomy. J Urol. 2004;172(2):776–7.
14. Fung AKY, Emad A. Robotic colonic surgery: is it advisable to commence a new learning curve? Dis Colon Rectum. 2013;56:786–96.
15. Fundamentals of laparoscopic surgery [internet]. 2014.http://www.flsprogram.org/index/why-take-the-fls-test/. Accessed 23 Apr 2014.
16. Dulan G, Rege RV, Hogg DC, Gilberg-Fisher KK, Tesfay ST, Scott DJ. Content and face validity of a comprehensive robotic skills training program for general surgery, urology, and gynecology. Am J Surg. 2012;203:535–9.
17. Chitwood WR, Nifong LW, Chapman WHH, Felger JE, Bailey M, Ballint T, et al. Robotic surgical training in an academic institution. Ann Surg. 2001;234(4):475–86.
18. Dulan G, Rege RV, Hogg DC, Gilberg-Fisher KM, Arain NA, Tesfay ST, et al. Developing a comprehensive, proficiency based training program for robotic surgery. Surgery. 2012;152:477–88.
19. Marecik SJ, Prasad LM, Park JJ, Pearl RK, Evenhouse RJ, Shah A, et al. A lifelike patient simulator for teaching robotic colorectal surgery: how to acquire skills for robotic rectal dissection. Surg Endosc. 2008;22:1876–81.
20. Halvorsen FH, Elle OJ, Dalinin VV, Mork BE, Sorhus V, Rotnes JS, et al. Virtual reality simulator training equals mechanical robotic training in improving robot-assisted basic suturing skills. Surg Endosc. 2006;20:1565–9.
21. Ali MR, Rasmussen J, BhaskerRao B. Teaching robotic surgery: a stepwise approach. Surg Endosc. 2007;21:912–5.
22. Yee JY, Mucksavage P, Sundaram CP, McDougal EM. Best practices for robotic surgery training and credentialing. J Urol. 2011;185:1191–7.
23. Herron DM, Marohn M, SAGES-MIRA Robotic Surgery Consensus Group. A consensus document on robotic surgery. Surg Endosc. 2008;22(2):313–25.
24. Weber PA, Merola S, Wasielewski A, Ballantyne GH. Telerobotic-assisted laparoscopic right and sigmoid colectomies for benign disease. Dis Colon Rectum. 2002;45:1689–96.
25. D'Annibale A, Pernazza G, Morpurgo E, Monsellato I, Pende V, Lucandri G. Robotic right colon resection:

evaluation of first 50 consecutive cases for malignant disease. Indian J Surg Oncol. 2012;3(4):279–85.

26. Park JS, Choi GS, Park SY, Kim HJ, Ryuk JP. Randomized clinical trial of robot-assisted versus standard laparoscopic right colectomy. Br J Surg. 2012;99(9):1219–26.

27. Spinoglio G, Summa M, Priora F, Quarati R, Testa S. Robotic colorectal surgery: first 50 cases experience. Dis Colon Rectum. 2008;51:1627–32.

28. Scarpinata R, Aly EH. Does robotic rectal cancer surgery offer improved early postoperative outcomes? Dis Colon Rectum. 2013;56:253–62.

29. Lee SW. Laparoscopic procedures for colon and rectal cancer surgery. Clin Colon Rectal Surg. 2009;22:218–24.

30. Prasad L, deSouza AL, Slawomir J, Park JJ, Abcarian H. Robotic pursestring technique in low anterior resection. Dis Colon Rectum. 2010;53(2):230–4.

31. Grabowski JE, Talamini MA. Physiological effects of pneumoperitoneum. J Gastrointest Surg. 2009;13:1009–16.

32. Neudecker J, Sauerland S, Neugebauer E, Bergamaschi R, Bonjer HJ, Cuschieri A, et al. The European Association for Endoscopic Surgery clinical practice guideline on the pneumoperitoneum for laparoscopic surgery. Surg Endosc. 2002;16:1121–43.

33. Chumillas S, Ponce JL, Delgado F, Viciano V. Pulmonary function and complications after laparoscopic cholecystectomy. Eur J Surg. 1998;164:433–7.

34. Kraut EJ, Anderson JT, Safwat A, Barbosa R, Wolfe BM. Impairment of cardiac performance by laparoscopy in patients receiving positive end-expiratory pressure. Arch Surg. 1999;134:76–80.

35. Demyttenaere S, Feldman LS, Fried GM. Effect of pneumoperitoneum on renal perfusion and function: a systematic review. Surg Endosc. 2007;21(2):152–60.

36. Nguyen NT, Perez RV, Fleming N, Rivers R, Wolfe BM. Effect of prolonged pneumoperitoneum on intraoperative urine output during laparoscopic gastric bypass. J Am Coll Surg. 2002;195(4):476–83.

37. Aly EH. Robotic colorectal surgery: summary of the current evidence. Int J Colorectal Dis. 2014;29:1–8.

38. Baik SH. Robotic colorectal surgery. Yonsei Med J. 2008;4(6):891–6.

39. Bholat OS, Haluck RS, Murray WB, Gorman PJ, Krummel TM. Tactile feedback is present during minimally invasive surgery. J Am Coll Surg. 1999;189(4):349–55.

40. Codd RJ, Evans MD, Sagar PM, Williams GL. A systematic review of peripheral nerve injury following laparoscopic colorectal surgery. Colorectal Dis. 2013;15(3):278–82.

41. Mills JT, Burris MB, Warburton DJ, Conaway MR, Schenkman NS, Krupski TL. Positioning injuries associated with robotic assisted urological surgery. J Urol. 2013;190(2):580–4.

42. Cheney FW, Domino KB, Caplan RA, Posner KL. Nerve injury associated with anesthesia. Anesthesiology. 1999;90(4):1062–9.

43. Shveiky D, Aseff JN, Iglesia CB. Brachial plexus injury after laparoscopic and robotic surgery. J Minim Invasive Gynecol. 2010;17(4):414–20.

44. Intuitive Surgical. Investor presentation Q1 2014. [document on the Internet]. http://investor.intuitive-surgical.com/phoenix.zhtml?c=122359&p=irol-IRHome. Accessed 7 May 2014.

45. Barbash GI, Giled SA. New technology and healthcare costs-the case of robot-assisted surgery. N Engl J Med. 2010;363:701–4.

46. Center for Medicare and Medicaid Services (US). Physician fee schedule search [Internet]. [updated 4 Apr 2014]. http://www.cms.gov/apps/physician-fee-schedule. Accessed 8 May 2014.

Emre Balık

Abstract

Four decades ago, the performance of the first laparoscopic cholecystectomy was a milestone in medicine. A decade later, the first laparoscopic colon resection was reported in the United States, and this progress ultimately led to the introduction of robotic surgery in 2000. There are many advantages of minimally invasive operative modalities. However, the widespread adoption of laparoscopic colorectal surgery has been delayed because of technical difficulties. Furthermore, operating in multiple quadrants and the lack of appropriate laparoscopic training for practicing colorectal surgeons have complicated the learning curve. Some of the limitations in terms of two-dimensional imaging, limited dexterity, and a long learning curve could possibly be overcome by robotic approaches. This chapter will describe robotic room setup, instrumentation, patient positioning, and trocar placement.

Keywords

Robotic surgery • Patient positioning • Trocar placement • Instrumentation

5.1　Introduction

Four decades ago, the performance of the first laparoscopic cholecystectomy was a milestone in medicine. A decade later, the first laparoscopic colon resection was reported in the United States, and this progress ultimately led to the introduction of robotic surgery in 2000. There are many advantages of minimally invasive operative modalities. However, the widespread adoption of laparoscopic colorectal surgery has been delayed because of technical difficulties. Furthermore, operating in multiple quadrants and the lack of appropriate laparoscopic training for practicing colorectal surgeons have complicated the learning curve. Some of the limitations in terms of two-dimensional imaging, limited dexterity, and a long learning curve could possibly be overcome by robotic approaches. This chapter will describe robotic

E. Balık, M.D. (✉)
Department of General Surgery, Koc University
School of Medicine, Rumelifeneri yolu, Sarıyer,
Istanbul 34450, Turkey
e-mail: Ebalik@Istanbul.edu.tr; emrebalik@yahoo.com;
emrebalik@me.com

© Springer International Publishing Switzerland 2015
H. Ross et al. (eds.), *Robotic Approaches to Colorectal Surgery*,
DOI 10.1007/978-3-319-09120-4_5

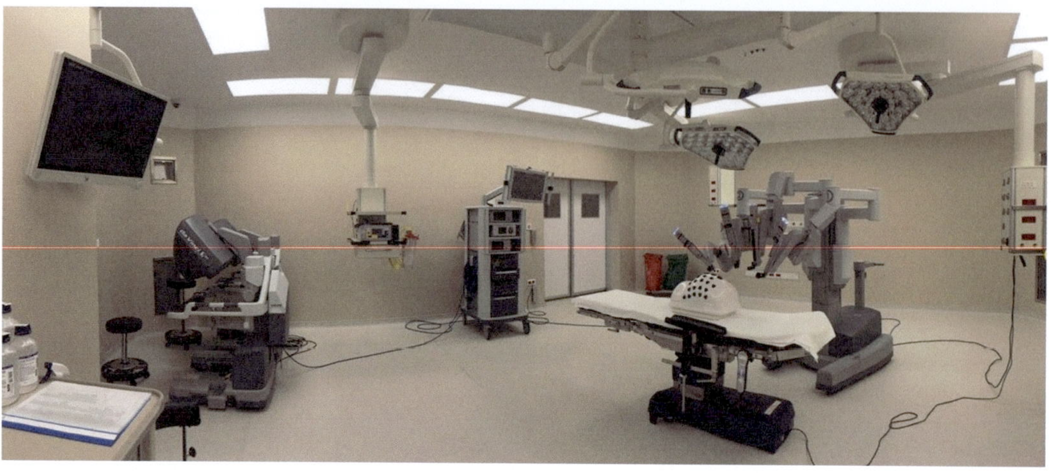

Fig. 5.1 Robotic Room

room setup, instrumentation, patient positioning, and trocar placement.

Robotic surgery systems have many technologic advantages. These include a stable camera platform, three-dimensional imaging system, better ergonomics, tremor elimination, ambidextrous capability, motion scaling, and instruments with multiple degrees of freedom [1–8]. This chapter will outline the details required for appropriate robotic positioning and trocar placement.

5.2 Robotic and Patient Positioning

The robotic surgery team consists of the surgeon, circulating nurse, surgical technician, and surgical assistants. Each member has to be knowledgeable in robotic-assisted, laparoscopic, and open surgery. The team members should develop good communication habits and preference cards for each procedure. Good outcomes are dependent on a team that communicates and adjusts accordingly for each procedure [5, 9]. It is critical that the entire team participate in a robotic course and see a more experienced robotic team in a surgery before beginning robotic surgery. Furthermore, it is important for the surgical team to remain consistent, and it is recommended to have a dedicated team to work together during the robotic surgery [5, 10, 11] (Fig. 5.1).

The surgeon will command and organize the whole group; however, each person on the team should feel that they are an integral part and that their participation leads directly to improve patient outcomes. The surgeon should not only be in full command of the robot procedure but also have knowledge and experience for the setup, basic services, and troubleshooting the system errors and be prepared for any emergency situations. The team members, nurses, and surgical technician have critical roles for robotic operations in regard to starting up the robot, draping, docking instruments, troubleshooting, and exchanging the instruments. We emphasize a "total team approach." The surgical assistant should have experience with trocar insertion, clipping, suction, and irrigation cutting and feel comfortable with vessel-sealing instruments [5, 9].

The operating room should be designed for robotic surgery to accommodate all of the robotic components. The robotic system needs more space than the standard laparoscopic system. The connections can be done easily, and each person can see each other and communicate in an easy way [5, 12, 13]. The room should be big enough to facilitate the docking of the robot for different types of surgery [2, 13, 14].

If the operation room is not dedicated to robotic surgery, there may be a need to have additional laparoscopic towers to accommodate the other instruments. Ideally the operating room

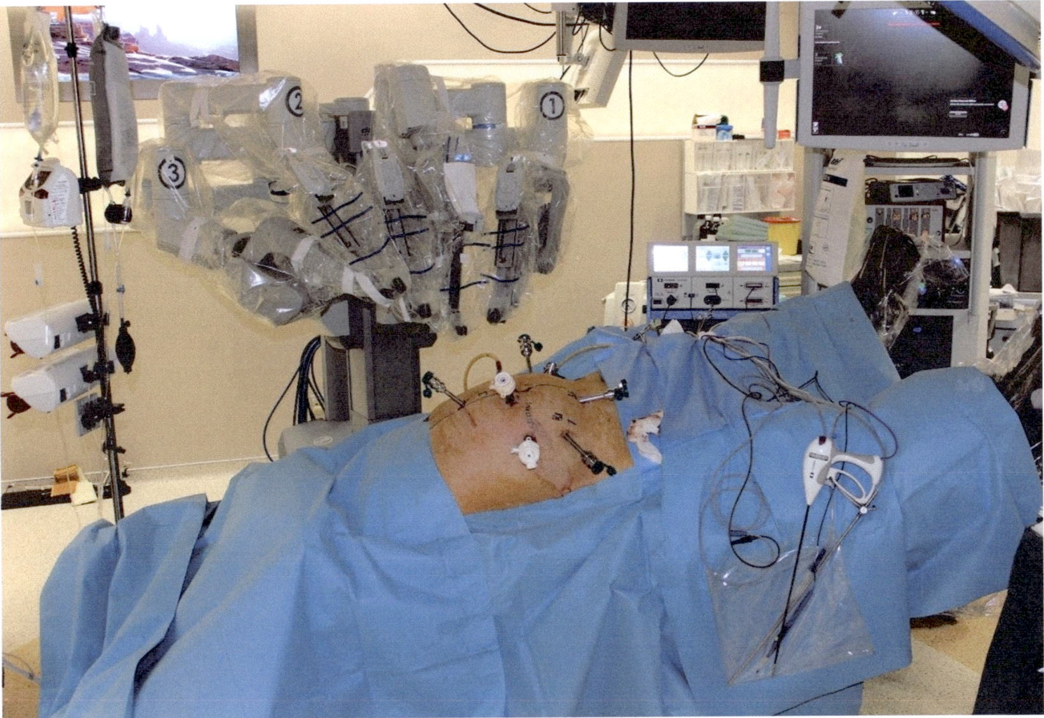

Fig. 5.2 Patient positioning

will accommodate a room for laparoscopic surgery and robotic surgery only [6, 15, 16].

5.3 Patient Positioning

For most surgical approaches, patients are placed directly onto a gel pad on the operating room table. The gel pad increases friction and prevents patients from sliding during the procedure. The patient is placed in a modified lithotomy position using yellow fin stirrups with thromboembolic stockings and intermittent pressure devices. The angle of the stirrups should allow the robotic arms to move without collision. We have found that flexion of less than 10° at the hip area is ideal. Both arms are padded and placed along the side of the patient's body. A block of foam is placed over the face as a protector. A safety strap or tape can be used to secure the patient to the table. We do not use any shoulder braces as these have been associated with brachial plexus injuries (Fig. 5.2).

5.4 Robotic System

The da Vinci Surgical System consists of three main parts: console, cart with the four arms, and video and insufflation systems [2, 17]. The surgeon performs the operation from the console with command of the four robotic arms. We often have to educate patients that the "da Vinci®" is a slave robotic system that does not have artificial intelligence and cannot perform the operation by itself. The standard system was released in 1999 and was originally with one camera and two instrument arms. A few years later, the S series was launched into the market. This system had some improved developments in terms of a motorized patient cart, color-coded fiber optic connections, more straightforward device connection, and quick click trocar attachments [3, 18, 19]. In 2007, the S system upgraded to a high-definition video system and named Si HD. Recently another surgeon console is adapted the Si system. The dual console connects two surgeon consoles to the same patient cart and is ideal

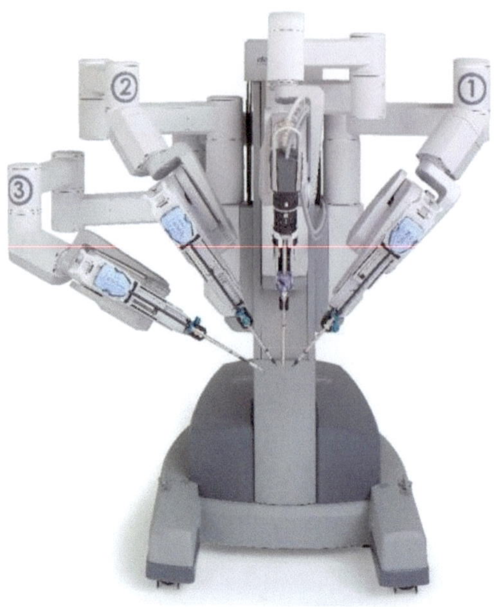
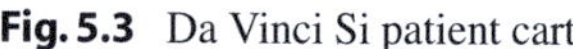

Fig. 5.3 Da Vinci Si patient cart

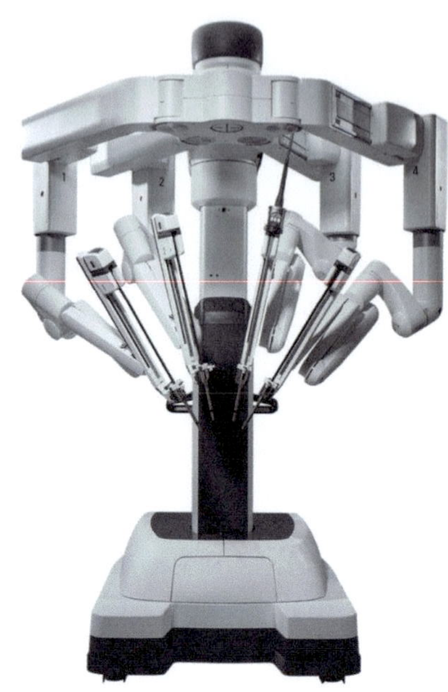

Fig. 5.4 Da Vinci Xi patient cart

for teaching purposes. It helps to coordinate surgery real time and also permits collaboration of different specialties at the same time during the operation. The "da Vinci" XI has been launched to the market in mid-2014. The XI system has many differences on the patient-side cart such as laser targeting system and long, thin, and more flexible arms. This new chart is more suitable for general surgery procedures such as complex procedures. This new technology allows for easier and faster docking and for multiple-quadrant approaches [20–24] (Figs. 5.3 and 5.4).

5.4.1 Surgeon Console

The surgeon console is the driver seat for controlling the robot. From here the surgeon obtains three-dimensional images of the surgical field through the stereo viewer, adjusts the system with the pod controls, and controls the instrument arms [9]. The stereo viewer displays the real-time high-resolution three-dimensional images of the surgical field, system status icons, and messages. The three-dimensional image is created by capturing two independent views from two 5 mm endoscopes fit-

ted into the stereo endoscope and displaying them into right and left optical channels [5, 10, 11, 25]. The system status icons and messages are displayed in specific locations within the stereo viewer and alert the surgeon to any changes or errors within the system. Directly adjacent to the stereo viewer are infrared sensors. These are activated at the surgeon console when the surgeon's head is placed between them. This prevents unwanted movement of robotic instruments inside of the patient's body as the robotic instruments are immediately deactivated when the doctor looks away from the stereo viewer and removes their head from between the infrared sensors. This feature is an exquisite security tool in robotic surgery [5, 11, 26].

The da Vinci standard and S models have right- and left-sided pod controls that can communicate significant system errors and turn on and off the system. The Si-HD model combines the right and left pod controls into a central touchpad on the armrest. In addition, the console can be adjusted in four different directions to facilitate better ergonomics and particular settings can be stored for each surgeon [5, 25, 27].

For all of the da Vinci models, the master controllers are the manual manipulators that the surgeon uses to control the instruments, arms, and endoscope. The controllers are grasped with the index finger and thumb. Movements are translated by a computer that scales, filters, and relays them to the instruments [5, 7, 28].

For activation of the instrument arms during the surgery, the surgeon must "match grips" by grasping the masters to match the position and grip of the EndoWrist instrument tips as seen within the body. This feature prevents accidental activation of the instrument arms and inadvertent tissue damage. When toggling between two instruments and taking control of an instrument that is retracting the tissue, the master is closed to prevent dropping the tissue. The foot switch panel allows the surgeon to control the camera for zoom-in or zoom-out positions and to activate energy sources if desired for each device in each arm. The clutch pedal allows the surgeon to change to the third arm or adjust the working distance between the master controllers. Quickly tapping of the clutch pedal once allows the designated master controller toggles between the powers of the current arm to the third robotic arm. Tapping the clutch pedal once again reverses the action. This feature allows the surgeon to toggle control of two different robotic arms using the same master controller. Depressing the clutch pedal disengages the master controls from the instrument arms, and the surgeon can readjust their arms to more comfortable position in the working space. Utterly depressing the camera pedal disengages the master controls from the instrument arms and instead engages the endoscope. The endoscope may then be moved or rotated to the appropriate area of interest within the body. The scope comes in 0 and 30°. There is a focus control lever on the standard and S systems for endoscope labeled "+/−" in the center of the foot switch panel. The coagulation pedal is connected to a compatible electrosurgical unit. With the dual power capabilities, one machine arm can be connected to bipolar energy while the other one is connected to monopolar energy. The Si model has a completely remodeled footboard with two tiers of pedals and levers on the side of the board. There are still clutch and camera pedals on the left side of the board. The brakes on the side of the panel are used to shift power between the two surgeons in dual-console mode. In addition, the foot switch panel on the right can be used to change the coagulation pedal to bipolar mode. This property prevents accidental electrosurgical activation of the wrong tool arm [5, 12, 22, 28].

5.5 Patient Cart

The patient cart for the standard and S system houses the camera and instrument arms. Each arm has several clutch buttons that assist with the gross movements of the arm and to enter or remove devices [2–4]. To activate the clutch, the buttons are depressed and the arm is moved. Otherwise, there will be resistance encountered, and the arm will return to the original position. Each arm has two port clutch buttons used for gross movements of the instrument arm. There is also a particular camera or instrument clutch button located at the top of each arm to adjust the final trajectory of the arm during docking and inserting or withdrawing endoscope/instruments. Each division requires several sterile accessories that are placed during the draping procedure [4].

The standard system was initially offered with a camera arm and two instrument arms. Later an optional third instrument arm became available for new standard systems. The third instrument arm is mounted on the same axis as the camera arm. Because of this reason, the team should be more careful and aware that the third arm can have collusion with the other arms or operating table. Each arm on the standard system is color coded, the camera arm is blue, and instrument arms are yellow, green, and red. With the standard system, the surgeon can only use one clutch at a time to move the tool arm. With S and Si systems, surgeon can use the port clutch and camera/instrument clutch simultaneously to maneuver the arm into position [2, 18, 29].

Similar to the standard system, S and Si systems have a camera arm and two instrument arms and are available with an optional third instrument arm. Each tool arm is numbered. These models also added LED light below the camera/instrument clutch and a touch-screen monitor. The LED light communicates the status of the arm to the surgical team using preset color scheme. The Xi system does not have specific camera arm. Each arm will act as a camera arm. The Xi system has laser-targeting mode. The laser-targeting specialty makes docking easier than the previous models [5, 11].

The touch-screen monitor is synchronized with the surgeon's view and displays all of the system status icons and messages. It can be used for endoscope alignment and telestration or to toggle between video inputs. The patient-side cart of the S and Si systems also features a motor drive, which assists in docking the patient cart to the operating table and trocars [5, 30].

5.6 Instruments

The actual robotic system has four arms for the surgical interventions. One arm is designed for the endoscope, and the other are for the surgical procedure. The endoscopic arm holds the endoscope and provides a stable image. In conventional laparoscopic surgery, the view is obtained by an assistant. This may cause unnecessary movements and low-quality vision also. In the robotic surgery, the surgeon commands the camera often eliminating the visual confusion caused by laparoscopy.

The robotic system does not contain an inherent smoke evacuator. Smoke occurs after every single cauterization. One of the trocars may be reserved for smoke evacuation. However, it is a time-consuming procedure and also one of the disadvantages of robotic surgery [31–33]. A suction/irrigator does exist; however, it will take up the use of one of the working arms. We usually use an assistant laparoscopic 5 mm port for this purpose.

With any surgery, hemostasis is paramount. The bleeding from a major vessel can directly contaminate the endoscope, and it causes of loss of vision. In this situation, the assistant should clean the lenses of the endoscope. The assistant should separate the endoscope from the robotic system, clean, and reinsert it immediately and rapidly. Sometimes this takes time and needs to convert to open surgery. In this case, the weight of the endoscope may cause a delay. Thus, a more secure dissection is required in robotic surgery [3, 14, 34]. More time is needed to control bleeding than the laparoscopic surgery or convert into an open surgery.

The tips of the instruments are designed to act like the dexterity of the human and wrist. This is a new technology and specific to the robotic surgery, and it is named EndoWrist function. The robotic instruments carry out precise motions, which are coming from the surgeon console [2, 14, 35, 36]. The instruments have 7 degrees of freedom with 180° of articulating and 540° of rotation simulating a surgeon's hand and wrist movements. The EndoWrist function allows the surgeon to perform secure intracorporeal anastomosis after bowel resections. This is one of the major advantages of robotic surgery. Laparoscopic intracorporeal anastomosis has often been a major hurdle for surgeons performing colorectal procedures and has led to the vast majority of anastomoses being performed by extracorporeal means. In addition, the EndoWrist function is also very useful for the pelvic dissection and around blood vessels. One can perform very delicate and precise dissection in very narrow confines of the deep pelvis [2, 3, 37, 38].

One of the major issues with pelvic surgery is dissection and transection of mesorectum, particularly in a narrow pelvis. This can often be a complicated and difficult procedure even in the open surgery. In laparoscopic surgery, the axis of the rectum and the axis of the instrument are often at oblique or tangential angles. The surgeon would prefer an acute- or right-angle approach to this dissection, but often it is not possible given the limitations of current widely applicable laparoscopic instruments. The robotic instrumentation, with its increased ability to rotate and provide acute angulation, allows for a right-angle approach during the transection of the mesorectum. The angulated instruments of the robotic system can act as a retractor also. The robotic instruments can create a bigger space than the classic laparoscopic instruments even in deeper pelvis [38–40]. However, the robotic instruments do have a usage limit. The robotic surgery system tracks the number of uses and data of usage will be tracked on the master console. An instrument arm will not function if an overused device is inserted [19, 20, 41].

The robotic surgery instruments are composed of an insertion and releasing part, instrument shaft, wrist, and a variety of tool tips. The standard robotic surgical tools are 52 cm with the gray label compared to the S systems being 57 cm with blue label. The tools are interchangeable between the systems. Nowadays, there are more than 40 EndoWrist® instruments available for colorectal surgery in 8 or 5 mm shaft diameters. The 8 mm devices operate on an "angled joint" compared to "snake joint." The angled joint allows the tip to rotate using a shorter radius compared to snake joint [20, 22, 23, 42–44].

5.7 General Considerations

5.7.1 Preparation of Robot

Preparing the operating room for robotic-assisted procedure is essential before the surgery starts. There should be a short checklist before the surgery [5, 11]:

1. Connect system cables, optical channels, focus control, and power cables, and turn on the system.
2. Position the instrument and camera arms so they have adequate room to move.
3. Drape the patient cart arms. The team should be in close coordination for draping. Draping should not be so tight. If it is too tight, then the arms cannot move correctly and the drapes may tear.
   (a) The instrument arms are draped to cover the arm completely, and the sterile instrument adapter is locked into the tool arm carriage. For the standard system, the sterile trocar mount is also locked into position while the S system has the trocar mount permanently attached, and the drape is placed over the mount.
   (b) The camera arm is draped in a similar way. For the standard system, a sterile endoscope trocar mount and camera arm sterile adapter are also placed at this time. The S system also requires a camera arm sterile adapter. Depending on when the S system was purchased, some use a sterile endoscope trocar mount, while others have the mount permanently attached. There are

different robotic camera arm trocar mounts for each trocar manufacturer.

4. Drape the endoscope by connecting the camera sterile adapter to the endoscope and then tape the drape to the sterile adapter. The camera head is connected, and the drape is inverted over the camera head and optical cables.
5. Connect the light source to the endoscope with the sterile light cable.
6. Align the endoscope and set endoscope settings (three-dimensional vs. two-dimensional, 0° vs. 30°)
7. Set the "soft spot" of the camera arm by aligning the trocar mount with the center of the patient cart column. Then extend the camera arm, so there is approximately 20″ between the back of the camera arm and patient cart. The S systems have a guide on the camera arm to assist with setting the soft spot. The Xi system also has laser targeting system.

5.7.2 Abdominal Access and Trocar Placement

Robotic surgery begins similar to laparoscopic surgery, abdominal access, and trocar placement. Verres needles or open-access methods (Hasson technique) can be used for the creation of pneumoperitoneum. The abdominal cavity is insufflated to 12–15 mmHg level [5, 7]. Any 12 mm disposable trocar can be used for first trocar placement, which is used for the robotic endoscope telescope. The camera trocar should be placed 15–20 cm from the targeted surgical field and allows optimal visualization of the surgical field. For the obese patients, optic trocar should be placed closer to the target area and a longer trocar is useful [5].

After the first trocar insertion, secondary trocars can be placed under laparoscopic vision. The latest model has laser targeting system which is mounted at the center of the boom and assists with alignment of cart to target anatomy. This latest improvement also helps to find accurate trocar sites and quicker docking. The robotic instrument arms are compatible with specific da Vinci 5 or 8 mm metal trocars that can be placed using blunt or sharp obturators. The robotic trocars need to be inserted to the thick black band/mark on the trocar at the level of the abdominal fascia [5, 10]. This acts as a pivot point for the trocar and robotic tool arm. It is recommended that robotic trocars be placed at least 10 cm away from the camera to avoid the instrument arm collision and facilitate intracorporeal suturing. Also, the angle created by the robotic and camera trocars should be greater than 90° to increase arm maneuverability [5, 7]. Other laparoscopic instruments may need to be available for lysis of adhesions prior to robot docking and the first assistant to use during the procedure. The important point is trocar places should be decided after completion of insufflation.

5.7.3 Patient Cart Docking

After pneumoperitoneum, the patient cart should be driven to the operating table for docking. One member of the surgical team drives the patient cart while another one guides the driver. The surgical table should be placed in the desired position (Trendelenburg, lithotomy, etc.) before docking the patient cart.

The standard system is pushed into position, and the brakes at the base of the cart are hand-tightened; also the S and Si systems have a motor drive to assist with the docking, but use of motor drive is not mandatory [5, 12, 13].

The camera arm is the first one connected to the patient by locking the camera trocar mount. It is important to use the camera setup joint buttons to move the camera arm into position and the camera grip to adjust the trajectory of the arm. Exclusively using the camera grip to move the camera arm may limit the range of motion of the camera during operation. The instrument arms are then attached to the robotic trocars and screwed into place using a twist-lock device. When using the S or Si system, snap-mounted devices are used to engage the robotic trocars. Port clutch should be used for gross movements of the instruments and final positioning. The

team should make sure to prevent a collision, contact, or pinching the patient's arm, body, or legs [5, 9, 13].

The surgical team should also recheck all instruments once again before beginning the surgical procedure. The team should check for proper working distance and make sure that the arms are not compressing the patient. After insertion of an endoscope to the camera trocar, the endoscope can be positioned to the surgical field using the camera clutch button. The working instruments (EndoWrist®) are added placing the instrument tip into the trocar and sliding the instrument housing into the adapter. The instrument is then moved to the surgical field by using instrument clutch button. Each device should be placed into the patient under endoscopic vision. To remove the instrument, the surgeon should straighten the instrument wrist and the assistant should squeeze the release levers and pull out the device. Close communication is mandatory for preventing inadvertent adjustment, movement, and complete removal of the device. As a safety measure, the system has security control that any new device can be inserted and placed to a depth 1 mm shorter than the previous instrument position [5, 9, 28].

5.8 Conclusion

A surgical robot is a computer-controlled device that can be programmed to aid the positioning and manipulation of surgical instruments. The goal of robotic colorectal surgery is to use a minimally invasive approach to perform procedures that are performed by laparotomy or are too complex for conventional laparoscopy. The potential advantages of robotic over conventional laparoscopy include three-dimensional imaging, mechanical improvement stabilization of instruments within the surgical field, and improved ergonomics. There are some limitations of clinical use of robots including cost, physician and nursing team training, and the need for more data.

5.9 Key Points

- The operating room setup is of paramount importance for robotic surgery.
- A dedicated and consistent surgical and nursing team is mandatory for a successful robotic surgery program.
- The team should be familiar with all types of the minimally invasive surgical operations.
- The team should be ready for emergency situations and should know the limitations of the robotic equipment.

References

1. Alasari S, Min BS. Robotic colorectal surgery: a systematic review. ISRN Surg. 2012;2012:293894.
2. Baik SH. Robotic colorectal surgery. Yonsei Med J. 2008;49(6):891–6.
3. Bertani E, Chiappa A, Ubiali P, Fiore B, Corbellini C, Cossu ML, et al. Role of robotic surgery in colorectal resections for cancer. Minerva Gastroenterol Dietol. 2012;58(3):191–200.
4. Bokhari MB, Patel CB, Ramos-Valadez DI, Ragupathi M, Haas EM. Learning curve for robotic-assisted laparoscopic colorectal surgery. Surg Endosc. 2011; 25(3):855–60.
5. Ty T, Higuchi MT. Robotic instrumentation, personnel and operating room setup. In: Su LM, editor. Atlas of robotic urologic surgery, Current clinical urology. London: Springer; 2011. p. 15–30.
6. Buyer's brief: robotic surgery. Healthc Financ Manage. 2013;67(6):53–4.
7. Vlcek P, Capov I, Jedlicka V, Chalupnik S, Korbicka J, Veverkova L, et al. [Robotic procedures in the colorectal surgery]. Rozhl Chir. 2008;87(3):135–7.
8. Volonte F, Pugin F, Buchs NC, Spaltenstein J, Hagen M, Ratib O, et al. Console-integrated stereoscopic OsiriX 3D volume-rendered images for da Vinci colorectal robotic surgery. Surg Innov. 2013;20(2):158–63.
9. Parekattil SJ, Moran ME. Robotic instrumentation: evolution and microsurgical applications. Indian J Urol. 2010;26(3):395–403.
10. Spinoglio G, Summa M, Priora F, Quarati R, Testa S. Robotic colorectal surgery: first 50 cases experience. Dis Colon Rectum. 2008;51(11):1627–32.
11. Roukos DH. The era of robotic surgery for colorectal cancer. Ann Surg Oncol. 2010;17(1):338–9.
12. Vitobello D, Fattizzi N, Santoro G, Rosati R, Baldazzi G, Bulletti C, et al. Robotic surgery and standard laparoscopy: a surgical hybrid technique for use in colorectal endometriosis. J Obstet Gynaecol Res. 2013;39(1):217–22.
13. Patel CB, Ragupathi M, Ramos-Valadez DI, Haas EM. A three-arm (laparoscopic, hand-assisted, and robotic) matched-case analysis of intraoperative and postoperative outcomes in minimally invasive colorectal surgery. Dis Colon Rectum. 2011;54(2):144–50.
14. Baek SK, Carmichael JC, Pigazzi A. Robotic surgery: colon and rectum. Cancer J. 2013;19(2):140–6.
15. Al-Naami M, Anjum MN, Aldohayan A, Al-Khayal K, Alkharji H. Robotic general surgery experience: a gradual progress from simple to more complex procedures. Int J Med Robot. 2013;9(4):486–91.
16. Baek SJ, Kim SH, Cho JS, Shin JW, Kim J. Robotic versus conventional laparoscopic surgery for rectal cancer: a cost analysis from a single institute in Korea. World J Surg. 2012;36(11):2722–9.
17. D'Annibale A, Pernazza G, Morpurgo E, Monsellato I, Pende V, Lucandri G, et al. Robotic right colon resection: evaluation of first 50 consecutive cases for malignant disease. Ann Surg Oncol. 2010;17(11):2856–62.
18. D'Annibale A, Morpurgo E, Fiscon V, Trevisan P, Sovernigo G, Orsini C, et al. Robotic and laparoscopic surgery for treatment of colorectal diseases. Dis Colon Rectum. 2004;47(12):2162–8.
19. Hottenrott C. Robotic surgery and limitations. Surg Endosc. 2012;26(2):580–1.
20. Jayne DG, Culmer PR, Barrie J, Hewson R, Neville A. Robotic platforms for general and colorectal surgery. Colorectal Dis. 2011;13 Suppl 7:78–82.
21. Keller DS, Hashemi L, Lu M, Delaney CP. Short-term outcomes for robotic colorectal surgery by provider volume. J Am Coll Surg. 2013;217(6):1063–9.e1.
22. Kim CW, Baik SH. Robotic rectal surgery: what are the benefits? Minerva Chir. 2013;68(5):457–69.
23. Koh DC, Tsang CB, Kim SH. A new application of the four-arm standard da Vinci(R) surgical system: totally robotic-assisted left-sided colon or rectal resection. Surg Endosc. 2011;25(6):1945–52.
24. Marescaux J. [State of the art of surgery. Robotic surgery and telesurgery]. Cir Cir. 2013;81(4):265–8.
25. Peterson CY, Weiser MR. Robotic colorectal surgery. J Gastrointest Surg. 2014;18(2):398–403.
26. Pedraza R, Ramos-Valadez DI, Haas EM. Robotic-assisted laparoscopic surgery of the colon and rectum: a literature review. Cir Cir. 2011;79(4):384–91.
27. Ma J, Shukla PJ, Milsom JW. The evolving role of robotic colorectal surgery. Dis Colon Rectum. 2011; 54(3):376. author reply-7.
28. Yu HY, Friedlander DF, Patel S, Hu JC. The current status of robotic oncologic surgery. CA Cancer J Clin. 2013;63(1):45–56.
29. Bell S, Carne P, Chin M, Farmer C. Establishing a robotic colorectal surgery programme. ANZ J Surg. 2015;85(4):214–6.
30. Marecik SJ, Prasad LM, Park JJ, Pearl RK, Evenhouse RJ, Shah A, et al. A lifelike patient simulator for teaching robotic colorectal surgery: how to acquire skills for robotic rectal dissection. Surg Endosc. 2008;22(8):1876–81.
31. Anvari M, Birch DW, Bamehriz F, Gryfe R, Chapman T. Robotic-assisted laparoscopic colorectal surgery.

Surg Laparosc Endosc Percutan Tech. 2004;14(6): 311–5.

32. Abdalla RZ. Robotic surgery, can we live without it? Arq Bras Cir Dig. 2012;25(2):74.

33. Ayloo S, Fernandes E, Choudhury N. Learning curve and robot set-up/operative times in singly docked totally robotic Roux-en-Y gastric bypass. Surg Endosc. 2014;28(5):1629–33.

34. Bianchi PP, Pigazzi A, Choi GS. Clinical Robotic Surgery Association Fifth Worldwide Congress, Washington DC, 3–5 October 2013: Robotic Colorectal Surgery. Ecancermedicalscience. 2014;8:385.

35. Abboudi H, Khan MS, Aboumarzouk O, Guru KA, Challacombe B, Dasgupta P, et al. Current status of validation for robotic surgery simulators: a systematic review. BJU Int. 2013;111(2):194–205.

36. Baek SJ, Kim CH, Cho MS, Bae SU, Hur H, Min BS, et al. Robotic surgery for rectal cancer can overcome difficulties associated with pelvic anatomy. Surg Endosc. 2015;29(6):1419–24.

37. Bianchi PP, Luca F, Petz W, Valvo M, Cenciarelli S, Zuccaro M, et al. The role of the robotic technique in minimally invasive surgery in rectal cancer. Ecancermedicalscience. 2013;7:357.

38. Casier R, Lenders C, Lhernould MS, Gauthier M, Lambert P. Position measurement/tracking comparison of the instrumentation in a droplet-actuated-robotic platform. Sensors. 2013;13(5):5857–69.

39. Dal Moro F. Robotic surgery and functional outcomes: a lesson from urology. Surg Laparosc Endosc Percutan Tech. 2014;24(4):392–3.

40. Dondelinger R. Robotic surgery systems. Biomed Instrum Technol. 2014;48(1):55–9.

41. Himpens J. Surgery in space: the future of robotic telesurgery (Haidegger T, Szandor J, Benyo Z. Surg Endosc 2011; 25(3):681–690). Surg Endosc. 2012; 26(1):286.

42. Jayne D. [Robotic colorectal surgery: current status and future developments]. Chirurg. 2013;84(8):635–42.

43. Robotic-assisted laparoscopic surgery. Med Lett Drugs Ther. 2010;52(1340):45–6.

44. New technology offers a gentle touch for cancer surgery. A new robotic surgical tool may detect tumors far more accurately than current minimally invasive techniques. Duke Med Health News. 2009;15(12):5–6.

Troubleshooting

6

Farrell Adkins and David J. Maron

Abstract

This chapter addresses common problems or errors that may arise during a complex robotic surgical case. A concise stepwise approach to solving such issues will limit the impact on the progression of a robotic surgical procedure as well as limit any impact on patient safety. The knowledge and experience of the surgeon and surgical team are paramount in addressing these problems.

Keywords

Surgical robot • Troubleshooting • Error

6.1 Introduction

Robotic surgical systems, developed to improve the dexterity and visualization of surgeons during complex laparoscopic procedures, require the seamless integration of numerous components. With multiple systems comprising three separate units (Surgeon Console, Vision Cart, and Patient Cart), there are several areas for the development of potential problems or issues that can derail even the most well-planned cases. Repeat exposure to robotic surgical cases with intimate knowledge of the various components and connections which drive the robotic surgical system is key to preventing or troubleshooting any problems that may arise. This chapter will explain common problems that arise either preoperatively or intraoperatively, as well as demonstrate basic steps to resolve them.

6.2 Issues with the Endoscope or Vision Systems

6.2.1 Problem: Unilateral Camera Fogginess (Fig. 6.1)

With its high-definition, three-dimensional (3D) optics, which requires the use of a binocular endoscope and camera, the da Vinci Surgical System can experience unique difficulties with image acquisition that result in unclear or "foggy" images obtained from one side of the

F. Adkins, M.D. • D.J. Maron, M.D., M.B.A. (✉)
Department of Colorectal Surgery,
Cleveland Clinic Florida, 2950 Cleveland
Clinic Boulevard, Weston, FL 33331, USA
e-mail: marond@ccf.org

© Springer International Publishing Switzerland 2015
H. Ross et al. (eds.), *Robotic Approaches to Colorectal Surgery*,
DOI 10.1007/978-3-319-09120-4_6

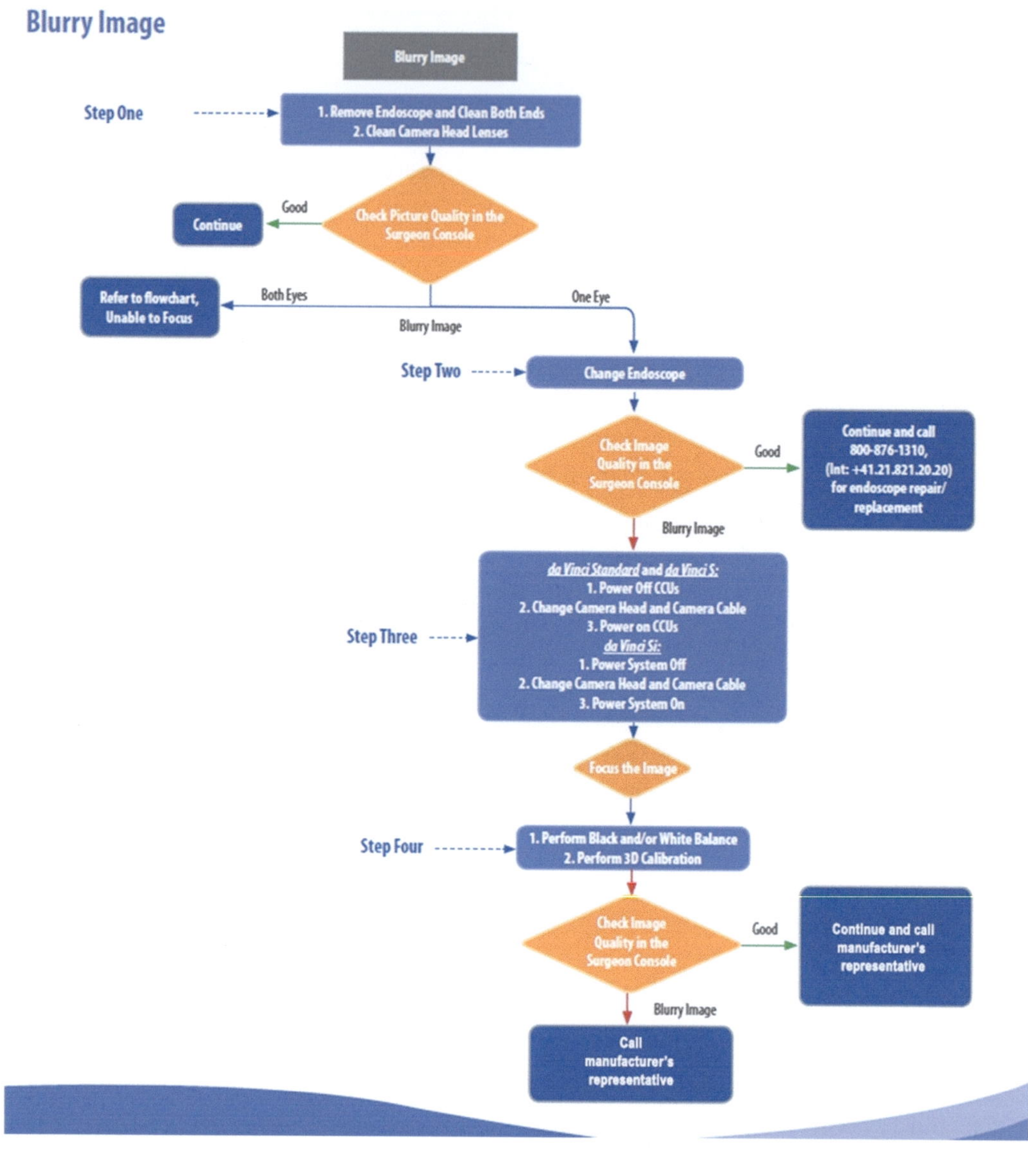

Fig. 6.1 Troubleshooting for a blurry image. *With permission from Intuitive Surgical Inc., Sunnyvale, CA*

system (right or left). This problem can arise at one of several points along the vision system: the endoscope lens, the camera, or the cable connecting the camera to the Vision Cart. Rapidly diagnosing the source of such a problem requires a dedicated, experienced robotic surgical team within the operating room and allows a robotic surgical case to begin or proceed with little interruption.

In order to troubleshoot a problem resulting in a unilateral unclear image, one must first determine which side (right or left) is having image difficulty as the camera is currently assembled. To determine this, toggle between the right- and left-side images displayed on the Vision Cart touchscreen, as this screen displays only a two-dimensional (2D) image acquired from one side of the system. This is done by accessing the menu in the lower left corner of the Vision Cart touch-screen and toggling between the right and left channels. Once it is determined that the image difficulty or "fogginess" is limited to one particular side, disconnect the endoscope from the camera, and rotate it by 180° prior to reconnecting it to the camera head. If this maneuver results in a switch of the image defect from the right to left channel (or vice versa) on the Vision Cart touchscreen, then the problem is most likely related to the endoscope itself. The endoscope should be removed from the camera and its lenses cleaned properly prior to reconnecting to the camera head. If simple cleaning alone fails to improve the image, then the endoscope may require repair or replacement, and an alternate endoscope should be obtained and used for the remainder of the robotic case [1, 2].

If rotating the endoscope 180° does not result in a switch of the image defect from one side to the other, then other sources for the unilateral image problem must be sought. At this point, the issue is likely related to either the camera itself or the cable connecting the camera to the Vision Cart. While the camera itself should be cleaned and reconnected to the endoscope first, either the camera or cable may need to be replaced with an alternate camera or cable to resolve the issue. This can be performed rapidly by the robotic surgical team in the operating room, as problems with the camera or cable are frequently first noticed during the preoperative setup of the surgical case, prior to draping.

6.2.2 Problem: Unbalanced Color or Image Brightness (Fig. 6.2)

At the start of a robotic surgical case, the surgeon seated at the Surgeon Console may note image differences between the right and left eye despite having clarity of the image itself. This is frequently perceived as unbalanced levels of brightness between the two sides or may be perceived as discoloration such as a red- or blue-tinged hue to the image on one particular side. This usually arises due to a failure to perform white balancing of the camera.

Resolution of this issue requires repeat white balancing of the camera. The camera should be removed from the Patient Cart, if attached, and a clean, white sheet of paper (not a gauze or laparotomy pad) should be placed 5–10 cm from the end of the endoscope. The vision setup button on the camera should then be pressed allowing the vision setup menu to be displayed on the Vision Cart touchscreen, and the White Balance option should be selected. Once white balancing is completed, a notation of "Successful" will be displayed on the touchscreen. Note that successful white balancing should only be performed with the Illuminator set to 100 %; otherwise, persistent issues with image color and balance may occur [1, 2].

6.2.3 Problem: Double Vision (Fig. 6.3)

Similar to problems with white balancing, a surgeon seated at the Surgeon Console at the beginning of a robotic surgical case may alternatively experience a sensation of double vision. The image presented to the surgeon appears to have two separate or somewhat overlapping images of objects within the visual field. This problem occurs due to incomplete or inaccurate three-dimensional (3D) calibration of the camera. Difficulties with 3D calibration result in incomplete alignment of the images produced by the separate right and left lenses of the camera. To resolve this issue, the camera should be removed from the Patient Cart, and the alignment target should be attached to the end of the endoscope. The vision setup button on the camera should then be pressed allowing the vision setup menu to be displayed on the Vision Cart touchscreen, and the Auto 3D Calibration option should be selected. At this point, separate magenta and green crosses will appear on the Vision Cart touchscreen, and the computer of the da Vinci Surgical System will automatically focus the images and align the two crosses. Once calibration is complete, an onscreen prompt will ask if calibration appears correct. If the image is not correct, the calibration process can be repeated.

Dark Image or Poor Color

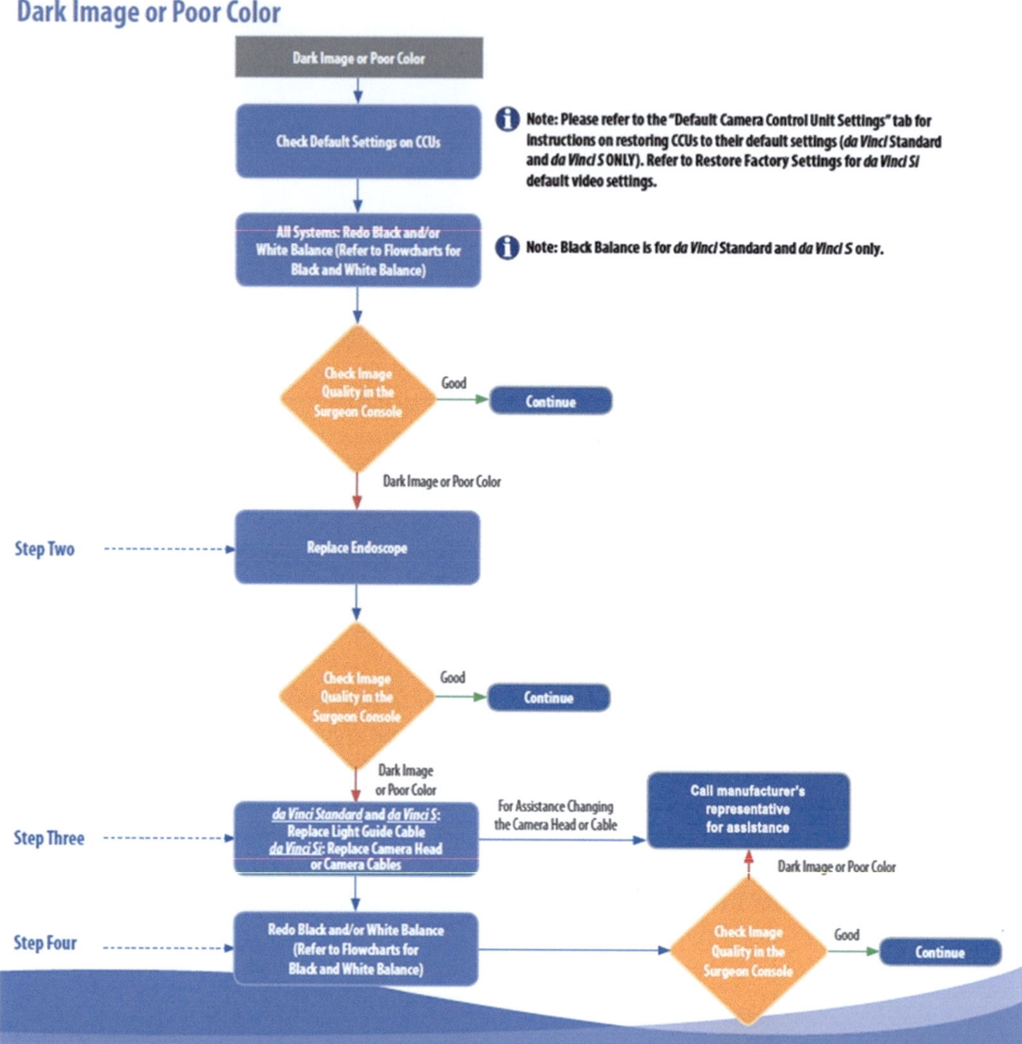

Fig. 6.2 Troubleshooting for a dark or poor color image. *With permission from Intuitive Surgical Inc., Sunnyvale, CA*

It is also important to note that if an angled endoscope is employed, 3D calibration will have to be repeated in both the angled up and angled down positions [1, 2].

6.2.4 Problem: Illuminator Lamp Issue/Error

The illuminator and lamp module contained within the Vision Cart provides a powerful source for lighting the surgical field when using the da Vinci Surgical System. In general, it is recommended that the lamp be changed after 1000 h of use. If the system is activated and the lamp module currently exceeds 1000 h of use, an error message will be displayed on the Vision Cart touchscreen indicating that this limit has been reached. At other points during a robotic surgical case, an error message will be received on the Vision Cart touchscreen which may read "Preventive maintenance recommended. Contact customer service" accompanied by shutdown of the illuminator. This is frequently due to an error in communication between the illuminator and the lamp module.

When these errors occur during a case, the instruments and camera should be immediately

Unable to Focus

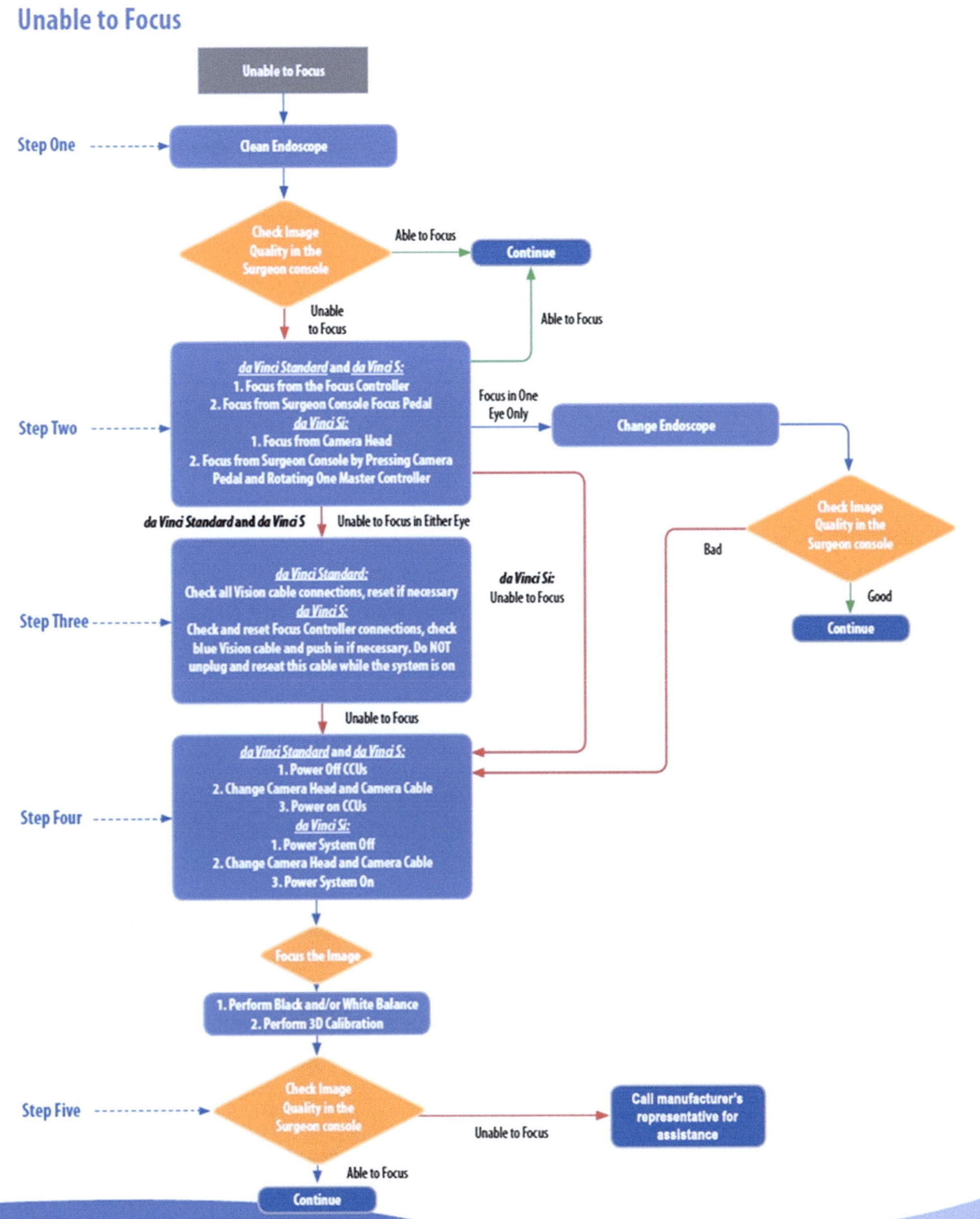

Fig. 6.3 Troubleshooting when unable to focus. *With permission from Intuitive Surgical Inc., Sunnyvale, CA*

removed from the Patient Cart arms to prevent patient injury. The da Vinci Surgical System should then be shut down, and total power to the Vision Cart can be interrupted using the power switch on the bottom right aspect at the back of the Vision Cart. This will eliminate any risk of electrical injury while further resolving this type of issue. After disconnecting the light cord, the lamp mod-

ule drawer can then safely be opened to expose the lamp module. The lamp module can be removed by sliding from the lateral aspect of the lamp module drawer. If the error message is related to exceeding recommended lamp hours, a simple exchange for a new lamp module should resolve the problem at this point. If it appears that the error message may be related to a communication issue between the lamp module and the illuminator, an attempt can be made to reseat the current lamp module within the lamp module drawer or exchanging the current lamp module for a new one. The lamp module drawer can then be closed, light cord reconnected, power to the Vision Cart restored, and system powered on [1, 2].

6.2.5 Problem: Image Grainy or Dark at Outer Edges

At various times throughout a robotic surgical case, the onscreen image may become distorted. Specifically, the image may take on a grainy appearance, which can partially impair visualization of structures or tissue planes. This commonly occurs when the brightness settings are too high. Resolution of this issue requires an adjustment of settings on the Vision Cart touchscreen or at the Patient Console touchpad. After selecting the video settings heading on the menu, ensure that the brightness level has not been set to the extreme far right of the slider bar in the orange portion of the bar. If so, reduce the brightness back to within the normal range of the control slider bar.

During the course of a robotic surgical case, the surgeon may perceive a darker halo or dimmer region at the outer edges of the surgical field as viewed through the Surgeon Console, a phenomenon referred to as vignetting. This results from viewing a surgical field that is wider than the light output from the camera. To reduce this perception requires ensuring that the camera is not set to wide mode. This can be adjusted on the Surgeon Console touchpad [1].

6.3 Issues with Instrumentation

6.3.1 Problem: Determining Instrument Usage

Prior to initiating any surgical case using the robotic system, it is important to check each instrument to be used during the case to determine the number of uses or "lives" left for each. Most 8 and 5 mm instruments have ten lives before requiring placement, meaning that ten separate cases can be performed given proper care and maintenance of the instrument. The robotic clip applier device can be fired 100 times, and in general, any training instruments usually have 30 lives.

In order to determine the number of lives remaining, the instrument is inserted in standard fashion into the appropriate cannula and secured onto the Patient Cart arm. Once in place, the Utilities menu can be used to select Inventory Management. This will display information for any instruments currently secured on the Patient Cart arms. The name for each instrument will be displayed as well as the number of lives remaining and total lives for the instrument. For example, a display of "Curved Bipolar Dissector 5/10" would indicate that from an original ten lives, currently five lives are remaining for this instrument.

It should be noted that the da Vinci Surgical System will remove a "life" from the instrument if the instrument is advanced through the cannula and control of the instrument is assumed by the surgeon seated at the Surgeon Console. In order to prevent such an event, an inventory check to determine the number of lives remaining should only be performed with the instrument secured to the Patient Cart arm but not fully inserted through the cannula. Once inserted, however, the da Vinci Surgical System will not remove additional lives from the instrument with each additional instrument removal or exchange. This holds true even if a system reset or shutdown is encountered as long as the sterile connector which seats the instrument on the Patient Cart arm remains in place [1].

6.3.2 Problem: Cannula Not Detected

The da Vinci Surgical System employs a system of sensors embedded within the cannula mount on each Patient Cart arm in order to sense the presence of a cannula within the cannula mount as well as the length of cannula currently in use (standard or long). This involves an interaction between the metallic rings at the neck of the cannula and proximity sensors within the cannula mount. Once a cannula is detected, the da Vinci Surgical System can determine how far a given instrument needs to be inserted in order to clear the tip of the cannula.

One frequent error that can occur during docking or during instrument exchanges is a "Cannula Not Detected" error. Resulting in an inability for the Surgeon Console to take control of the instrument in a given Patient Cart arm, this error occurs when the interaction between the cannula and the cannula mount on the Patient Cart arm has been disrupted. This frequently arises as a result of interference by the rubber piece, which covers the cannula mount as part of the drape for the Patient Cart arm. If this rubber piece becomes bunched within the cannula mount, the cannula cannot be properly sensed by the proximity sensors. Alternatively, this error can occur if the drape becomes bunched on the posterior aspect of the cannula mount resulting in an inability to completely close the wings on the posterior aspect to fully engage the cannula mount. To prevent such errors from occurring during docking, care should be taken to ensure that the cannula is engaged in a parallel orientation to the mount and all portions of the drape are smoothly in place to allow for proper interaction [1].

6.4 System Errors

6.4.1 Problem: Recoverable, Non-recoverable, and Arm-Specific Faults

System errors within the da Vinci Surgical System are classified as either recoverable or non-recoverable faults based on the degree of severity of the problem. Recoverable faults will stop the function of the da Vinci Surgical System until the error is corrected, at which time system function will resume. When a recoverable fault occurs, an Error Status window will be displayed on the Vision Cart touchscreen as well as on the Surgeon Console touchpad indicating that such a fault has occurred and a brief description of the fault as well as a corresponding error code number for reference. Examples of recoverable faults include excessive force on surgical arms, collisions between surgical arms, power fluctuation, or functioning on low battery backup power. Once the fault has been resolved, system function can be immediately recovered by pressing the Fault Override button on the Error Status window.

A non-recoverable fault represents an error within the system that is more severe and will require a complete system restart in order to recover system function. As with a recoverable fault, when a non-recoverable fault occurs, an Error Status window will be displayed with a corresponding error code number for reference. All instruments should then be removed for the safety of the patient and the entire system shut down. The system should then be restarted by pressing a system power button [3].

At times, an arm-specific error may occur to one of the arms of the Patient Cart. The da Vinci Surgical System allows for disabling of an individual arm if such an error should occur. This permits further progression and completion of a robotic surgical procedure until such time as further troubleshooting or maintenance can be performed to the given arm. If an arm-specific error occurs, an Error Status window will appear on the Vision Cart touchscreen or on the Surgeon Console touchpad indicating which arm is involved as well as an error code number for reference. To disable the indicated arm, press the Disable Arm button on the Error Status window. The indicated arm will not be able to function again until the system is reset [3].

For any recoverable or non-recoverable fault that occurs and is unable to be resolved by standard measures, contact with customer support for the da Vinci Surgical System will be required. This may require information in the system Event Log which can be accessed via the Vision Cart touchscreen or Patient Console touchpad via the Utilities menu and Event Log submenu [3].

6.5 Summary

Problems are not uncommon and may arise during the preoperative or intraoperative course of any robotic surgical procedure. Thorough knowledge of the components and relevant connections that make up the affected system within the surgical robot allows for such problems to be addressed in a concise stepwise fashion. This limits the impact that such problems may have on the initiation or progression of a robotic surgical procedure. An emphasis should be placed on the development of a dedicated robotic surgical team with training and experience to recognize and respond to the myriad of problems and errors that can develop.

components of the surgical robot can limit development of problems during the preoperative setup for the procedure, as well as quickly respond to intraoperative issues that may arise.

6.6 Key Points

- The surgical robot is a complex instrument with numerous components presenting multiple opportunities for the development of problems or errors throughout the course of a robotic surgical case.
- A dedicated, experienced robotic surgical team with thorough knowledge of the various

References

1. Intuitive Surgical. da Vinci Si system troubleshooting online module [Internet video]. http://www.davincisurgerycommunity.com. Accessed 2014.
2. Intuitive Surgical. Troubleshooting flow chart [Corporate Publication]. Intuitive Surgical. 2010.
3. Intuitive Surgical. da Vinci Si system safety features online module [Internet video]. http://www.davincisurgerycommunity.com. Accessed 2014.

Anatomy Considerations in Robotic Surgery

7

Kevin R. Kasten and Todd D. Francone

Abstract

From Ancient Greece through modern surgical practice, anatomical knowledge has remained of utmost importance. Surgery, more than any other field, relies heavily on this framework to both diagnose and treat patients. Despite the fundamental basis for anatomic knowledge in surgery, many teaching institutions are placing less and less emphasis on gross anatomy coursework. For those without a strong fund of anatomic knowledge, unfamiliarity with minimally invasive visualization of structures may produce angst. As critical structures in abdominal procedures appear different in open, laparoscopic, and robotic approaches, one should always establish familiar orientation depending upon modality used. This chapter seeks to demonstrate relevant colorectal anatomy from a robotic perspective.

Keywords

Robot • Anatomy • Colorectal • Proctectomy • Rectum

7.1 Introduction

Twenty-five years following the first laparoscopic right colectomy in the United States, utilization of this technique accounts for fewer than 25 % of benign abdominal procedures around the world [1, 2]. Initially, growth was tempered by concern for complications and poor long-term outcomes in cancer. Unfortunately, despite publication of multiple randomized controlled trials demonstrating equivalency with open surgery, utilization rates for laparoscopy in cancer resection continue below 12 % in the United States [3]. While recent data suggests strong growth in the

K.R. Kasten, M.D.
Division of Colon and Rectal Surgery,
Brody School of Medicine at East Carolina University, Greenville, NC, USA

T.D. Francone, M.D., M.P.H. (✉)
Department of Colon and Rectal Surgery,
Lahey Hospital & Medical Center,
41 Mall Road, Burlington, MA 01805, USA

Tufts University Medical Center, Boston, MA, USA
e-mail: todd.d.francone@lahey.org

© Springer International Publishing Switzerland 2015
H. Ross et al. (eds.), *Robotic Approaches to Colorectal Surgery*,
DOI 10.1007/978-3-319-09120-4_7

use of minimally invasive techniques for cancer, growth remains less robust for benign disease [3]. Suggested reasons for slow adoption of minimally invasive surgery in colorectal compared with general surgery include complexity of procedures, high risk of procedure conversion, cost, and difficulty with visualization and organ manipulation to successfully complete indicated procedures. With similar complaints plaguing laparoscopic prostatectomy, urologic surgeons embraced the improved benefits of superior 3D optics, multi-arm endowrist articulation, and control of three instruments. Over the last decade, the robotic approach has not simply supplanted, but replaced laparoscopic prostatectomy [4]. As such, more colorectal and general surgeons are following the lead of robotic colorectal pioneers and utilizing this technology for pelvic dissections.

For surgeons learning and applying the robotic approach in practice, surgical anatomy remains absolutely crucial. While 3D visualization provides many advantages, the loss of haptic feedback compared to open and laparoscopic procedures cannot be understated. In this text we demonstrate important aspects of robotic colorectal surgery, including visualization, instrument placement, and procedures to ensure patient safety. As always, patient morbidity and mortality are tantamount. If a procedure cannot be completed safely using the robotic modality, an alternative technique must be selected.

7.2 Basics of Robotic-Assisted Laparoscopic Colectomy

When embarking on a new technique, it is easy for a surgeon to change too much. We recommend the opposite. Minimizing the amount of alteration in your approach can optimize success with robotic-assisted surgery. As with laparoscopy, various approaches to robotic-assisted laparoscopic colorectal resection are available (medial to lateral, lateral to medial, inferior to superior, superior to inferior). The lateral to medial dissection initiates mobilization of the colon from the lateral peritoneal attachments along the "white" line of Toldt, as traditionally taught in open cases. In contrast, the medial to lateral approach involves incision along the colonic mesentery with early ligation of vascular pedicle. The division of the lateral peritoneal attachments occurs once the majority of the mobilization is completed. This approach produces several advantages and is preferred by the authors for the following reasons:

1. Early pedicle ligation theoretically prevents tumor shedding and dispersion throughout the mesentery while manipulating the colon—basis of the Turnbull no-touch technique.
2. In the setting of abdominal or pelvic sepsis, as seen in diverticulitis or Crohn's disease, generally, a high ligation away from the infectious processes will subsequently allow for easier and quicker visualization and consequently safer dissection of the colon and mesentery away from other vital structures (posterior and lateral).
3. Preservation of the lateral attachments permits dissection without a redundant and floppy colon and mesentery while performing the rest of the procedures.

A robust knowledge and understanding of vital structures, anatomic planes (retroperitoneal and peritoneal), nervous system anatomy, and lymphatic drainage allows fluid transition from one approach to another. The best approach is the one most comfortable to the surgeon. Keeping the approach similar should ideally increase the recognition of essential visual cues during the dissection, which is critical in the absence of haptic perception with the current technology.

From a robotic-assisted standpoint, the surgeon must choose an approach that (1) maximizes visualization with a more limited range of camera movement and (2) minimizes risk of injury from robotic arm movement/immobilization that may occur off the screen.

Correct positioning for the intended procedure is critical for success. Once the robot is docked, patient position is set unless the robot is undocked and adjusted. As with most minimally invasive techniques, gel pads or bean bags should be affixed to the operating table with safety straps to

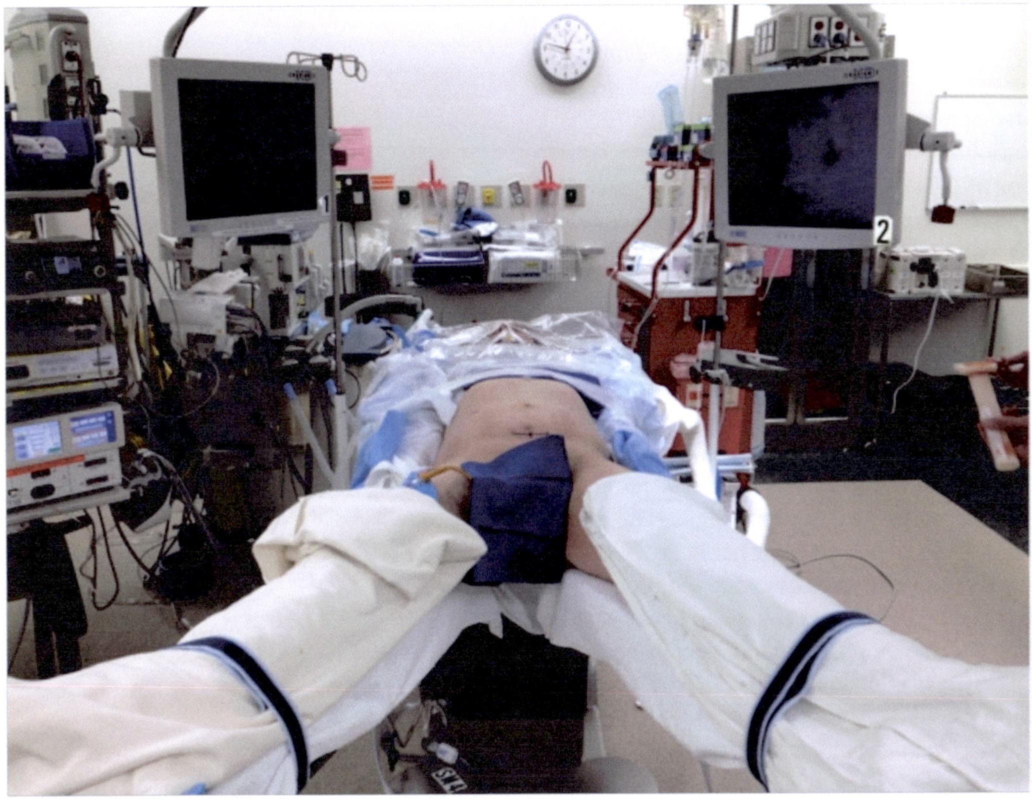

Fig. 7.1 Patient setup. Patient is placed in the split-leg position for most cases. In cases requiring a synchronous perineal approach such as an intersphincteric dissection, the patient is placed in the modified lithotomy position

ensure minimal patient movement during positioning. Appropriate padding at pressure points including the hands, wrists, elbows, and heels should coincide with positioning (modified lithotomy, supine, split leg). We advocate the split-leg position for almost all patients, including those undergoing ileocolic or right colon resections (Fig. 7.1). Positioning in this manner affords the surgeons numerous advantages such as:

1. Exposure to the anus/rectum for intraoperative colonoscopy if needed. This can be particularly useful for a tumor not preoperatively tattooed and localized or when colonoscopy and laparoscopy are used together as adjuncts for resection-sparing colonic polypectomy.
2. In inflammatory disease processes such as Crohn's, an occult fistula may not be appreciated despite preoperative imaging until intraoperative exploration. Operative intervention may then necessitate both right- and left-sided mobilization as well as possible utilization of per-anus anastomotic stapling device.
3. Operator positioning between the legs during more difficult dissections.

Depending upon the surgeon's robot docking schema, split-leg positioning may not be feasible. Familiarize yourself with side (parallel) and pelvic docking to ensure appropriate case-specific robot positioning. Both docking positions are utilized in pelvic dissection; however, for right or left colectomies, including low anterior resections, the side docking position is preferred. Room layout is crucial to provide adequate space for the entire operative team, which facilitates docking and undocking of the robot. Carefully planned operative layout and robot docking allow for efficient, effective docking. Although studies demonstrate increased operative times with robotics versus laparoscopy, most added time comes from docking the system. These times can be significantly reduced with appropriate team development, planning, and practice [5, 6].

Robotic-assisted surgery is an enhanced version of laparoscopy, and as such, port placement is vital. If ports are inappropriately placed, exposure and anatomic definition is inferior. Additionally, instrument collision due to poorly placed ports will significantly hinder progression of the case. The current Si da Vinci robot has excelled in urology and gynecologic surgery due to superiority when focused on single quadrant surgery, in particular the pelvis. Colorectal surgery differs from those specialties as it often requires multi-quadrant dissection. The current da Vinci models are somewhat bulky with arms that often collide when moving from one quadrant to another. Several schemata have been recommended for right and left colectomies as well as pelvic dissections; however, port placement will vary based on the surgeons' preferred approach and technique.

After prepping and draping, diagram your proposed port placement on the abdomen as a guideline. Following insufflation, port placement is confirmed or adjusted based on pneumoperitoneum. Remember, if you have extra body surface area to space ports out, use it to avoid collisions. Entrance to the abdomen is completed via open (Hasson), optiview, or closed (Veress) technique per the operating surgeon's preference. Our preference is to place a 12-mm camera port 2 cm cranial and 2 cm right lateral from the umbilicus for left-sided dissections or supraumbilical in right-sided dissections. A supraumbilical port can be used for left-sided dissections, as diagrammed in placement schema (Figs. 7.2, 7.3, 7.4, and 7.5). A 5-mm laparoscopic camera, 8-mm robotic camera, or 12-mm robotic camera can be used to complete intraperitoneal diagnostic exploration and guide robotic instruments into the peritoneal cavity. An initial laparoscopic overview is performed in every procedure. We argue its elevated importance in robotic-assisted colon surgery for several reasons. Firstly, the surgeon must inspect the abdomen and pelvis for evidence of (1) occult metastatic disease, (2) altered anatomy, or (3)

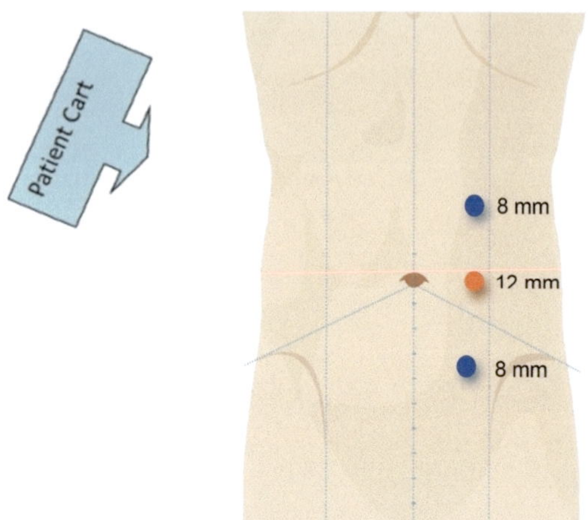

Fig. 7.2 Three-arm technique for robotic right colectomy. Extraction site is through the midline or surgeon preference

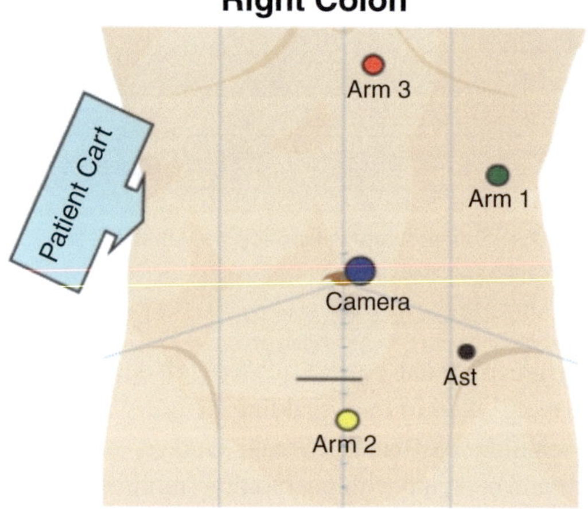

Fig. 7.3 Four-arm technique for robotic right colectomy. Extraction site is through the midline or surgeon preference

inability to safely perform the procedure with robotic assistance. Secondly, the surgeon can evaluate port placement and anatomical markings and determine if robotic assistance will benefit or harm the operation. The larger robotic camera is quite cumbersome and heavy, not to mention costly to repair if dropped, so we discourage its use for this portion of the case. In contrast, the opening of a 5-mm laparoscope and other laparoscopic equipment may add unnecessary cost to the procedure. By avoiding the use of unnecessary

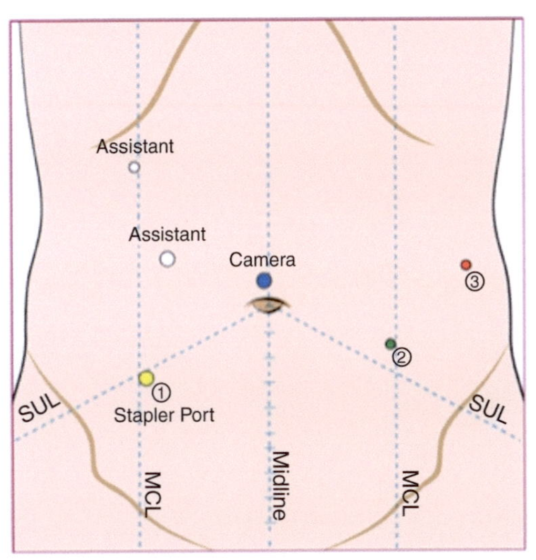

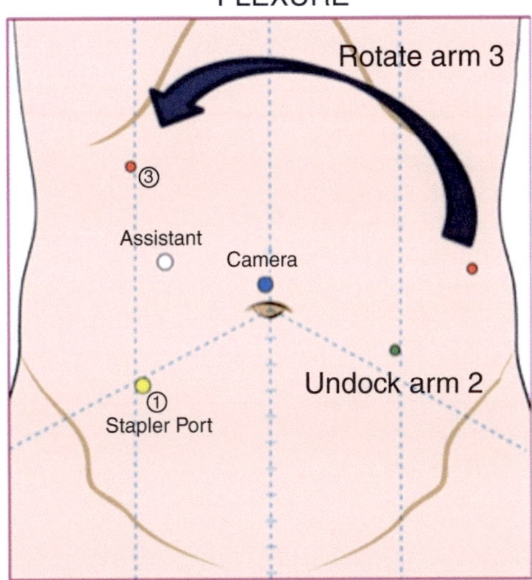

Fig. 7.4 Port placement for a robotic low anterior resection. When approaching the splenic flexure, arm #3 is moved from the left side of the abdomen to the right side. Arm #2 is undocked to avoid unnecessary collisions

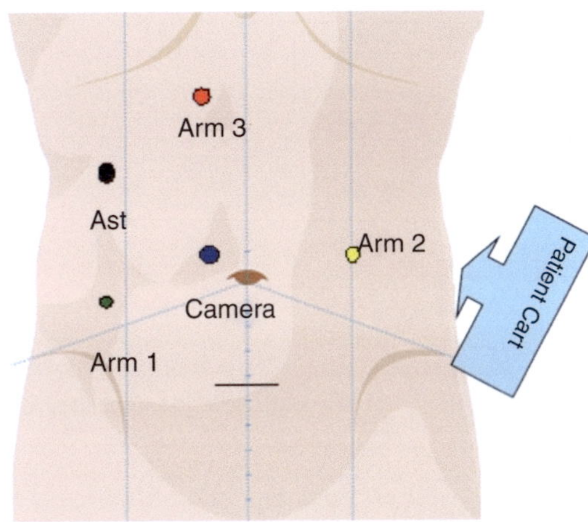

Fig. 7.5 Port placement for a robotic sigmoidectomy. Notice that the camera port is slightly off midline. This allows dissection of the splenic flexure and upper pelvis utilizing arm #3 (which is also moved slightly more medial)

equipment, expenses are lowered. We prefer to utilize the 5-mm laparoscopic camera as it is easier to maneuver, especially when visualizing ports in the upper quadrants. Once all ports are placed, the camera visualizes careful insertion of robotic instruments, all pointed toward the pelvis.

PEARL: *As with all minimally invasive techniques, placement of ports and instruments into the peritoneal cavity is performed under direct vision in order to minimize unnecessary injury to the underlying viscera.*

7.3   The Right Colon

7.3.1   Brief Anatomy Review

The right colon is supplied by the ileocolic artery branching off the superior mesenteric artery, which travels just infero-caudally to the third portion of the duodenum. The ileocolic artery is present in 100 % of patients, while the middle colic artery is present in 98 % of patients. In contrast, the typically depicted right colic artery branching off the superior mesenteric artery actually only occurs in 11 % of cases (Fig. 7.6). Often, the distal right colon is perfused by the middle colic vessel. The middle colic vessel is also the primary blood supply to the proximal two-thirds of the transverse colon. It branches off the superior mesentery artery just inferior to, and then overlies, the pancreas (Fig. 7.7a).

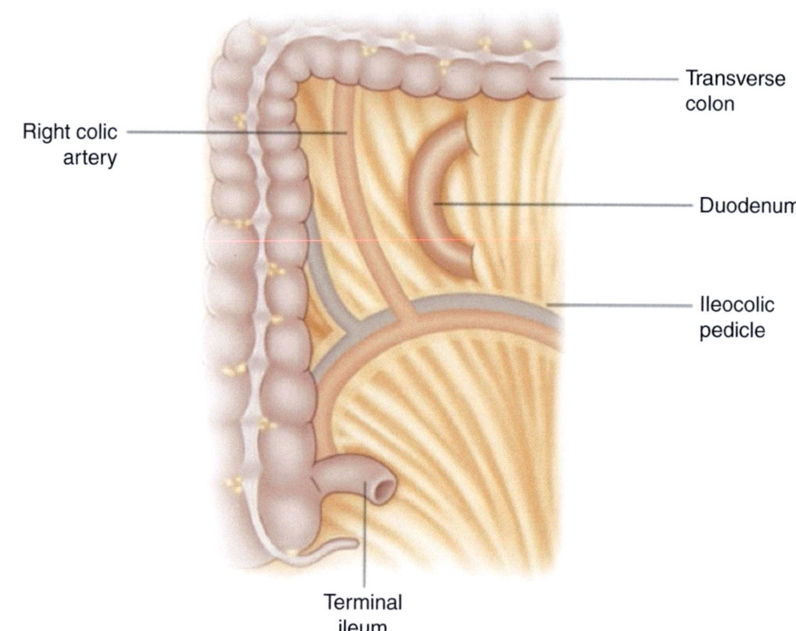

Fig. 7.6 The ileocolic artery is present in 100 % of patients; the right colic artery most commonly arises from the ileocolic artery rather than the SMA. *With permission from Landmann RG and Francone T. Surgical Anatomy. In: Minimally Invasive Approaches to Colon and Rectal Disease: Techniques and best practices. Ross HM, Lee SW, Mutch MG, Rivadeneira DE, Steele SR. Springer, New York, 2015: pp. 25–50*

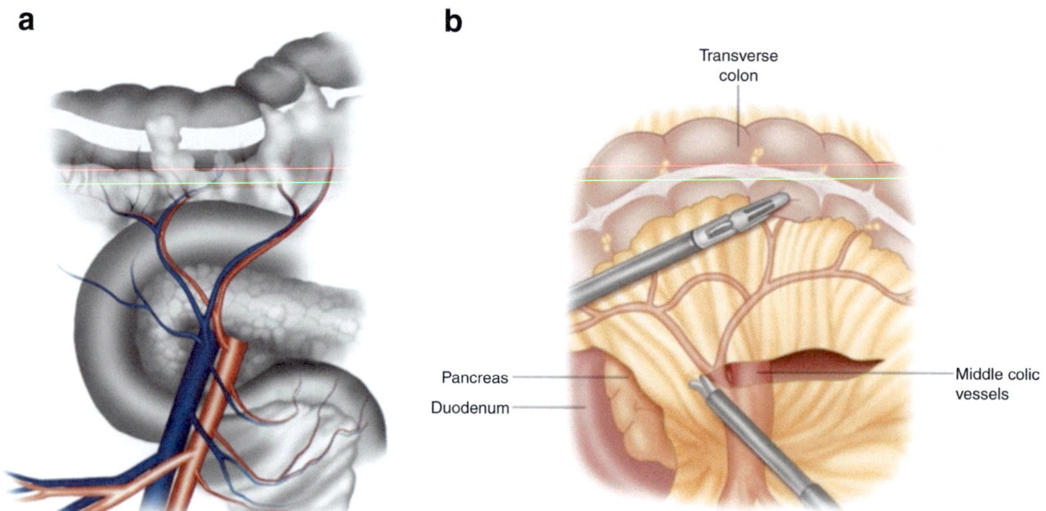

Fig. 7.7 (**a**) Superior mesenteric artery and its branches. (**b**) Note the typical "Y" appearance of the middle colics. *With permission from Landmann RG and Francone T. Surgical Anatomy. In: Minimally Invasive Approaches to Colon and Rectal Disease: Techniques and best practices. Ross HM, Lee SW, Mutch MG, Rivadeneira DE, Steele SR. Springer, New York, 2015: pp. 25–50*

The common middle colic artery is very short, quickly branching into a left and right vessel, giving it the classic "Y" appearance upon retraction of the transverse colon mesentery ventrally (Fig. 7.7b). When dissecting the right branch of the middle colic artery, one must also consider the right branch of the middle colic vein. The middle colic vein may give a communicating branch to the gastroepiploic vein which courses behind the transverse colon mesentery. When mobilizing the transverse colon mesentery, this communicating or bridging vein can be disrupted causing difficult to control hemorrhage.

After completion of diagnostic laparoscopy, the patient is placed in slight Trendelenburg position combined with left inclination. It is often beneficial to limit the amount of Trendelenburg incline with robotic surgery such that positioning does not favor exposure to one quadrant and limit it in another. This is particularly critical when performing a robotic splenic flexure mobilization, where too much Trendelenburg can prevent adequate exposure in the left upper quadrant but superb exposure in the pelvis. The camera port and the arm #1 port are typically placed first to position the patient and assess case feasibility. The surgeon retracts the omentum superiorly over the transverse colon, along with mobilizing the small bowel out of the pelvis and into the left upper quadrant. Once completed, additional ports are inserted under direct visual guidance. With the patient positioned in the split-leg position, the robot is docked over the patient's right chest. A three- or four-arm technique can be used to perform the right colectomy (Figs. 7.2 and 7.3). In the four-arm technique, arm #3 is typically an assistant port used to hold up mesentery or omentum for facilitation of dissection. Arms #1 and #2 are utilized more frequently to perform dissection, either lateral to medial or vice versa.

7.3.2 Lateral to Medial Dissection

This approach is generally the easier dissection to learn and perform. There are several critical anatomic landmarks that once appreciated can lead to a safer, more expedient, and appropriate oncologic resection (sometimes termed total mesocolic excision). With the exclusion of a right colectomy for pathological enlargement of the appendix (i.e., mucocele, cystadenoma, cystadenocarcinoma, or carcinoid), grasping this tubular structure can help significantly in retraction. Otherwise, either the terminal ileum or cecum can be gently and carefully grasped to mobilize the enteral structures anteriorly and toward the left upper quadrant. Arm #3 is typically utilized to grasp and retract the mesentery leftward in a ventral and cephalad direction, exposing the lateral attachments of the colon and mesentery to the retroperitoneum (white line of Toldt). Division of this attachment allows entry into a loose alveolar plane, whereby dissection can proceed distally along the ascending colon to the hepatic flexure. Arm #1 or #2 may be used for this portion of the procedure depending on exposure and surgeon preference. At the ileocecal valve, care is taken to identify and preserve the ureter as it crosses the right iliac artery bifurcation (Fig. 7.8). Further care is taken to stay within the appropriate plane as straying laterally leads to dissection of Gerota's fascia with subsequent medial mobilization of the kidney.

Fig. 7.8 The right ureter enters into the pelvis slightly more lateral crossing over the right external iliac artery

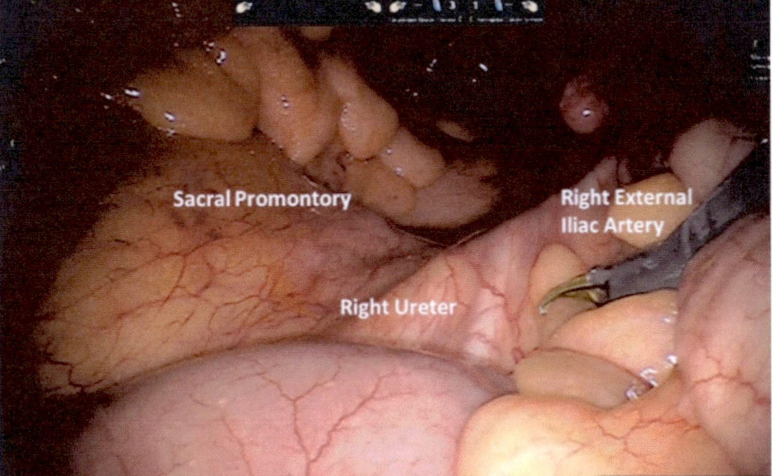

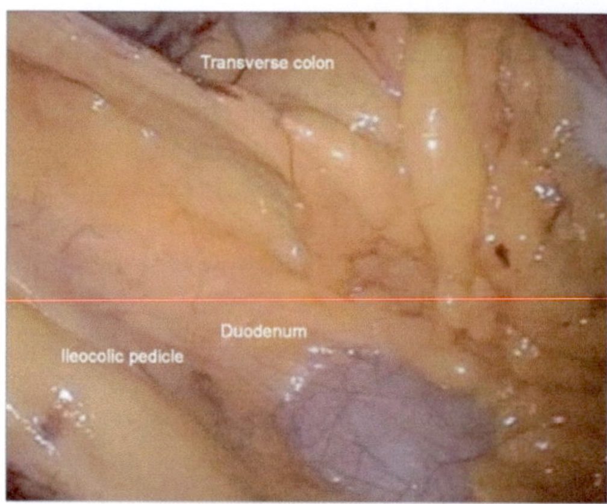

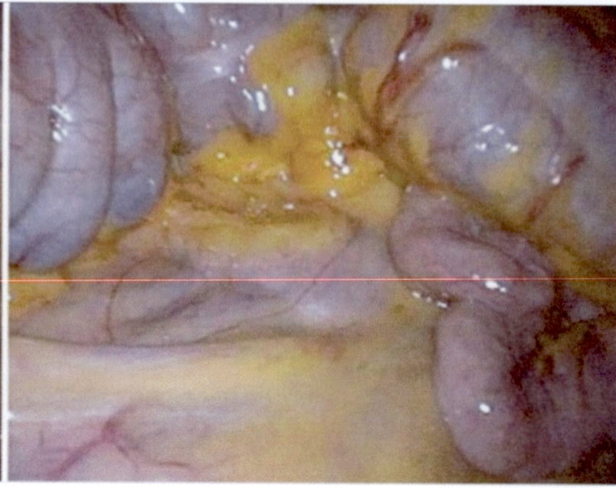

Fig. 7.9 The ileocolic artery courses infero-caudally to the duodenum; in thinner patients, the duodenal sweep can often be identified prior to the initiation of the dissection. *With permission from Landmann RG and Francone T. Surgical Anatomy. In: Minimally Invasive Approaches to Colon and Rectal Disease: Techniques and best practices. Ross HM, Lee SW, Mutch MG, Rivadeneira DE, Steele SR. Springer, New York, 2015: pp. 25–50*

Mobilization within the correct plane of the mesocolon from the retroperitoneum centrally (or medially) toward the takeoff base of the ileocolic pedicle will expose the anterior surface of the duodenum and pancreas. The mesentery of the terminal ileum is then divided from the retroperitoneum to the level of the right iliac artery. At this point, the base of the ileocolic pedicle is easily visualized and divided using energy (vessel sealer), stapler, or clips. When using a vessel-sealing device, the authors suggest having an endoloop or clips readily available should bleeding ensue.

7.3.3 Medial to Lateral Dissection

The key to a proficient medial to lateral dissection, using either laparoscopic or robotic approach, is entry into the avascular plan between the colonic mesentery and the retroperitoneum. Before beginning, the surgeon should make an attempt to identify the pertinent anatomy (ileocolic pedicle, ureter, and duodenum) involved in dissection to prevent untoward events. This is often easier in thinner patients than the morbidly obese where identification of the duodenal sweep or C-curve can be observed with superoanterior retraction of the transverse colon. Carefully grasping the cecum, or its mesentery, close to the base and lifting toward the anterolateral abdominal wall display the ileocolic artery cours-

ing infero-caudally to the duodenum (Fig. 7.9). This motion creates a tenting or "bowstring" effect with a distinct crease coursing parallel to the vessel (Fig. 7.10). Arm #3 can be used for cecal retraction, freeing arms #1 and #2 to develop the correct plane. Care is taken with the robot to not avulse vessels due to lack of haptic feedback. Once bowstringing is noted, the peritoneum is scored parallel to the vessel, allowing pneumoperitoneum to fill the avascular space and facilitate development of the appropriate plane. Some mobilization of the mesocolon from the retroperitoneal structures may be necessary and can be performed with gentle, blunt sweeping motions dorsally. Particular attention must be given medially and posteriorly where the C-loop of the duodenum lies and can be easily injured with the dissecting instrument or energy device (Fig. 7.11a, b). When in the correct plane, it is generally not necessary to identify the ureter or iliac vessels located in the inferolateral aspect of the dissection. However, in the presence of penetrating disease, either benign with perforating Crohn's disease or malignant with penetrating neoplastic mass, the surgeon must be aware of the surrounding anatomy.

As the avascular plane is developed, there is a consistent thinning out or paucity of adiposity in the mesenteric fat on both sides of the ileocolic pedicle (Fig. 7.10). Careful dissection through this mesentery creates a window around the pedicle at

Fig. 7.10 Grasping the cecum or its mesentery and lifting anterolateral to the abdominal wall will create a tenting or "bowstring" effect with a distinct crease coursing parallel to the vessel

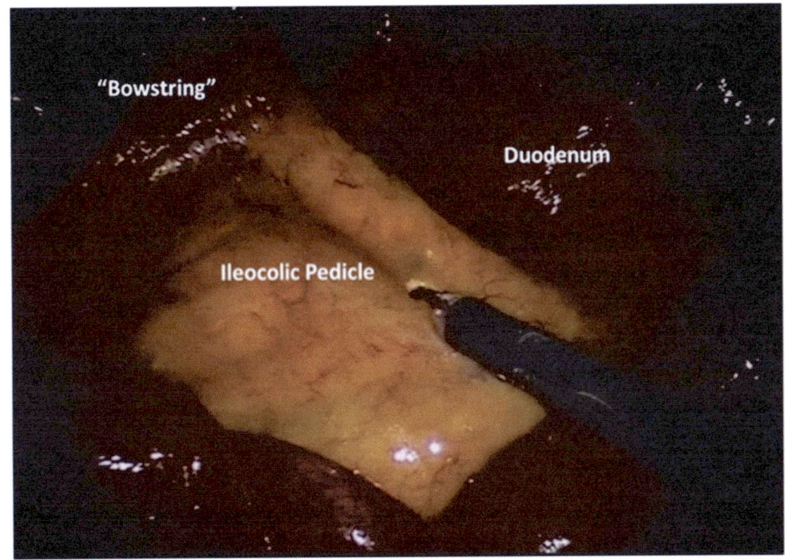

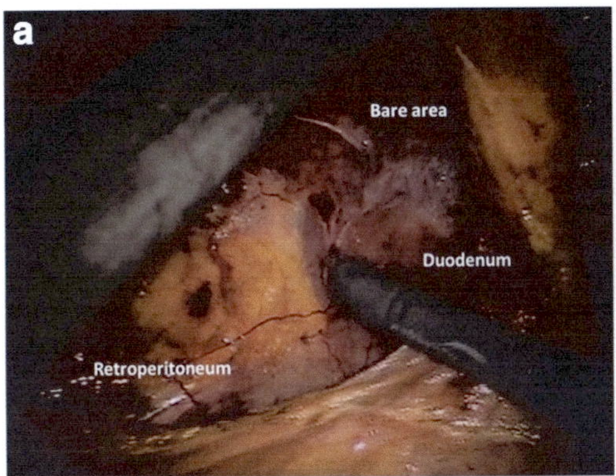

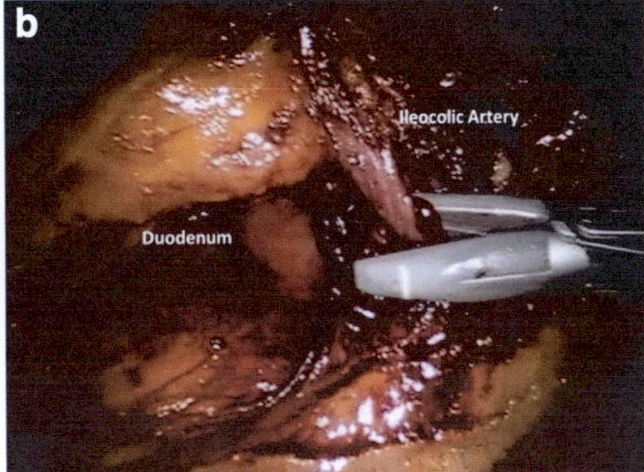

Fig. 7.11 (**a**) Medial dissection is initiated by sweeping the retroperitoneum down and away; immediate identification of the duodenum is critical in order to avoid injury. (**b**) When dividing the ileocolic artery, the surgeon must always be mindful of the duodenum

which point the vessel can be divided (Fig. 7.11a). Once critical structures are well visualized and out of harm's way, a high or central ligation is performed. Surgeon's preference dictates method of ligation and division, with options including endoscopic stapling devices, energy devices, or application of clips with intermediary division. As noted previously, when using a vessel-sealing device, the authors suggest ready availability of endoloop or clips should bleeding ensue.

PEARL: *When dissecting under the ileocolic pedicle, always beware of the duodenum coming into surgical view (Fig. 7.11b).*

Once ligation is completed, medial to lateral dissection continues by careful elevation of the mesentery followed by gentle, blunt sweeping of the retroperitoneum downward. A thin, white line of Toldt is visualized separating mesocolon from retroperitoneal structures (Fig. 7.12). A key point in performing this maneuver is to gently push or sweep the peritoneal reflection line down rather than pull other structures up. In general, arm #3 is stationary and used to retract the mesocolon up, while arms #1 and #2 continue the dissection. If the surgeon maintains the correct plane, risk of bleeding, elevation of the right kidney, and damage to the duodenum should not occur.

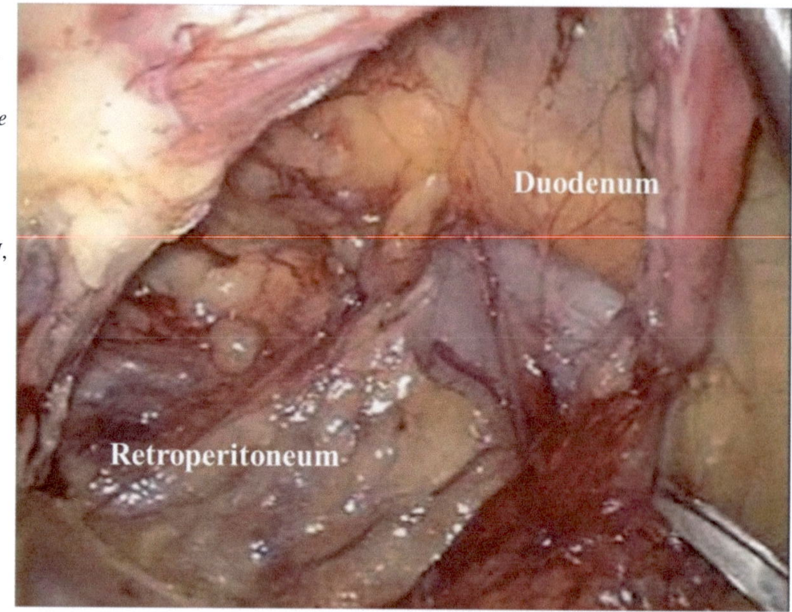

Fig. 7.12 Medial to lateral mobilization highlighting duodenum and white line of Toldt. *With permission from Landmann RG and Francone T. Surgical Anatomy. In: Minimally Invasive Approaches to Colon and Rectal Disease: Techniques and best practices. Ross HM, Lee SW, Mutch MG, Rivadeneira DE, Steele SR. Springer, New York, 2015: pp. 25–50*

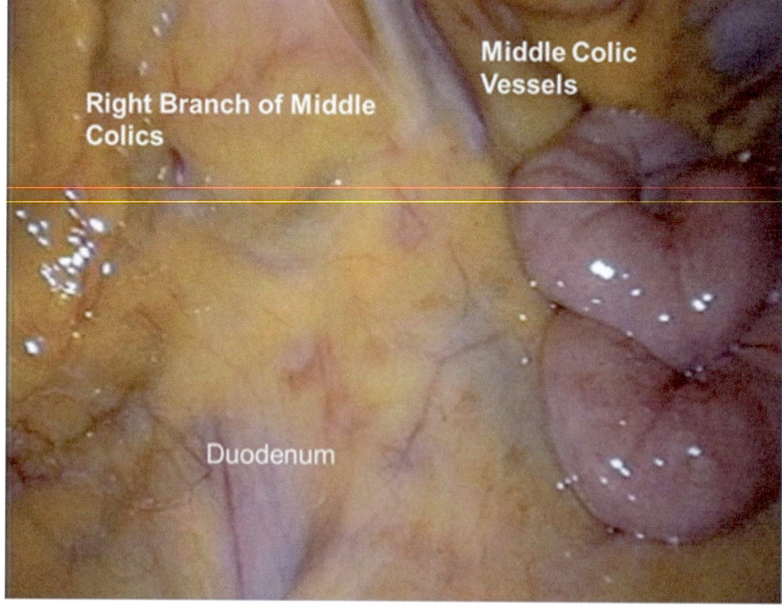

Fig. 7.13 Transverse colon anatomy and middle colic vessels. *With permission from Landmann RG and Francone T. Surgical Anatomy. In: Minimally Invasive Approaches to Colon and Rectal Disease: Techniques and best practices. Ross HM, Lee SW, Mutch MG, Rivadeneira DE, Steele SR. Springer, New York, 2015: pp. 25–50*

Difficulty visualizing this plane is often attributable to incomplete maintenance of tension/counter-tension.

Upon reaching the lateral sidewall, dissection is carried superiorly toward the hepatic flexure. Caution must again be taken as the right colic and the right branch of the middle colic artery may be encountered during this part of the operation. Identification of the middle colic vessels usually occurs with ventral retraction of the transverse colon mesentery. It is often first identified inferior to the pancreas but with further exploration is found to overlie the pancreas with its main branch coming off the superior mesenteric vessel (Fig. 7.13). In both laparoscopic and robotic-assisted procedures, the surgeon must beware of inadvertently disrupting these vessels, especially the pancreaticoduodenal and gastroepiploic branches, which lie close to this

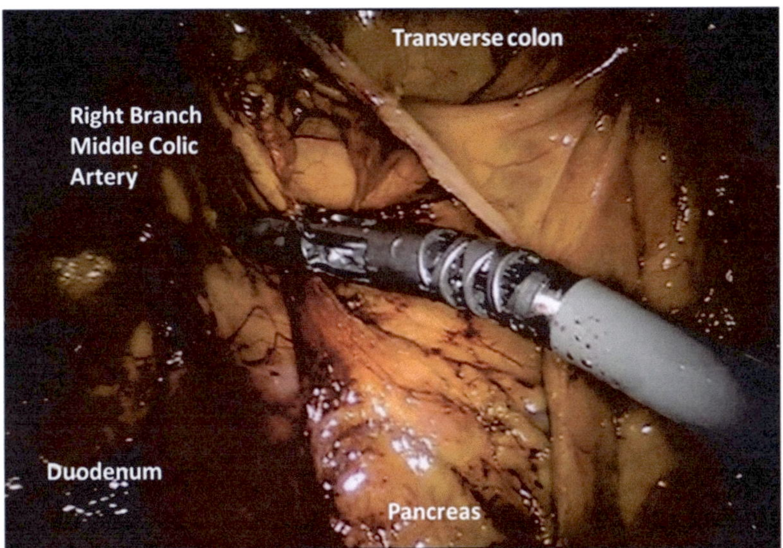

Fig. 7.14 The right branch of the middle colic vessels is often divided during a right colectomy

region and can result in troublesome bleeding that is difficult to control.

The right branch of the middle colic is often divided during a right colectomy (Fig. 7.14). As mentioned previously, anterosuperior retraction of the transverse colon mesentery often demonstrates the takeoff of the right and left branches from the main branch giving the classic "Y" pattern of the middle colic vessels (Fig. 7.7b). Similar to ligation of the ileocolic pedicle, the right branch of the middle colic is isolated then divided. In addition, the right colic vein may also be visualized in this area, lateral to the right branch of the middle colic and coursing from the pancreas toward the hepatic flexure. If encountered, this vessel should be carefully ligated to prevent bleeding during completion of right colon mobilization. Once both pedicles are safely controlled, dissection of the mesentery may proceed, ensuring that the terminal ileum and cecal mesentery, as well as the transverse colon mesentery, have been adequately mobilized.

At this point, the right colon remains affixed by lateral avascular attachments to the abdominal sidewall, hepatic flexure attachments, and gastrocolic attachments of the omentum to the transverse colon. These can generally be easily divided by either a dissecting energy device (ultrasonic or bipolar type) or energized, monopolar cautery/ Metzenbaum scissors. It is the authors' preference to start the dissection at the pelvic brim.

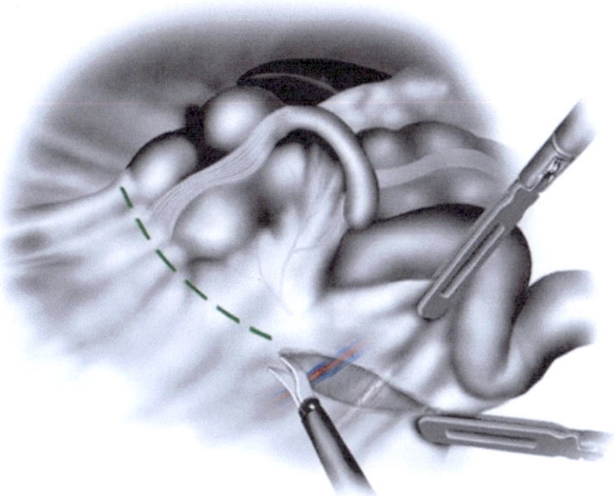

Fig. 7.15 Inferiorly along the terminal ileal mesentery, there is a reflection noted at the attachment to the retroperitoneum. This fold is medial to the ureter, overlies the right iliac vessels in the right pelvis, and is also superolateral to the sacral promontory. *With permission from Landmann RG and Francone T. Surgical Anatomy. In: Minimally Invasive Approaches to Colon and Rectal Disease: Techniques and best practices. Ross HM, Lee SW, Mutch MG, Rivadeneira DE, Steele SR. Springer, New York, 2015: pp. 25–50*

The cecum or terminal ileum is gently retracted anteromedially with arm #3, while arms #1 and #2 divide the lateral attachments. Dissection proceeds proximally toward the hepatic flexure. Inferiorly along the terminal ileal mesentery, there is a reflection noted at the attachment to the retroperitoneum (Fig. 7.15). This fold is medial to the ureter, overlies the right iliac vessels in the right pelvis, and is also superolateral to the sacral promontory. If performed appropriately with anterior retraction of the terminal ileum, the surgeon should enter into the previously dissected plane between the mesocolon and the retroperitoneum. Retract the ileum anteriorly, and dissect along this fold to further mobilize the terminal ileal mesentery toward the duodenum and pancreas. Proper mobilization along this plane will ensure adequate small bowel mobilization to reach the transverse colon and perform a tension-free anastomosis.

The hepatocolic and gastrocolic attachments are divided, rendering the right colon a midline structure. Specimen may then be extracted though a midline incision when performing an extraperitoneal anastomosis. For right colectomies, the distal extent of dissection is generally around the falciform ligament or in line with the middle colic vessels. It is often best to start at this point and work retrograde toward the hepatic flexure. With arm #3 retracting the omentum ventrally, arms #1 and #2 dissect into the lesser sac with visualization of the posterior wall of the stomach and colonic mesentery. The key to mobilizing the transverse colon is careful dissection of the omental layers one at a time. At a certain point, the omentum will then be fully mobilized, and attention is directed toward the hepatocolic ligament. An avascular plane is developed between this and the proximal transverse colon mesentery. Caution must be taken when developing the plane as one can easily injure the duodenal sweep lying posteriorly or inadvertently tear the right colic vein. At the level of the gallbladder, the surgeon should expect to enter the previous medial to lateral dissection plane. Where previously dissected planes meet, the surgeon should encounter purple-hued tissue. The lateral attachments can be easily divided with excellent exposure of the surrounding structures. This creates a fully mobilized right colon that easily approaches the midline.

PEARL: *Prior to undocking the robot, the surgeon must ensure proper mobility of the speci-men, including terminal ileum. If mobility is required, there exists a fold medial to the right ureter and superolateral to the sacral promontory, which signifies an attachment of the terminal ileal mesentery to the retroperitoneum.*

7.4 Transverse Colectomy

A segmental transverse colon resection is rarely required. More often, the transverse colon is resection in conjunction with either the left or right colon. In theory, a transverse colectomy would likely place the robot over the right or left shoulder with a half-moon port set up in the lower abdomen. The authors have not performed a specific robotic transverse colectomy but have used the system to resect part of the transverse colon during a right or left colectomy. As mentioned numerous times before, port placement becomes crucial for the success of this procedure (Figs. 7.2, 7.3, 7.4, and 7.5).

If a total colectomy is necessary, then the procedure is performed similar to a combined left and right colectomy with robot re-docking midway through the case. When performing a total colectomy, it is our preference to approach the right colon first with entry into the lesser sac (Fig. 7.16a, b). The dissection is continued to the hepatic flexure and as far as possible toward the splenic flexure. Elevation of the transverse colon provides exposure of the middle colic vessels, with care being taken to not tear this pedicle (Fig. 7.17). The assistant ports are key in this maneuver. The surgeon may benefit from a second assistant port through the anticipated extraction site which is especially useful in the morbidly obese with limited exposure. It is best to individually isolate and ligate the left and right branches of the middle colic artery, when possible. Upon ligation of the vascular pedicle, when the surgeon is dissecting the transverse mesocolon from the pancreas, he/she will encounter the right gastroepiploic vein overlying the pancreas. This should be identified and preserved prior to division of the middle colic vein.

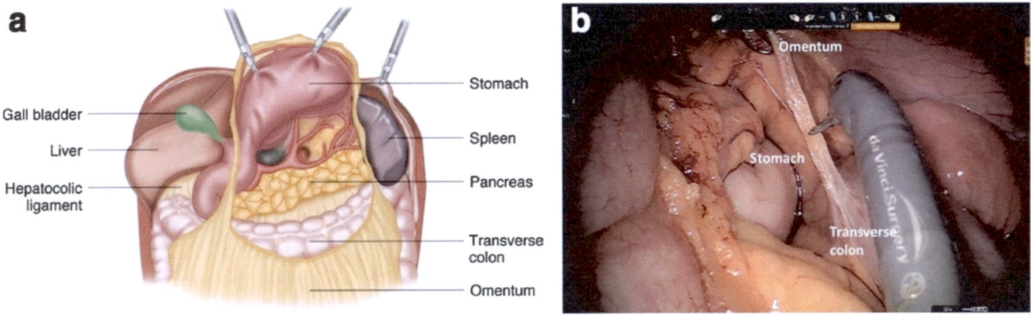

Fig. 7.16 (**a**) Accessing the lesser sac through the omentum (gastrocolic ligament). (**b**) Early entry into the lesser sac is key to facilitating mobilization of the transverse colon

Fig. 7.17 The classic "Y" pattern of the middle colic vessels is not always straightforward. Often, both the right and left branches course to the patient's right. The right branch courses over the head of the pancreas and the duodenum; the left branch makes a sharp upward turn and then veers to the left, as depicted in the picture above

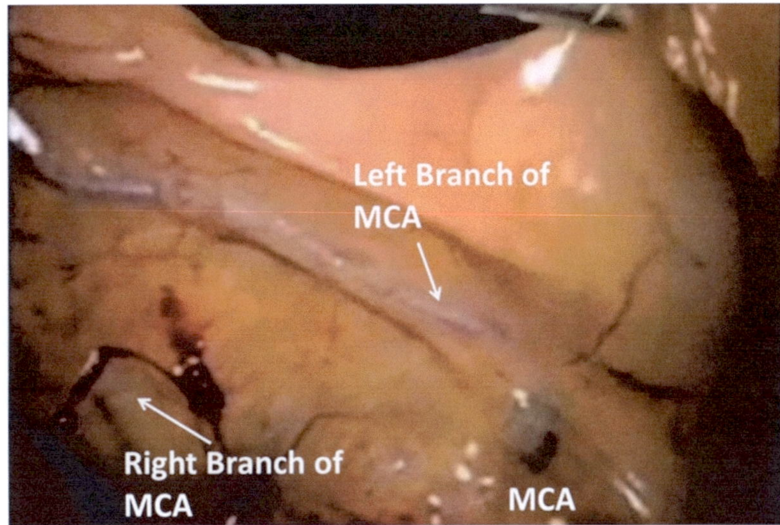

7.5 The Left Colon

7.5.1 Brief Anatomy

7.5.1.1 Inferior Mesenteric Artery

As the IMA supplies hindgut structures such as the distal transverse, descending, and sigmoid colon, understanding its branches assists robotic mesenteric dissection and colon resection (Figs. 7.18 and 7.19). The IMA gives off its first branch near the L3 vertebrae just prior to bifurcation of the aorta into the common iliac arteries. The first branch of the IMA is the left colic artery, which occurs 2–3 cm distal to the IMA origin.

The left colic divides further into two branches, the ascending and descending vessels, with the ascending vessel feeding the distal transverse and descending colon. The descending branch of the left colic supplies the distal descending and proximal sigmoid colon. The sigmoid also receives blood supply from individual distal sigmoidal branches of the IMA, along with the superior rectal artery. The IMA essentially terminates into the superior rectal artery which supplies the upper rectum in addition to the distal sigmoid colon. Just below the sacral promontory, its splits into a left and right branch, which courses down the lateral rectum within the endopelvic fascia. Of note, the splenic flexure is vascularized

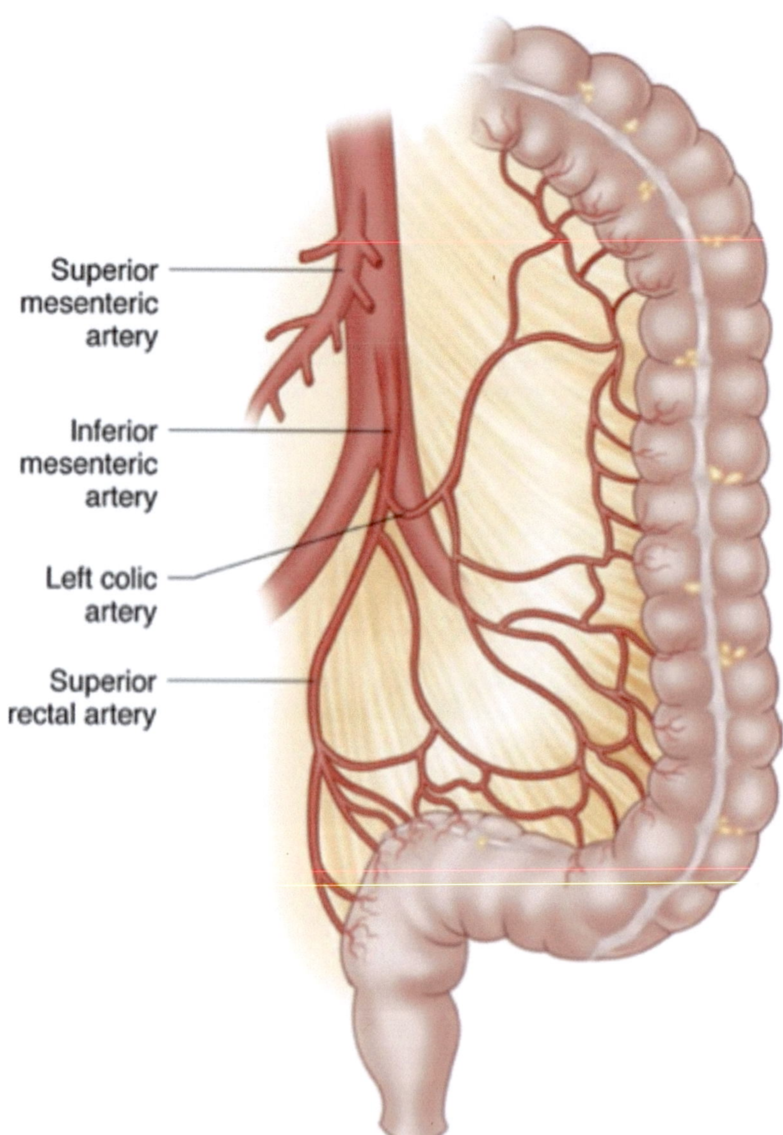

Fig. 7.18 The IMA courses over the left common iliac artery and vein and gives rise to its terminal branch, the superior rectal artery. *With permission from Landmann RG and Francone T. Surgical Anatomy. In: Minimally Invasive Approaches to Colon and Rectal Disease: Techniques and best practices. Ross HM, Lee SW, Mutch MG, Rivadeneira DE, Steele SR. Springer, New York, 2015: pp. 25–50*

by branches of both the middle and left colic arteries. Vascular anatomy can be variable, but the most common anatomical arrangement occurs between the ascending and descending branches of the left colic and the middle colic via the marginal vessels.

7.5.1.2 Ureter

The surgeon must identify the left ureter, which lies upon the psoas muscle under the peritoneum. If dissection is carried deep to the IMA pedicle and downward, the surgeon is likely to elevate the ureter and gonadal vessels off the psoas and

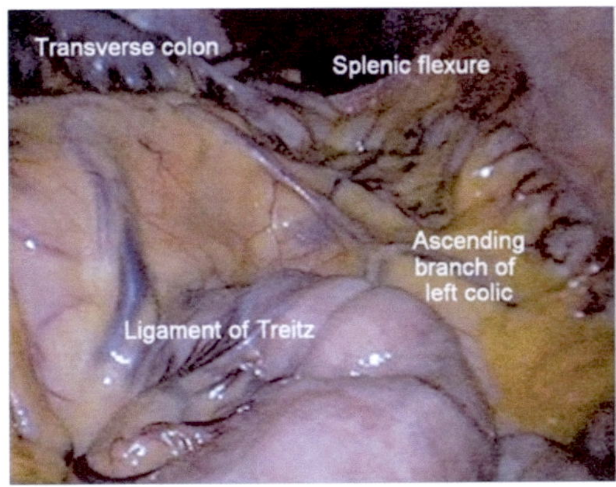

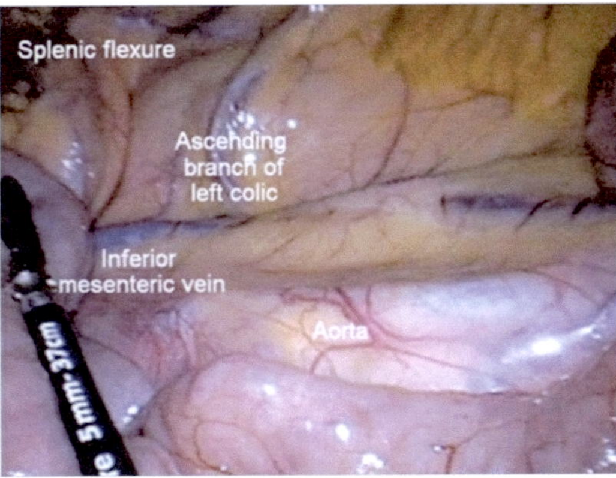

Fig. 7.19 Left colon anatomy. *LBMC* left branch of middle colic, *ABLC* ascending branch of left colic, *SF* splenic flexure. *With permission from Landmann RG and Francone T. Surgical Anatomy. In: Minimally Invasive Approaches to Colon and Rectal Disease: Techniques and best practices. Ross HM, Lee SW, Mutch MG, Rivadeneira DE, Steele SR. Springer, New York, 2015: pp. 25–50*

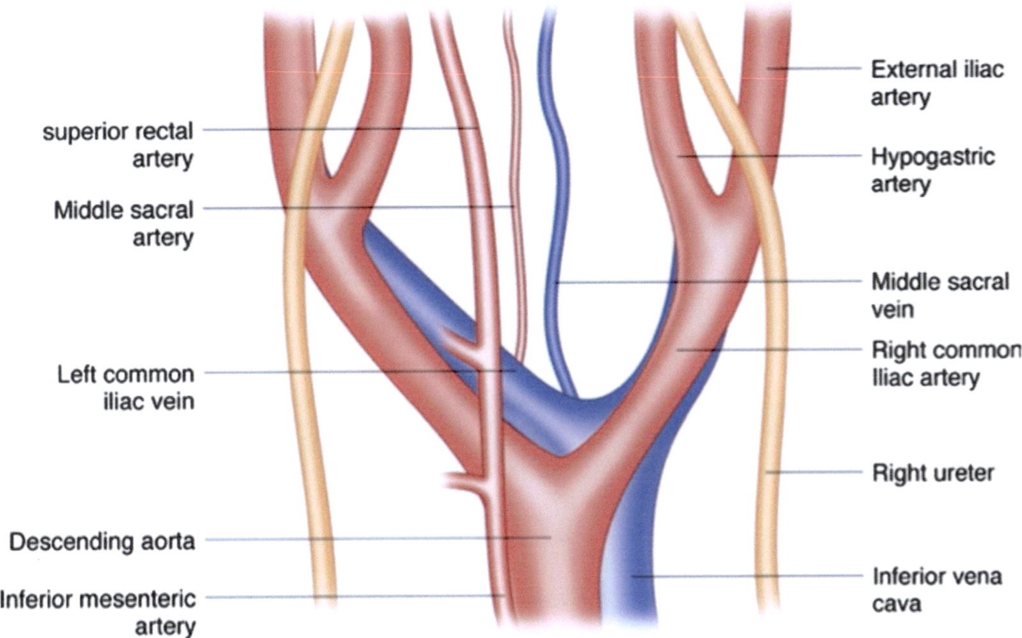

Fig. 7.20 Course of the ureters. *With permission from Landmann RG and Francone T. Surgical Anatomy. In: Minimally Invasive Approaches to Colon and Rectal Disease: Techniques and best practices. Ross HM, Lee SW, Mutch MG, Rivadeneira DE, Steele SR. Springer, New York, 2015: pp. 25–50*

into the surgical field. To maintain orientation, remember the right and left ureters track straight from the renal pelvis to the pelvic brim, crossing over the iliac vessels and maintaining a 5-cm lateral distance from the IVC and aorta. Classic teaching suggests the right ureter courses over the right external iliac artery (Figs. 7.8 and 7.20), while the left ureter courses more medially over the common iliac artery (Fig. 7.20). As ureters enter the pelvis, they course inferiorly and poste-

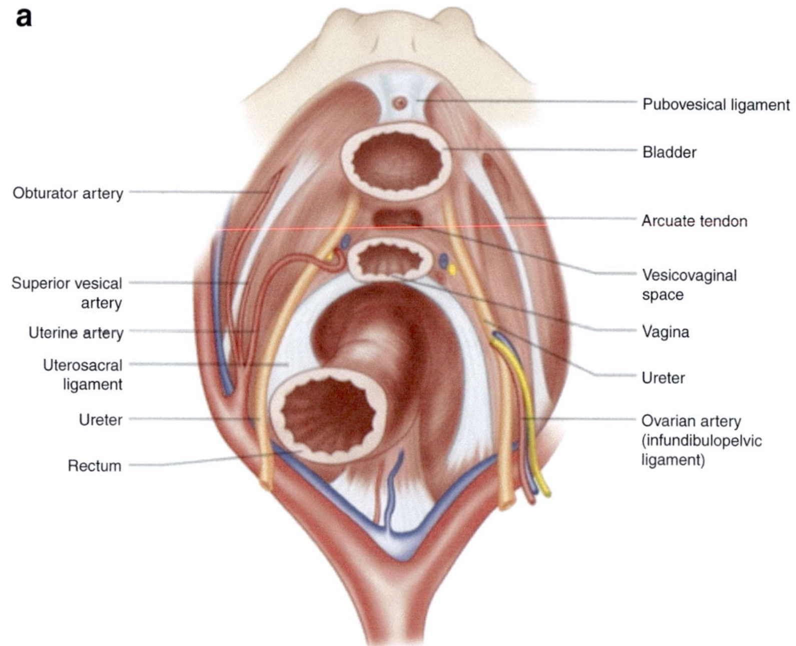

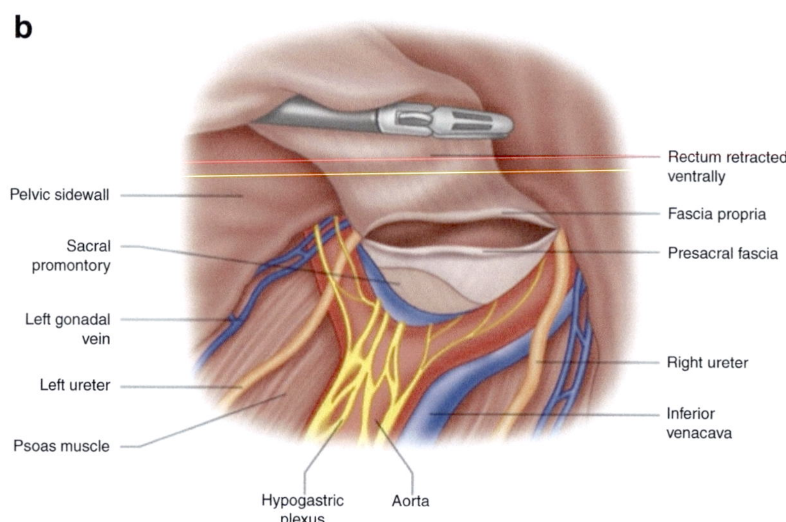

Fig. 7.21 Entry into the (**a**) pelvis and (**b**) presacral space. Notice the course of the ureter and the nerves at this level. *With permission from Landmann RG and Francone T. Surgical Anatomy. In: Minimally Invasive Approaches to Colon and Rectal Disease: Techniques and best practices. Ross HM, Lee SW, Mutch MG, Rivadeneira DE, Steele SR. Springer, New York, 2015: pp. 25–50*

riorly along the lateral pelvic sidewalls before entering the posterolateral surface of the bladder and extending to form the trigone (Fig. 7.21).

When completing robotic dissection, the ureters are usually encountered at the pelvic brim where they overlie the iliac vessels. If the ureter is visualized within the pelvis, dissection has been carried too far lateral of the vas deferens in males or the uterine artery in females. As with any technique, open, laparoscopic, or robotic, the surgeon must be comfortable with multiple approaches to surgical dissection (medial to lateral, lateral to medial). If the surgeon is unable to identify the ureter with confidence, an alternative approach must be utilized to clearly identify and prevent injury to the ureter. It is the authors' preference to perform a medial to lateral approach followed by lateral to medial when the ureter is difficult to identify.

7.5.1.3 Gonadal Vessels

When identifying the IMA and ureter, the gonadal arteries are also often identified. They arise from the aorta below the renal artery and course obliquely toward the pelvis, crossing the ureter midway between renal pelvis and pelvic inlet. Testicular vessels enter the deep inguinal ring after crossing halfway between the inguinal ligament and sacroiliac joint. In women, ovarian vessels enter the broad ligament at the pelvic brim. Disruption of these vessels, while not always immediately noticeable, can cause significant hemorrhage.

7.6 Left Colectomy

As with right colectomy, left colectomy requires dissection in multiple quadrants. Even without mobilization of the splenic flexure, port placement must allow dissection in at least two different quadrants: the left upper and lower quadrant. One cannot understate the importance of proper port placement in order to avoid unnecessary collision of the arms and assure successful completion of the dissection. Figures 7.4 and 7.5 demonstrate port placement for a left colectomy and sigmoidectomy, which also allows adequate dissection of the splenic flexure. Unlike laparoscopic surgery, once the robot is docked, the table cannot be moved or adjusted. During diagnostic laparoscopy, the surgeon should make every attempt to expose the left upper and lower quadrants without requiring too much Trendelenburg positioning. Steep Trendelenburg results in small bowel within the left upper quadrant, preventing adequate exposure of the IMV pedicle and the splenic flexure (Fig. 7.22). Right-sided tilt is

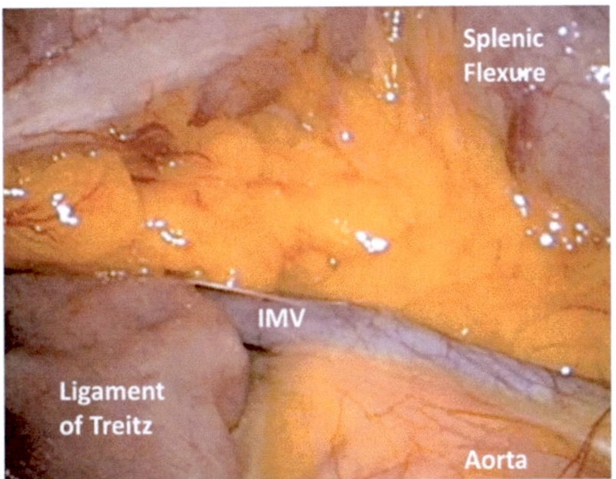

Fig. 7.22 Displacement of the small bowel into the right upper quadrant will allow for adequate exposure of the inferior mesenteric vein (IMV) and splenic flexure

acceptable, although too much angle can make your medial to lateral dissection difficult.

Once the patient is adequately positioned in slight Trendelenburg with table tilted slightly right down, docking is completed from the pelvis or the patient's left side. Familiarity with both approaches is suggested; however, the surgeon should choose one major approach to simplify setup for her team. As noted earlier, it is our preference to dock the robot over the left hip. Upon sitting at the console, evaluate the surrounding anatomy, taking note of the right ureter, iliac vessels, and other pelvic organs in relation to the sigmoid colon and sacral promontory. Due to lack of haptic feedback, visual cues will guide the dissection. Take care to remain oriented throughout all portions of the operation, and when in doubt, return to a global view of the pelvis, and regain your bearings.

As in a laparoscopic medial to lateral approach, begin by carefully elevating the sigmoid mesocolon using arm #2 to outline the inferior mesenteric artery (IMA) pedicle (Fig. 7.23a, b). This pedicle courses over the sacral promontory before it splits into right and left superior rectal arteries. Scoring parallel and inferior to this pedicle allows for entry of carbon dioxide into the appropriate plane (Fig. 7.23c), further illuminating the avascular plane between sigmoid mesocolon and posterior structures such as presacral fascia, autonomic nerves, and iliac vessels (Fig. 7.24).

Fig. 7.23 (a) Mobilization of the left colon under the IMA (*green arrow* depicts elevation of the pedicle and *dashed arrow* depicts direction of dissection). Notice the relationship of the ureter to the gonadal vessels. (**b**) The outline of the inferior mesenteric artery (IMA) can be visualized by gentle ventral retraction of the pedicle as it courses over the sacral promontory (SP). The space between the IMA and the sacral promontory has been termed the critical angle and marks the avascular plane between the retroperitoneum and the colon mesentery. (**c**) Scoring parallel to the IMA allows for entry of CO_2 into the avascular areolar plane indicating the appropriate plane. *With permission from Yuko Tonohira. With permission from Landmann RG and Francone T. Surgical Anatomy. In: Minimally Invasive Approaches to Colon and Rectal Disease: Techniques and best practices. Ross HM, Lee SW, Mutch MG, Rivadeneira DE, Steele SR. Springer, New York, 2015: pp. 25–50*

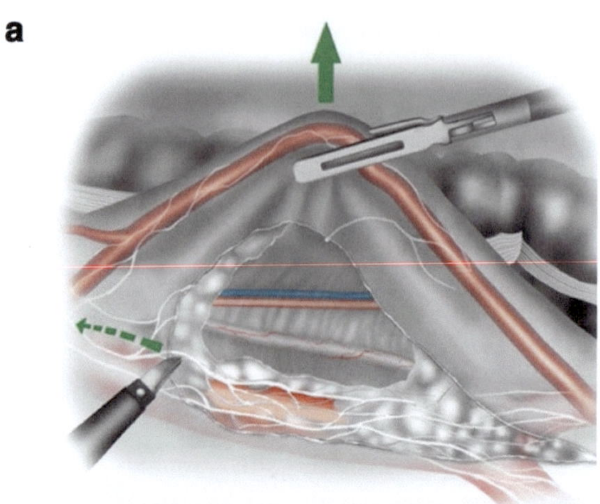

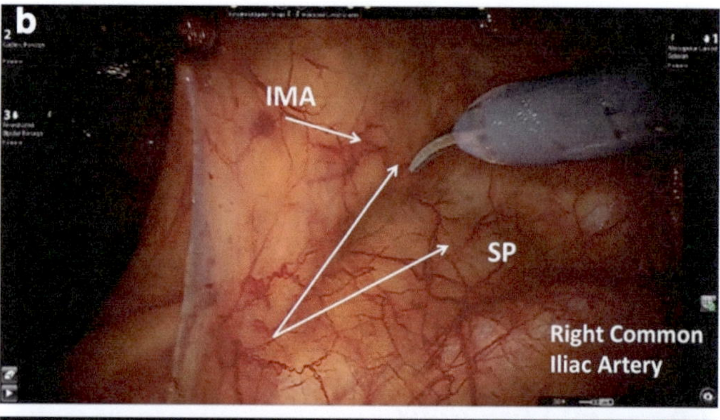

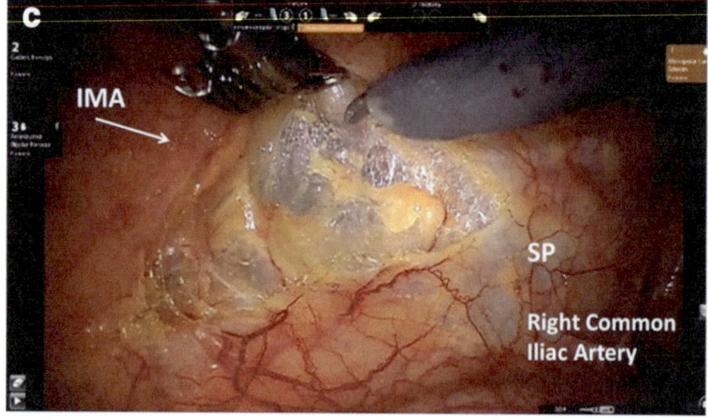

Arms #1 and #3 are then free to perform the medial lateral dissection. After several procedures, you quickly realize arm #2 is limited in the left lumbar and left upper region of the peritoneal cavity. As such, this arm is mainly utilized for retraction in an up-down or ventral-dorsal axis. Knowing the limitations of the port in the quadrant of dissection will also limit collisions. For example, arm #2 has limited use in mobilizing the splenic flexure and is often undocked in order to provide arm #3 and arm #1 adequate space to perform the dissection.

While one robotic arm elevates the sigmoid mesentery, the remaining arms carefully dissect underneath the IMA pedicle toward the sidewall. Care is taken to identify and avoid the left ureter, left gonadal vessels, and the hypogastric nerve plexus (Fig. 7.25a, b). If these structures are not

Fig. 7.24 Pelvic anatomy highlighting the ureter, gonadal vessels, sacral promontory, hypogastric nerves, and avascular alveolar space between the fascia propria and the presacral fascia

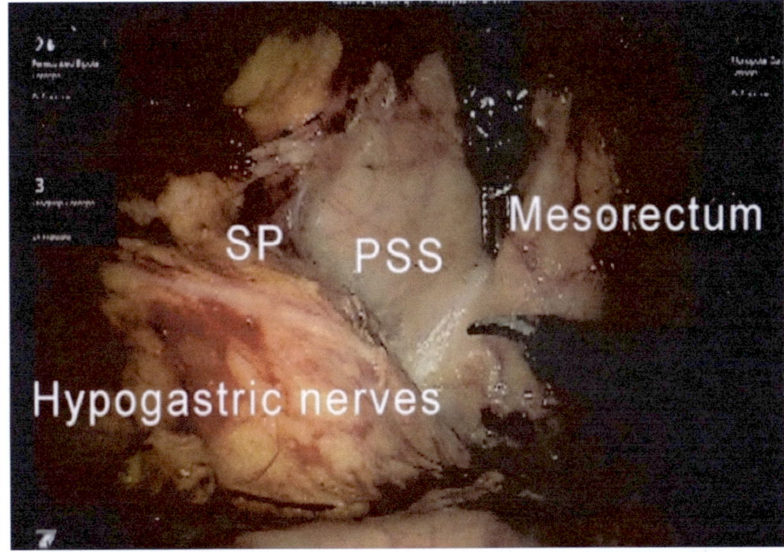

Fig. 7.25 Care is taken to identify and avoid the left ureter, left gonadal vessels, and the hypogastric nerve plexus. On the left, the ureter courses more medial and will cross over the left common iliac artery as it enters the pelvis

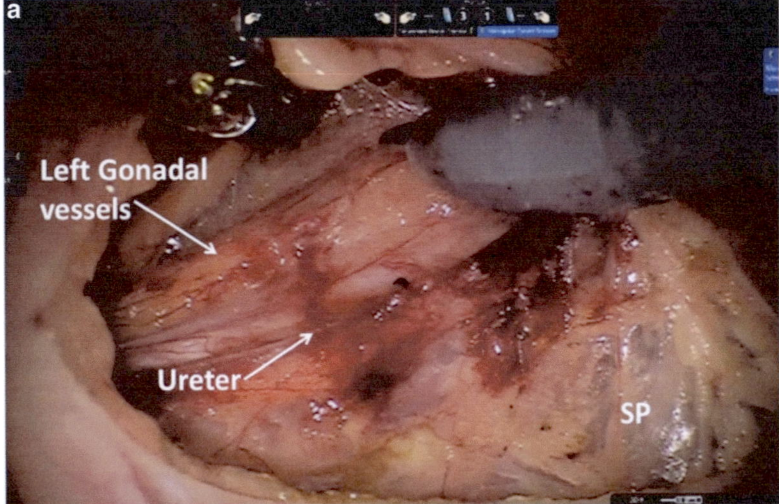

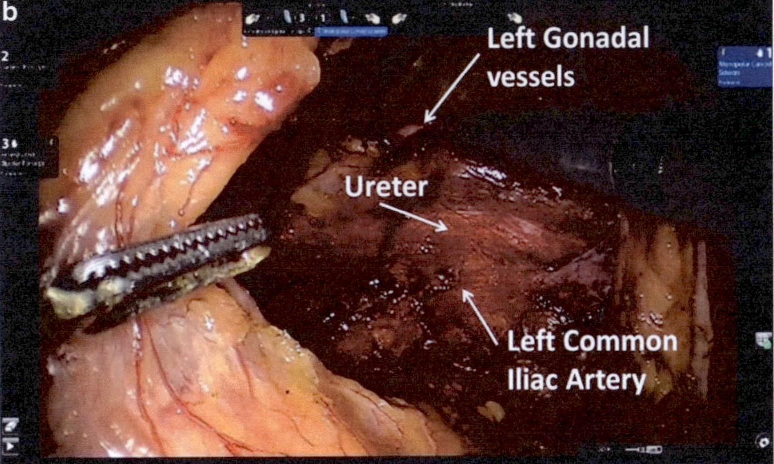

clearly identified, the approach should be altered until these retroperitoneal structures have been properly visualized and kept out of harm's way. Following identification and protection of the ureter, the IMA pedicle may be divided. However, it is the author's preference to continue the medial to lateral dissection between the base of the IMA and the base of the IMV (Fig. 7.26). Complete mobilization of the medial to lateral plane allows isolation and a clear understanding of the anatomy giving a "T" appearance to the IMA pedicle (Fig. 7.27). At this point, the surgeon may decide to divide the IMA proximal or distal to the take-off of the left colic or divide the IMV if splenic flexure mobilization is required. Early division of the IMV allows some leniency when mobilizing the splenic flexure from a medial lateral approach as the IMV can be easily avulsed during dissection, resulting in uncontrollable and possibly lethal hemorrhage (Fig. 7.28). The IMV is identified at the inferior tail of the pancreas near the splenic flexure. Care should be taken to identify the duodenum at the ligament of Treitz to prevent incidental traction or cautery injury. The focus then becomes completion of splenic flexure mobilization. It is the author's preference to utilize the vessel sealer for division of both the IMA and IMV; however, other methods can be utilized and should be available in case of need such as a stapler, clips, or endoloop.

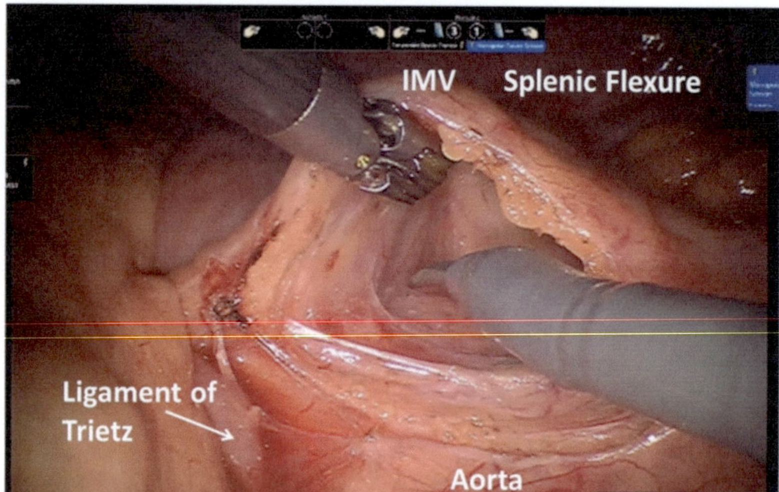

Fig. 7.26 Continued medial to lateral mobilization between the IMA and IMV will facilitate mobilization of the splenic flexure

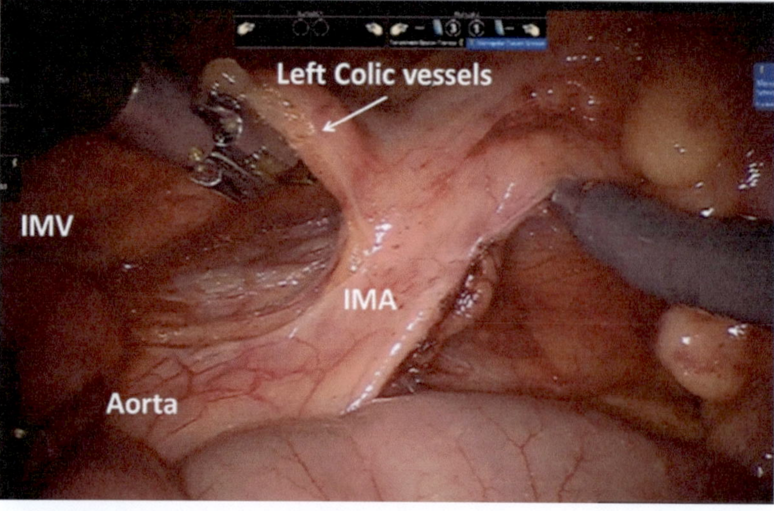

Fig. 7.27 Mobilization cephalad and caudal to the takeoff of the IMA will give a "T" appearance; this allows proper identification of the left colic artery such that it may be preserved when necessary

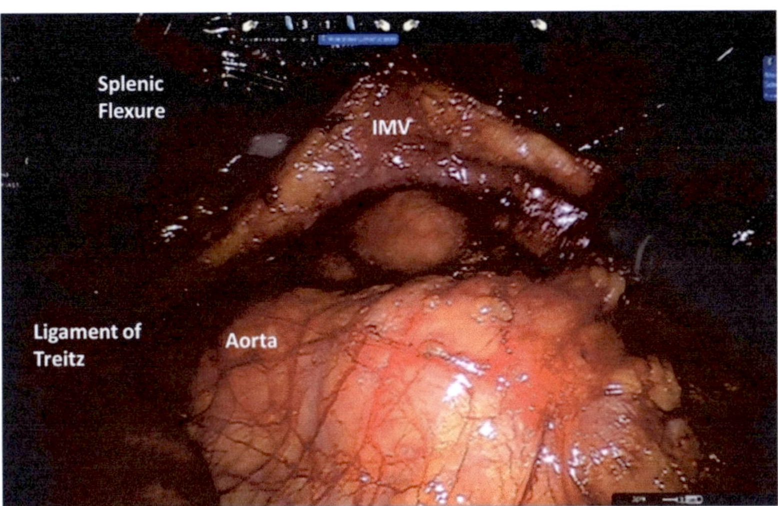

Fig. 7.28 The IMV is identified at the inferior tail of the pancreas near the splenic flexure. *With permission from Landmann RG and Francone T. Surgical Anatomy. In: Minimally Invasive Approaches to Colon and Rectal Disease: Techniques and best practices. Ross HM, Lee SW, Mutch MG, Rivadeneira DE, Steele SR. Springer, New York, 2015: pp. 25–50*

Once the IMA is divided, medial to lateral dissection is completed. The more complete one's medial to lateral dissection, the less dissection required when dividing the lateral attachments (Fig. 7.29a). Once the abdominal sidewall is reached, dissection is carried cephalad to the superior pole of the kidney (Fig. 7.29b). Remember, depending upon port placement, this portion of the operation may become more difficult. The surgeon must assure appropriate arm positioning such that inadvertent damage to intra-abdominal structures does not occur. As one approaches the left upper quadrant, arm #2 becomes less helpful and will cause unnecessary collisions or tearing of tissues if attempting to retract tissue outside its range of motion.

7.6.1 Splenic Flexure

A sufficient medial to lateral mobilization, completed to the inferior border of the pancreas, leaves only the lateral splenocolic ligaments remaining. If splenic flexure mobilization is unnecessary, then simple division of the lateral sidewall attachments with monopolar will free the descending and sigmoid colon to allow for resection and anastomosis (Fig. 7.29). If the splenic flexure is to be mobilized, start at the left sidewall, and divide attachments toward the splenic flexure. Here, arm #1 performs the dissection with either a monopolar or vessel-sealing device, while arm #3

retracts the proximal colon to provide adequate tension/counter-tension. Remember to utilize your assistant port when mobilizing the splenic flexure as this helps with adequate tension/counter-tension and exposure. The dissection is carried as far cephalad as possible. Once exposure becomes difficult, dissection may be redirected to the transverse colon and lesser sac.

There are usually two layers connecting omentum to transverse colon at the splenic flexure. Taking each layer individually with cautery or other energy devices prevents inadvertent gastric injury. Additionally, the surgeon is better able to distinguish colonic mesentery from congenital attachments of posterior omentum to the mesocolon. With entry into the lesser sac (Fig. 7.16), division of splenocolic attachments is facilitated. Arm #3 is used for ventral retraction of the omentum, while the assistant port provides caudal retraction. Arm #1 is then free to dissect along the correct plane. The dissection is continued medially until the splenic flexure is rendered a midline structure and the designated colon reaches to the pelvis without tension.

Entry into the lesser sac to complete dissection of the flexure may require more than one approach. If unable to enter the lesser sac from the lateral to medial approach or if dense adhesions prevent adhesion from an anterior approach, the use of a posterior approach may prevent injury to the pancreas. Elevate the transverse colon to the anterior abdominal wall, and enter the avascular plan

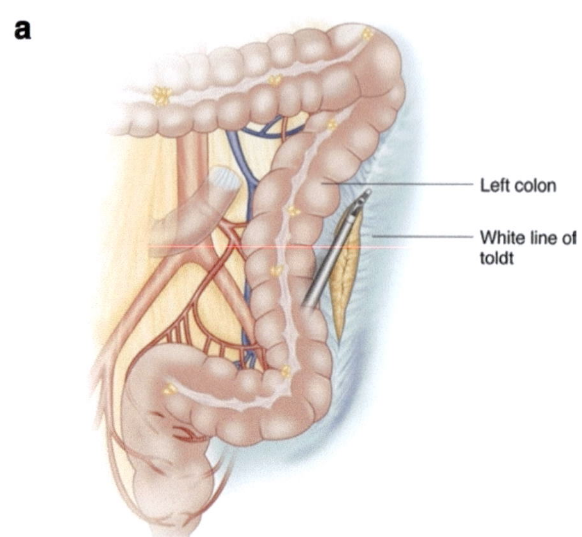

Fig. 7.29 When dividing the lateral attachments, dissection is carried from the pelvis toward the splenic flexure; often, arm #2 becomes limited in its use due to increased collisions

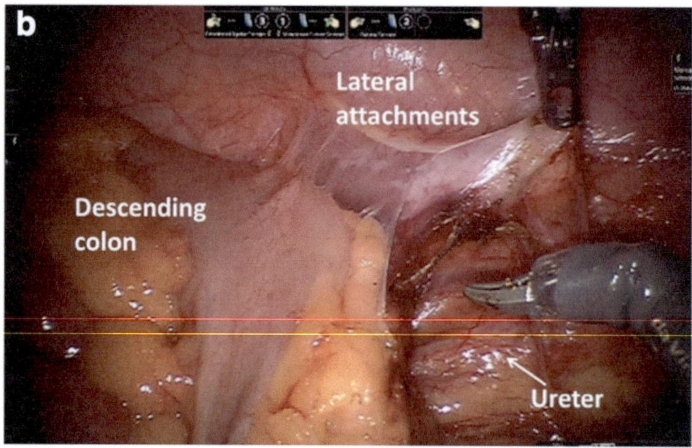

above the ligament of Treitz, found above the duodenum and near the transverse mesocolon. Entry through this space places you within the lesser sac and is also a good way to approach the left branch of the middle colic if performing a more extensive resection. If the descending colon is your conduit, take care not to injure this branch or the marginal artery of Drummond.

7.7 The Pelvis

7.7.1 Brief Anatomy

Without an intimate understanding of pelvic anatomy, it becomes easy to lose orientation during robotic-assisted laparoscopic procedures. Disorientation greatly increases risk for inadvertent injury. As such, knowledge of pertinent anatomy prior to minimally invasive rectal dissection is exceedingly important.

7.7.1.1 Pelvic Compartments

The four compartments (posterior, lateral, anterior, and middle) contain vascular structures, ureters, neurologic structures, and the rectum (Fig. 7.30). The posterior compartment contains the rectum, mesorectum, fascia propria, and presacral fascia. The presacral fascia covers autonomic nerves, presacral veins, and the middle sacral artery, while the fascia propria overlies the rectum and mesorectum as a continuation of the endopelvic fascia. The anterior border of the posterior compartment is marked by the rectogenital

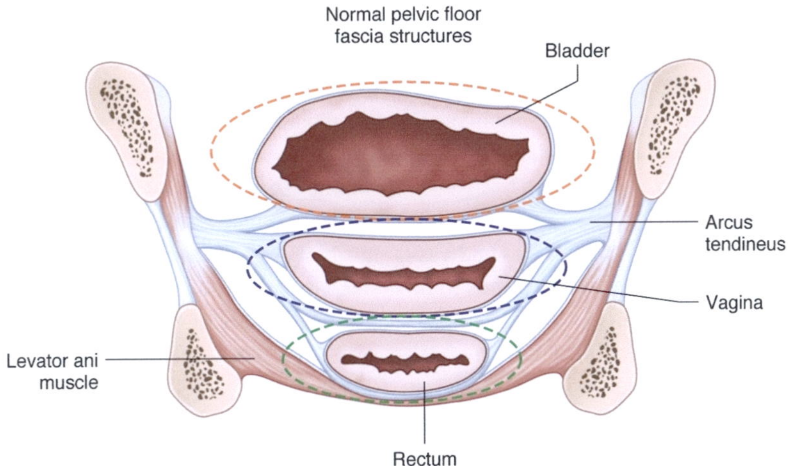

Fig. 7.30 *Dashed green line* depicts the posterior rectum, while the *blue* and *orange* lines represent the middle and anterior compartments; the middle compartment is only present in females. *With permission from Landmann RG and Francone T. Surgical Anatomy. In: Minimally Invasive Approaches to Colon and Rectal Disease: Techniques and best practices. Ross HM, Lee SW, Mutch MG, Rivadeneira DE, Steele SR. Springer, New York, 2015: pp. 25–50*

Fig. 7.31 Anterior plane of dissection highlighting Denonvilliers fascia. *With permission from Landmann RG and Francone T. Surgical Anatomy. In: Minimally Invasive Approaches to Colon and Rectal Disease: Techniques and best practices. Ross HM, Lee SW, Mutch MG, Rivadeneira DE, Steele SR. Springer, New York, 2015: pp. 25–50*

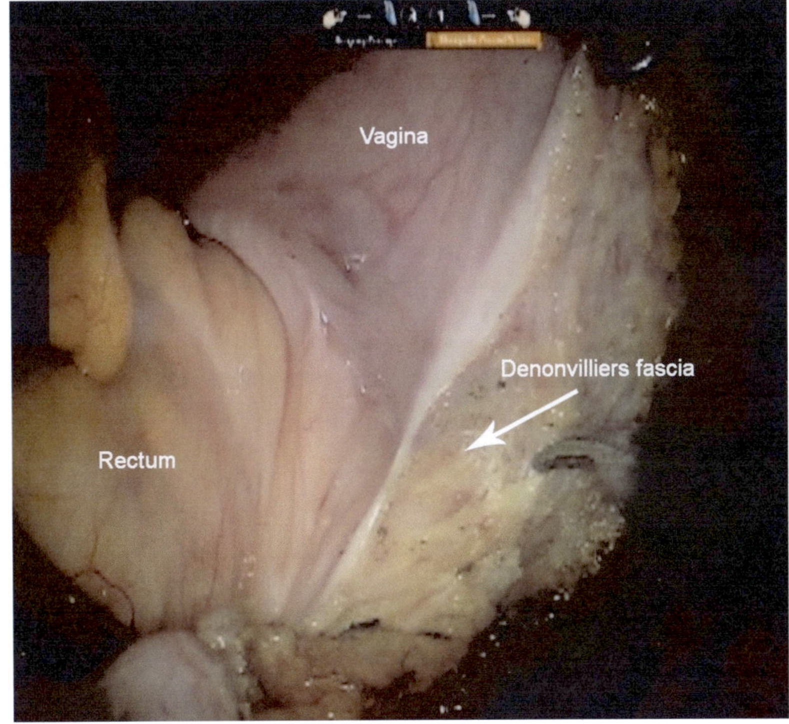

septum, defined by Denonvilliers fascia separating the vagina or prostate from the extraperitoneal rectum (Fig. 7.31). Care is required during dissection to prevent bladder injury and damage to hypogastric nerves required for sexual function. The bladder and paravisceral fat pad are within the anterior compartment, with the nerve-vessel plate interposed between these two structures. In women, the middle compartment includes endopelvic fascia overlying the vagina, uterus, and tuberosacral ligament. Lateral compartments include branches of the inferior mesentery artery, internal ilia, and distal ureters as they enter the bladder. These structures are best delineated intra-abdominally prior to entering the pelvis.

7.7.1.2 Innervation

While no less important than the ureters and vascular supply in the pelvis, innervation tends to be overlooked by most surgeons. Robotic-assisted laparoscopic surgery allows for clear visualization of parasympathetic and sympathetic nerve bundles that supply the left colon and rectum. Sympathetic nerves arise from L1–L3, with fibers of the inferior mesenteric and inferior hypogastric plexuses traveling along the IMA and superior rectal artery. Fusion of these two bundles into the hypogastric plexus at the sacral promontory innervates the lower rectum (Fig. 7.32a, b). From here, two larger bundles form and enter the pelvis along the lateral pelvic sidewall, terminating at the lateral stalks of the mesorectum. S2–S4 supply nerve roots to the pelvic splanchnic nerves, commonly referred to as nervi erigentes, which provide parasympathetic innervation to the rectum and anal canal. The nervi erigentes travel with hypogastric nerves on the lateral sidewall of the pelvis, eventually giving rise to the periprostatic plexus. In males, this plexus is responsible for the bulbourethral glands, ejaculatory ducts, urethra, prostate, seminal vesicles, and vas deferens (Fig. 7.33). While damage to these nerves in males carries significant consequences, interruption in females leads to vaginal dryness, dyspareunia, bladder dysfunction, and rectal dysfunction. With enhanced 3D visualization and endowrist movement, surgeons utilizing robotics can safely identify and protect these important neurovascular bundles, potentially reducing patient complication rates.

7.7.2 Low Anterior Resection

This procedure combines the previously described left colectomy with pelvic dissection. As noted above, knowledge of pelvic anatomy is tantamount to the prevention of complications from inadvertent injury. Advanced optics and endowrist movements provide a significant advantage over laparoscopy for this procedure. Additionally, extension of pelvic dissection to the pelvic floor is required for robotic-assisted laparoscopic abdominoperineal resection. The advantages of robotic surgery allow for minimally invasive procedures to be performed in a hostile, narrow, or morbidly obese pelvis more easily than in open or standard laparoscopic procedures.

Several port placements have been suggested with the most commonly used arrangements detailed in Figs. 7.4 and 7.5. For thinner patients, the port set up in Fig. 7.5 may be used for both splenic flexure mobilization and pelvic dissection; however, most patients will require utilization of the port system described in Fig. 7.4. Here, arm #3 is docked in the RUQ for use in the medial to lateral and splenic flexure mobilization. When the pelvic dissection is initiated, arm #3 is moved to the left lumber region. Of note, arm #3 will often collide with the camera and may have difficulty reaching into the deep pelvis. With arms #2 and #3 on the left, collisions are minimized, if not eliminated, while working in the deep pelvis.

It is the preference of the authors to perform medial to lateral dissection and splenic flexure mobilization prior to proceeding with the pelvic dissection. Developing the correct medial to lateral plane with division of the IMA facilitates dissection into the pelvis. The critical maneuver at this juncture is the development of the space immediately posterior to the fascia propria of the rectum, which separates the mesorectum from presacral fascia (Fig. 7.23a). Care is taken to stay out of the presacral fascia, which covers the presacral veins, middle sacral artery, nerve bundles, and the sacrum. Incision of the lateral peritoneum during anterior and upward traction on the rectum will illuminate this plane when CO_2 enters the space, helping to prevent starting within the presacral fascia (Fig. 7.23c). This is often described as the "cotton candy" layer due to its characteristic appearance of fluffy, white areola tissue (Fig. 7.24). Dissection should be carefully continued within this plane toward the levator ani and puborectalis muscles, posteriorly and laterally. In most cases, this portion of the operation is bloodless due to an avascular plane.

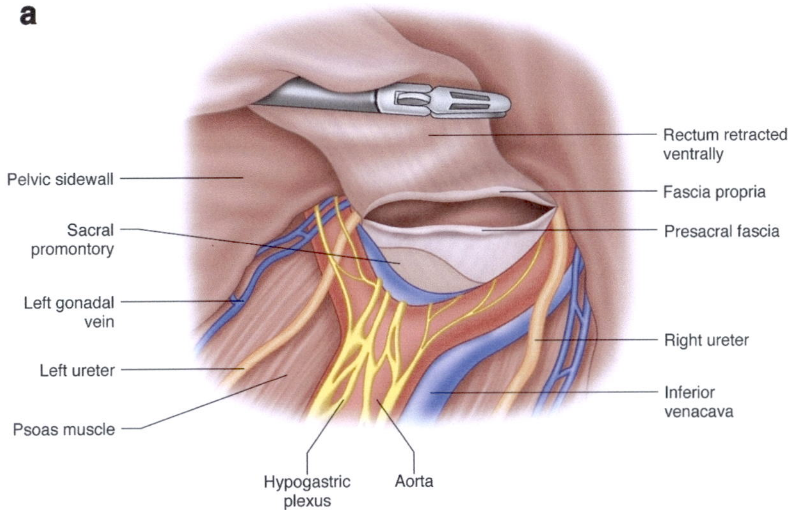

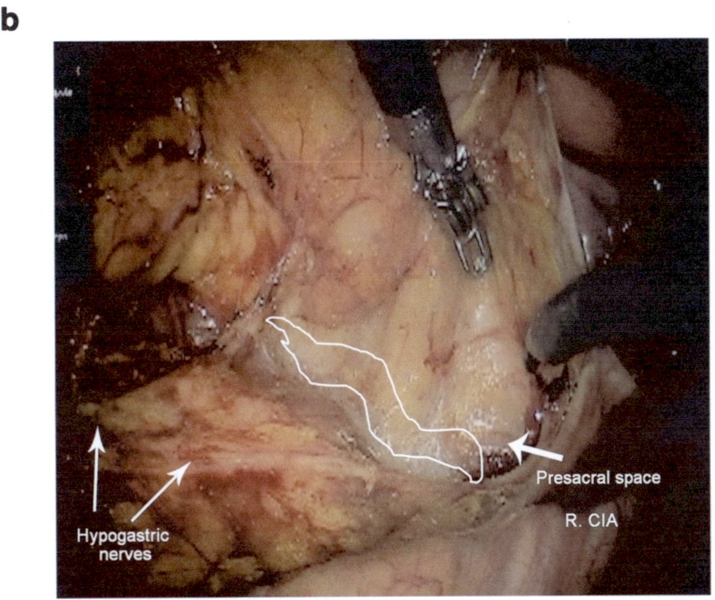

Fig. 7.32 (**a**) Entry into the presacral space. Notice the course of the ureter and the nerves at this level. (**b**) Pelvic anatomy highlighting the sacrum, hypogastric nerves, and avascular alveolar space between the fascia propria and presacral fascia. *With permission from Landmann RG and* *Francone T. Surgical Anatomy. In: Minimally Invasive Approaches to Colon and Rectal Disease: Techniques and best practices. Ross HM, Lee SW, Mutch MG, Rivadeneira DE, Steele SR. Springer, New York, 2015: pp. 25–50*

PEARL: *It is often helpful to have the first assistant stationary with retraction of the rectum out of the pelvis. This may be facilitated by wrapping the rectum with a vaginal packing allowing the assistant to hold the rectum without tearing the mesorectum causing bleeding and disruption of your oncologic margins. Arms #2 and #3 are then free to provide adequate tension/counter-tension at the level of dissection. Arm #1 provides the energy source.*

In open and laparoscopic cases, it is customary to extend the posterior dissection to the left and right lateral aspects of the mesorectum followed by mobilization of the anterior plane (Fig. 7.34). This is often accomplished by completing the

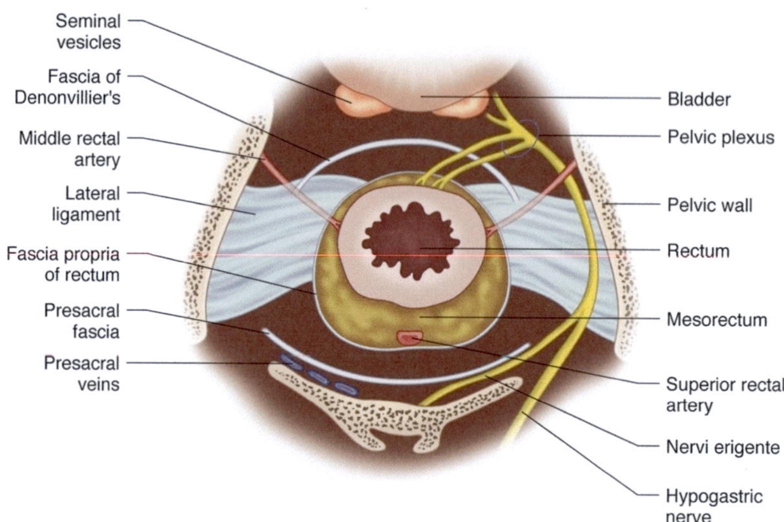

Fig. 7.33 Schematic representation of the prostate, nerves, rectum, and pelvic structures. *With permission from Landmann RG and Francone T. Surgical Anatomy. In: Minimally Invasive Approaches to Colon and Rectal Disease: Techniques and best practices. Ross HM, Lee SW, Mutch MG, Rivadeneira DE, Steele SR. Springer, New York, 2015: pp. 25–50*

division of the right lateral peritoneal reflection toward the pouch of Douglas and anterior peritoneal reflection. During this dissection, condensations of pelvic fascia known as the lateral stalks (or ligaments) are encountered. Although vessels may traverse these "stalks," they are relatively small and are not considered to be representative of the middle rectal artery. Even so, care must be taken when performing this portion of the dissection and can often be accomplished with a monopolar energy source. Once the right side is fully mobilized, the left is performed in a similar fashion.

After developing the posterior and lateral planes, the anterior dissection is then performed. Continuation of the lateral and posterior dissection can often lead the surgeon in the right plane. Commonly, there is an "open-C" type or "opening-zipper" configuration of this fascia at this level that will demarcate the appropriate dissection plane (Fig. 7.35). In this instance, starting from a known to unknown dissection will help identify the appropriate dissection plane with loose alveolar tissue as the definitive marker. The vagina or prostate and seminal vesicles will be visualized anteriorly as dissection proceeds caudally along Denonvilliers fascia (Figs. 7.31 and 7.36).

An alternative approach to the pelvic dissection is worthwhile mentioning given the lateral dissection plane can often be ambiguous due to previous inflammation, radiation, or simply a bulky mesorectum. As a result, the dissection can unintentionally be carried too far to the right and left resulting in injury of the nervi erigentes, pelvic sidewall vasculature, or even the ureter. When performing this dissection, one has to give careful consideration to the width and contour of the pelvis and follow the plane accordingly. When needed, the anterior plane may be developed following mobilization of the posterior mesorectum. This is often helpful in clarifying the correct dissection plane along the lateral stalks with an exaggerated "C" type or open "zipper" configuration. Arms #2 and #3 are often used for retraction on the prostate or vagina, while the assistant port is used to provide adequate cephalad tension on the rectum.

PEARL: *The surgeon should make use of all three robotic arms during rectal dissection, especially the lateral and anterior portions. Proper tension/counter-tension is essential for the development of the avascular plane, especially deep within the pelvis.*

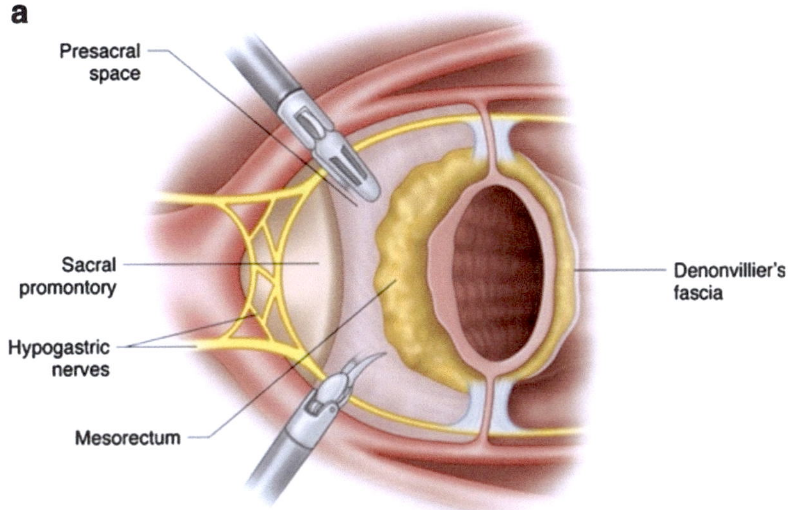

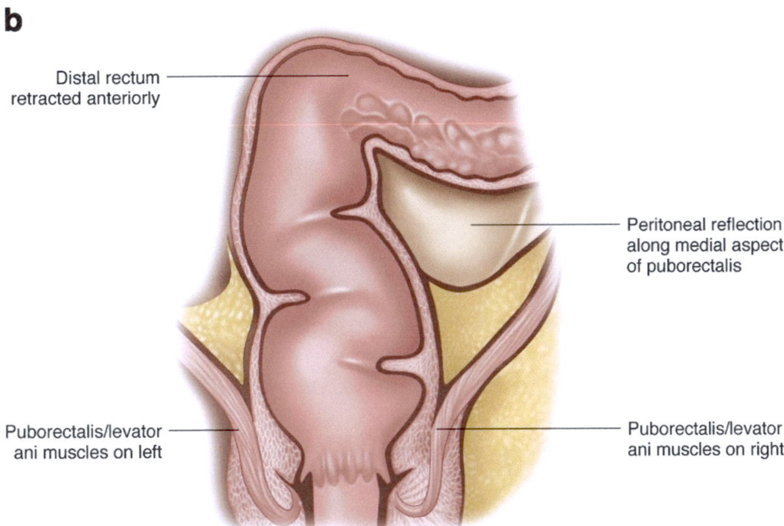

Fig. 7.34 (**a**) Cross-sectional view of the pelvis at the sacral promontory. *With permission from Landmann RG and Francone T. Surgical Anatomy. In: Minimally Invasive Approaches to Colon and Rectal Disease: Techniques and best practices. Ross HM, Lee SW, Mutch MG, Rivadeneira DE, Steele SR. Springer, New York, 2015: pp. 25–50.* (**b**) Posterior dissection. Note the fibers of the puborectalis and levator ani posterior bilateral with the distal rectal canal retracted anteriorly. Note the peritoneal reflection (*white line*) along the medial border of the puborectalis leading to the intersphincteric space

During distal-most dissection, robotic assistance may allow for identification of the distal mesorectal canal (Fig. 7.37). The surgeon will see a paucity of mesorectal fat at the pelvic floor and may continue distal dissection through the pelvic floor in an intersphincteric fashion (Fig. 7.38). While this extent of dissection is not necessary in most cases of low anterior resection, knowledge of surrounding anatomy allows the surgeon to clearly identify surgical planes and maximize the benefits of robotic colorectal surgery.

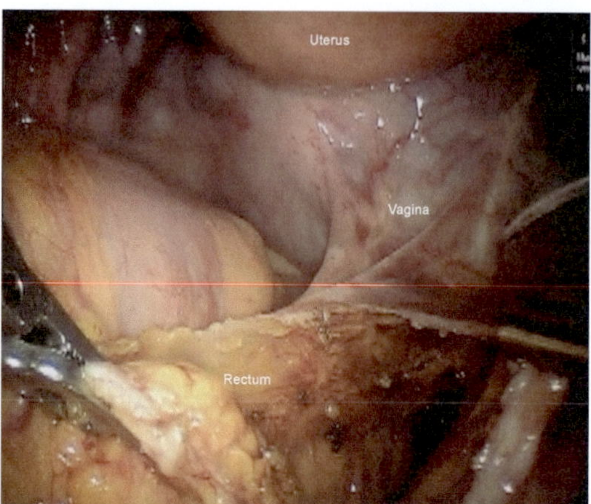

Fig. 7.35 Reverse "C-shaped" plane during distal antero-lateral dissection along right pelvic sidewall. *With permission from Landmann RG and Francone T. Surgical Anatomy. In: Minimally Invasive Approaches to Colon and Rectal Disease: Techniques and best practices. Ross HM, Lee SW, Mutch MG, Rivadeneira DE, Steele SR. Springer, New York, 2015: pp. 25–50*

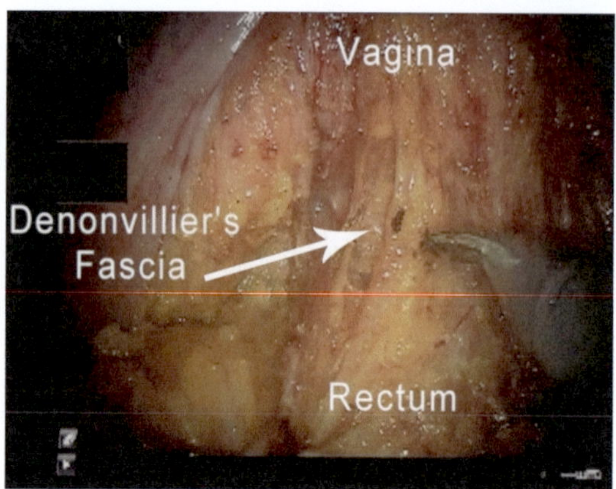

Fig. 7.36 Denonvilliers fascia can often be a difficult plane to identify; careful tension/counter-tension between the rectum and the genitourinary structure will help develop the appropriate plane. *With permission from Landmann RG and Francone T. Surgical Anatomy. In: Minimally Invasive Approaches to Colon and Rectal Disease: Techniques and best practices. Ross HM, Lee SW, Mutch MG, Rivadeneira DE, Steele SR. Springer, New York, 2015: pp. 25–50*

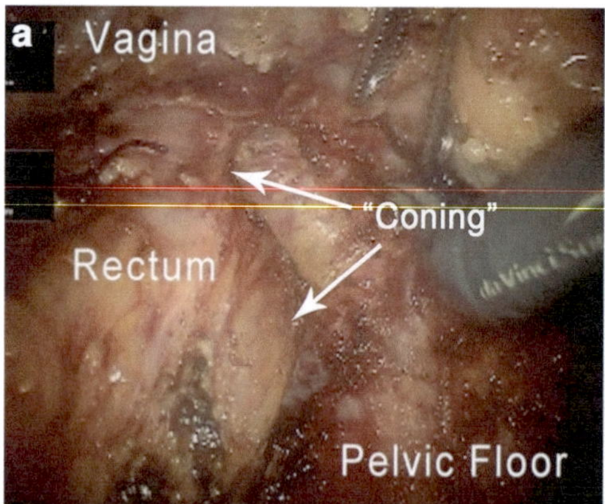

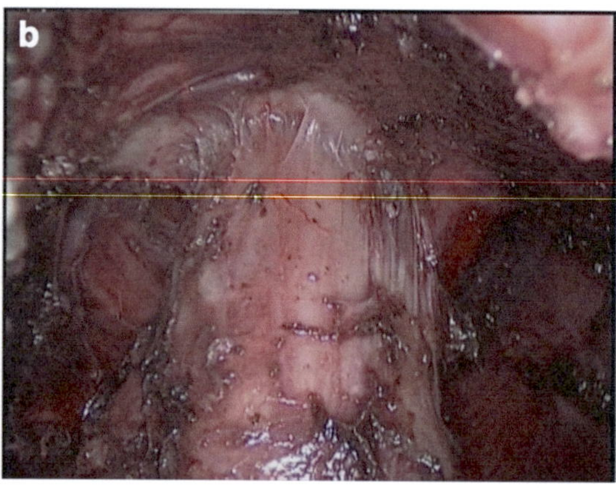

Fig. 7.37 (**a**) During a total mesorectal excision, the dissection may be extended to the level of the pelvic floor. *With permission from Landmann RG and Francone T. Surgical Anatomy. In: Minimally Invasive Approaches to Colon and Rectal Disease: Techniques and best prac-* tices. *Ross HM, Lee SW, Mutch MG, Rivadeneira DE, Steele SR. Springer, New York, 2015: pp. 25–50.* (**b**) At this point the mesorectum is thinned and the typical "coning" is seen

7.7.3 Perineal Dissection

If an abdominoperineal resection is required, dissection must continue below the levator ani muscles (Fig. 7.39). Following this, perineal dissection begins. The anal canal and lower rectum are dissected and removed through the ischiorectal fossa and urogenital diaphragm. If the tumor is extensively invasive, removal of a female patient's vagina, vulva, and urethra may be required. The entire specimen may then be removed via an abdominal or perineal incision.

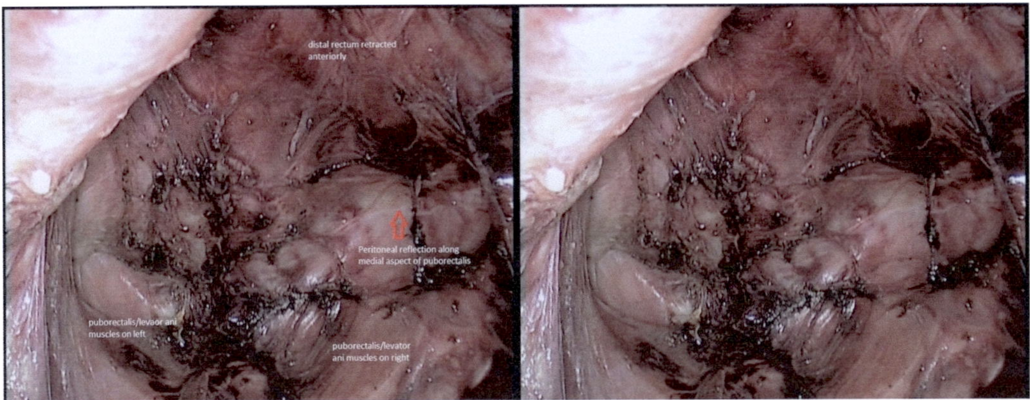

Fig. 7.38 Posterior dissection. Note the fibers of the puborectalis and levator ani posterior bilateral with the distal rectal canal retracted anteriorly. Note the peritoneal reflection (*white line*) along the medial border of the puborectalis leading to the intersphincteric space

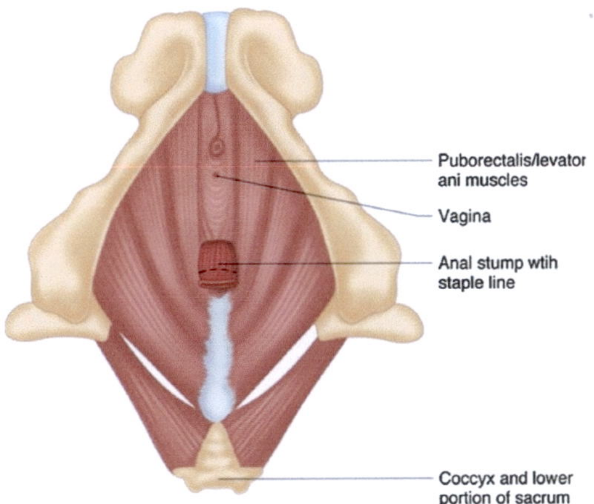

Fig. 7.39 Anatomy of the pelvic floor demonstrating the perineal musculature

7.7.4   Challenges

7.7.4.1 Presacral Bleeding

PEARL: *As in any situation with excessive bleeding, direct pressure is the first step in maintaining control of the bleeding and the operation. Consider contacting a partner for assistance when necessary.*

Presacral bleeding may be difficult to control given retraction of the vessels into the sacral foramen and the high hydrostatic pressure of the presacral venous system. The presacral veins are avalvular and communicate with the basiverte-bral veins. Control of presacral vein bleeding is quite difficult when performing both open and laparoscopic dissections. When performing a laparoscopic dissection, it would be prudent to consider conversion to either a hand-assist or open approach to ensure adequate exposure and overall safety of the patient if hemorrhage is uncontrolled. Before conversion, the hemorrhage should be controlled by tamponade of the pelvis with packing and direct pressure with a laparoscopic instrument. Definitive control is then attained with pressure, tacks, or muscle patch.

7.7.4.2 Uterine Retraction

It may be difficult at times to gain appropriate exposure to the anterior rectum and Denonvilliers fascia in a woman with a large uterus and poor suspension from the broad ligaments (Fig. 7.40). In these cases, several options exist, with the authors generally preferring the last:

1. Endo-uterine manipulator—this is placed per vagina and held in place by an assistant or retractor.
2. Dynamic manual retraction via a grasper or fan retractor—this generally is performed by the assistant who is also manipulating the camera. This does provide for some limited dynamic control/retraction if needed.
3. Static retraction and suspension—these are performed by placing a transabdominal fixation stitch (i.e., 2-0 Prolene on a Keith needle)

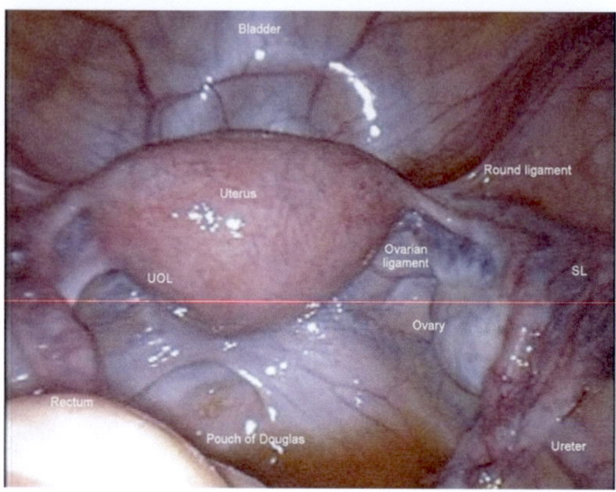

Fig. 7.40 Uterine anatomy highlighting pouch of Douglas. *SL* suspensory ligament of the ovary, *UL* utero-sacral ligament, *UOL* utero-ovarian ligament, *FT* fallopian tube, *OL* ovarian ligament

through the abdominal wall, then anterior to posterior through the broad ligament, around the fundus, and then again in a posterior-to-anterior fashion through the contralateral broad ligament and again out the abdominal wall. At this point, both ends of the suture are pulled taut and tied down while the uterus is being suspended ventrally. Rather than the broad ligament, some surgeons may prefer going directly through the uterine fundus, minimizing potential for uterine artery hemorrhage.

This last option provides significantly more retraction and exposure. Additionally, it frees up the assistant to utilize a laparoscopic grasper for dynamic retraction.

7.8 Key Points

- A thorough understanding of anatomy is imperative for proper exposure during minimally invasive operations, especially robotic-assisted procedures. Every effort must be made to gain a clear understanding of the anatomy prior to proceeding with dissection.

- Excellent exposure, meticulous technique, and proper assistance cannot be overstated. They are essential components to providing appropriate care to the patient, improving outcomes, and minimizing complications.

- Tension/counter-tension is an essential maneuver in developing and maintaining correct exposure of planes during any minimally invasive colon and rectal procedure. This maneuver is more challenging with current robotic minimally invasive techniques as haptic perception is absent. Appropriate tension is gauged with visual cues such as a taut mesentery or whitening of tissues representing constriction of blood flow.

- Retroperitoneal structures are always at risk during laparoscopic colectomy and must be identified and avoided throughout the dissection: right colectomy (duodenum), transverse colectomy (pancreas and mesenteric vessels), left colectomy (ureter/gonadal vessels, autonomic nerves), and pelvic dissection (ureter, hypogastric nerves).

References

1. Excellence. NNIfHaC. NICE implementation and uptake report: laparoscopic surgery for colorectal cancer. March 2010.
2. Robinson CN, Chen GJ, Balentine CJ, et al. Minimally invasive surgery is underutilized for colon cancer. Ann Surg Oncol. 2011;18(5):1412–8.
3. Rea JD, Cone MM, Diggs BS, Deveney KE, Lu KC, Herzig DO. Utilization of laparoscopic colectomy in the United States before and after the clinical outcomes of surgical therapy study group trial. Ann Surg. 2011;254(2):281–8.
4. Ramamoorthy S, Obias V. Unique complications of robotic colorectal surgery. Surg Clin North Am. 2013;93(1):273–86.
5. Lasser MS, Patel CK, Elsamra SE, Renzulli 2nd JF, Haleblian GE, Pareek G. Dedicated robotics team reduces pre-surgical preparation time. Indian J Urol. 2012;28(3):263–6.
6. Einarsson JI, Hibner M, Advincula AP. Side docking: an alternative docking method for gynecologic robotic surgery. Rev Obstet Gynecol. 2011;4(3–4):123–5.

Robotic Approaches

8

Vincent Obias and Lee J. Milas

Abstract

Minimally invasive colorectal surgery has evolved from a laparoscopic procedure to various stages of purely laparoscopic, purely robotic, and hybrid techniques. This has been driven primarily by the location of the patient's disease process, the advances in surgical skill, and the availability of enhanced technologically advanced equipment. The clinical goals have not changed. They include improved short-term outcomes, better quality of life, acceptable long-term oncologic outcomes, reduced operative times, and containing costs.

Keywords

Robotic surgery • Approaches • Minimally invasive surgery • Colorectal surgery • Enhanced technology • Full robotic approach • Sigmoid colectomy • Right hemicolectomy • Robotic rectal surgery • Natural orifice robotic surgery

Minimally invasive colorectal surgery has evolved from a laparoscopic procedure to various stages of purely laparoscopic, purely robotic, and hybrid techniques. This has been driven primarily by the location of the patient's disease process, the advances in surgical skill, and the availability of enhanced technologically advanced equipment. The clinical goals have not changed. They include improved short-term outcomes, better quality of life, acceptable long-term oncologic outcomes, reduced operative times, and containing costs [1–8].

V. Obias, M.D. (⊠)
Division of Colon and Rectal Surgery, George Washington University Hospital, 2150 Pennsylvania Ave NW, Washington, DC 20037, USA
e-mail: vobias@gmail.com

L.J. Milas, M.D.
Department of General Surgery, The George Washington University School of Medicine, Yardley, PA, USA

8.1 Robotic Colon and Rectal Surgery

Robotic colon surgery was developed to overcome some of the technical limitations of laparoscopic surgery. However, robotic systems have some disadvantages as well. Most notably, robotic techniques have limited intracorporeal range of motion impacting procedures that require a larger operative field such as colectomy. Since colectomy requires access to multiple quadrants of the abdomen, a laparoscopically assisted hybrid technique or multiple dockings of the robotic cart are necessary. Other options include utilizing different ports and redocking of only 1 or 2 arms versus fully redocking the robotic bedside cart.

8.2 Full Robotic Approach

8.2.1 Right Hemicolectomy

The patient is placed in a supine position with both arms tucked at their side. Pneumoperitoneum is established via a needle through the umbilicus. The placement of the trocars for the robotic arms and the assist port vary based on the surgeon's preference and are well described by Rawlings et al. [9] and Baik [10]. The position of the robotic cart is to the right of the patient, either at the upper right side of the patient (Rawlings, right upper oblique) or at the level of the endoscope (Baik, right vertical). The surgical table is maneuvered left side down to allow the small bowel to fall away from the surgical field. Manual movement of the endoscope can be performed to carefully examine the abdominal and pelvic contents; otherwise, it can be done robotically after the robotic cart is docked. The surgical dissection and excision generally proceed in a medial to lateral direction and are described in detail in following chapters. Extracorporeal anastomosis has been described by Baik et al. and is most commonly performed because it's familiar to laparoscopic facile surgeons and it decreases operative time as well [10]. Rawlings et al. have reported robotic intracorporeal ileotransverse anastomosis for right hemicolectomy [9].

My preferred trocar placement is to place the camera at the umbilicus, the number 3 arm subxiphoid, the number 1 arm in the left upper quadrant, and the number 2 arm in the suprapubic position. With this setup, the surgeon can do basic mobilization with an extracorporeal anastomosis or an intracorporeal anastomosis with extraction of the colon through a suprapubic extraction site. For low-BMI patients (BMI < 30), I prefer a single-port setup through the umbilicus and use 2–8 mm instruments and an 8 mm camera.

8.3 Sigmoid Colectomy

The patient is placed in a supine, modified lithotomy position with adjustable stirrups. Bolsters are sometimes placed at both shoulders to prevent sliding toward the head of the bed with movement of the operative table, and both arms are tucked to the patient sides. Pneumoperitoneum is established via a needle, and the camera port is placed periumbilically. Careful inspection of the abdominal and pelvic contents is performed as described above. The placement of the trocars for the robotic arms and the assist port vary based on the surgeon's preference and are well described by Rawlings et al. [9] and Baik [10]. The position of the robotic cart is to the left of the patient, either at the lower left side of the patient (Rawlings, left lower oblique) or at the level of the camera (Baik, left vertical). The patient is placed right side down. Baik describes a technique placing the patient in Trendelenburg position through the entire procedure, including mobilization of the splenic flexure. The robotic cart remains docked throughout, and there is no movement of the location of the robotic arms. Rawlings describes a technique starting in right side down in reverse Trendelenburg position for mobilization of the splenic flexure, and then the robotic arms are removed. The patient is then placed in the right side down Trendelenburg position, and the robotic arm locations are altered to facilitate dissection of the inferior mesenteric artery and the upper rectum. The technique reported by Baik appears to have the advantage of limited manipulation of the robotic system, but mobilization of the splenic flexure may be surgically more challenging in the Trendelenburg position. The operative time differential between these techniques has not been elucidated. The procedure details will be described in the following chapter. Some surgeons have advocated a hybrid approach for the ease of left colon mobilization, which is described below.

My preferred port placement for a sigmoid colectomy is to place the camera at the umbilicus, the number 1 port/stapler port in the right lower quadrant, the number 3 arm in the right upper quadrant/midclavicular line just two fingerbreadths below the costal margin, and the number 2 arm in the left upper quadrant just a few cm above the level of the camera. Sometimes, if a large amount of pelvic dissection is needed, I will place another 8 mm port in the LLQ where the number 3 arm will be moved after mobilization of the left colon/splenic flexure is done. Extraction is via the umbilicus or left lower quadrant if a port is placed there.

8.4   Robotic Rectal Surgery

In rectal cancer surgery, total meso-rectal excision (TME) is the standard, regardless of the surgical technique. Laparoscopic rectal surgery is limited due to the narrow anatomy of the pelvis or in the presence of locally advanced disease. High conversion rates to an open surgical approach have been demonstrated from the laparoscopic approach [11, 12].

8.4.1   Robotic Low Anterior Resection

A low anterior robotic resection is a challenging procedure because it requires dissection in the upper left quadrant for mobilization of the splenic flexure and ligation of the IMA, as well as left lower quadrant resection for TME. This would require undocking and movement of the heavy, cumbersome robotic cart and relocating the weighty robotic arms. The hybrid procedure was developed to overcome the limitations of the robotic system. Many surgeons prefer the full robotic approach and will be addressed as well. Technical development of the surgical robotic system, lighter and longer robotic arms with increase mobility, will help to overcome current system constraints [13–21].

8.4.2   Hybrid Low Anterior Resection

The patient is placed supine in a modified lithotomy position with their legs in modified lithotomy. Bolsters are placed at both shoulders to limit shifting toward the head of the bed, with both arms tucked at patient's side. Pneumoperitoneum is established by a needle. The endoscope is placed supraumbilically. Careful inspection of the abdominal and pelvic contents is performed as previously described. The placement of the trocars for the robotic arms and the assist port vary based on the surgeon's preference and are well described by Baik [10]. The patient is placed right side down and in Trendelenburg. A surgeon on the right side of the patient performs conventional laparoscopic IMA ligation and mobilization of the splenic flexure and the left colon down to the rectosigmoid junction. The robotic cart is brought in from the perineal area, between the patient's legs. The robotic arms are placed as per surgeon preference. The dissection is described in details in the following chapters. A suprapubic robotic trocar site is extended 4 cm for specimen extraction. Based on tumor anatomy, coloanal anastomosis and abdominoperineal resection can be performed.

8.4.3   Full Robotic Rectal Surgery

Hellan et al. [22] and Luca et al. [23] have all documented their robotic rectal TME techniques. The robotic cart is docked to the lower left of the patient. The procedure follows in two distinct steps with the endoscope place supraumbilical. The first step entails ligation of the IMA and IMV and mobilization of the splenic flexure and the left colon down to the rectosigmoid junction (as with the hybrid procedure). The placement of the robotic arms is per surgeon preference. The second step concerns the rectal TME and requires disengaging the robotic arms with relocation to a new or shared port site. The patient is not moved, and this does not require undocking of the robotic cart.

My preferred technique is to do a fully robotic technique. We start by finding the middle of the abdomen after insufflation and placing the camera 2 cm to the right of midline. We place the number 1 arm/stapler trocar in the RLQ. The number 3a arm is placed in the right upper quadrant in the midclavicular line, two fingerbreadths below the costal margin. The number 2 arm is placed in the left midclavicular line a few fingerbreadths above the level of the camera. The number 3b arm is placed in the LLQ. We begin by dissecting under the IMA, identifying the ureter, and taking the IMA high at its base with the robotic vessel sealer. We then do a medial to lateral dissection separating the descending colon from the retroperitoneum. The splenic flexure can be fully mobilized when the number 3a arm is used. Once the left colon and splenic flexure are fully mobilized, the number 3a arm is now moved to the LLQ 3b port, and the number 3a port can be used as an assistant port. We then do an appropriate TME for the cancer associated with the level of the cancer. Stapler is used through RLQ port, and the colon is brought out through the LLQ widened port. After transection of the bowel, we next use Firefly and ICG to make sure we have good perfusion of our anastomosis before we place our purse string. We then do an EEA anastomosis and leak test.

8.5 Natural Orifice Robotic Surgery

Natural orifice surgery has become an increasingly attractive option in the advancement of minimally invasive colorectal surgery. Whether the approach is robotic or laparoscopic, specimen extraction typically involves an abdominal incision of variable length (4–5 cm) either by extending a trocar incision or by adding a new incision into the abdominal wall. Clinical evidence indicates that abdominal incisions are associated with increased somatic pain, are prone to infection, and have an increased risk of incisional hernia [24–27]. Natural orifice specimen extraction (NOSE) is an alternative approach, whereby the resected specimen is delivered through an ana-

tomic orifice, namely, the vagina or the rectum. The hypothesized benefits of this technique are less cutaneous trauma, less postoperative pain, faster recovery, and decreased length of hospital stay.

Robotic techniques have likewise been adapted to include natural orifice specimen extraction. Choi et al. documented their robotic-assisted NOSE in colorectal cancer [28]. Thirteen patients underwent the procedure, 11 low anterior resections and 2 anterior resections. The lower anterior resections were conducted with a hybrid technique, with the ligation of the IMA and IMV, mobilization of the splenic flexure, and left colon completed laparoscopically, followed by robotic TME. All underwent complete intracorporeal resection and anastomosis of the colon or rectum. The specimen was collected in a plastic bag introduced through the anus for removal or in women with a tumor in the upper rectum or distal sigmoid colon, through a transverse colpotomy for removal. In the transvaginal cases, the colpotomy was closed robotically via intracorporeal suturing after specimen retrieval. The investigators reported that in their group of seven females, two underwent transvaginal extraction, with all of the remaining patients underwent transrectal extraction. They documented three postoperative complications, in two patients. One had an anastomotic bleed, and one had anastomotic leak, following an inferior mesenteric arterial bleed. All circumferential margins were negative, and one distal resection margin was positive. They did not find an increased occurrence of rectovaginal fistula, nor did they note intraoperative adjacent organ injury that was seen laparoscopically with transvaginal NOSE. This may be related to improved visualization and manipulation of the robotic hands in the narrow pelvis, thereby potentially giving robotics a surgical advantage for transvaginal and possibly transrectal NOSE.

Natural orifice extraction has also been employed for excision of colorectal pathology not employing laparoscopy or robotic techniques. Hellan and Maker reported a case of a 5 cm GIST tumor 3 cm above the dentate line in a 70-year-old woman, who had refused an abdominoperitoneal resection with end colostomy [29]. She agreed to and underwent a transvaginal approach. In lithotomy position, the posterior wall of the vagina was incised and then extended into the left perineum similar to an episiotomy. The tumor was displaced anteriorly by pushing through the anal canal. The $5 \times 5 \times 8$ cm mass was successfully delivered transvaginally. The muscular propria of the rectum was tumor-free, yet the tumor cells were within 0.1 mm. from the surgical margin. The authors noted that although local excision of anorectal tumors about 3 cm from the dentate line is generally approached transanally, it was felt that this tumor was too large and would risk not obtaining a tumor-free margin. Fu et al. previously reported successful transvaginal excision of rectal carcinoma about 4 cm from the dentate line in 18 women [30]. Only 1 of the 18 developed rectovaginal fistula.

8.6 Comments Regarding Patient Selection for Various Robotic Surgical Techniques

Preoperative patient selection involves assessment of the patient and the surgical technique [31–35]. Key components of deciding which surgical technique to employ are the size, location, and the colorectal disease process. This dictates which approach will best provide a surgical cure and subsequent long-term survival. Not every tumor- or disease-specific surgical approach is a suitable option for an individual patient. Patient comorbidities may limit surgical options. Morbid obesity presents significant challenges, but is not an absolute contraindication to robotic surgery. A BMI of greater than 33 kg/m^2 has been used as an exclusion criteria in cited studies. A patient with severe osteoarthritis or advanced age may not be able to maneuver into the lithotomy position or accommodate the robotic cart between their legs. The presence of significant cardiovascular or pulmonary disease may limit the patient's ability to tolerate Trendelenburg position or pneumoperitoneum. Conversely, natural orifice specimen extraction may be beneficial in the setting of significant patient morbidities, thereby avoiding an abdominal incision and possible compromise of respiratory function in a patient with COPD. Therefore, each patient and disease process must be examined from a risk-benefit standpoint in order to plan the safest surgical plan.

References

1. Weber PA, Merola S, Wasieleswski A, Ballantyne G. Telerobotic-assisted laparoscopic right and sigmoid colectomies for benign disease. Dis Colon Rectum. 2002;45:1689–94.
2. D'Annibale A, Morpurgo E, Fiscon V, et al. Robotic and laparoscopic surgery for treatment of colorectal diseases. Dis Colon Rectum. 2004;47:2162–8.
3. Delaney CP, Lynch AC, Senagore AJ, et al. Comparison of robotically performed and traditional laparoscopic colorectal surgery. Dis Colon Rectum. 2003;46:1633–39.
4. Rawlings AL, Woodland JH, Vegunta RK, et al. Robotic versus laparoscopic colectomy. Surg Endosc. 2007;21:1701–8.
5. de Souza AL, Prasad LM, Park JJ, et al. Robotic assistance in right hemicolectomy: is there a role? Dis Colon Rectum. 2010;53:1000–6.
6. Park JS, Choi GS, Park SY, et al. Randomized clinical trial of robotic-assisted versus standard laparoscopic right colectomy. Br J Surg. 2012;99:1219–26.
7. Park SY, Choi GS, Park JS, et al. Robot-assisted right colectomy with lymphadenectomy and intracorporeal anastomosis for colon cancer: technical considerations. Surg Laparosc Endosc Percutan Tech. 2012;22:1219–26.
8. D'Annibale A, Pernazza G, Morpurgo E, et al. Robotic right colon resection: evaluation of first 50 consecutive cases for malignant disease. Ann Surg Oncol. 2010;17:2856–62.
9. Rawlings AL, Woodland JH, Crawford DL. Telerobotic surgery for right and sigmoid colectomies: 30 consecutive cases. Surg Endosc. 2006;20:1713–8.
10. Baik SH. Robotic assisted colorectal surgery. In: Baik SH, editor. Robot surgery. Rijeka: InTech; 2010. p. 73–94. www.intechopen.com.
11. Guillou PJ, Quirke P, Thorpe H, et al. Short-term endpoints of conventional versus laparoscopic-assisted surgery in patients with colorectal cancer (MRC CLASICC trial): multicenter, randomized controlled trial. Lancet. 2005;365:1718–26.
12. Jayne DG, Guillou PJ, Thorpe H, et al. Randomized trial of laparoscopic-assisted resection of colorectal carcinoma: 3-year results of the UK MRC CLASICC trial group. J Clin Oncol. 2007;25:3061–8.
13. Baik SH, Ko YT, Kang CM, et al. Robotic tumor-specific mesorectal excision of rectal cancer: short-term outcome of a pilot randomized trial. Surg Endosc. 2008;22:1521–5.

14. Baek JH, Pastor C, Pigazzi A. Robotic and laparoscopic total mesorectal excision for rectal cancer: a case-matched study. Surg Endosc. 2011;25:521–5.

15. Quah HM, Jayne DG, Eu KW, et al. Bladder and sexual dysfunction following laparoscopically assisted and conventional open mesorectal resection for cancer. Br J Surg. 2002;89:1551–6.

16. Kim JY, Kim NK, Lee KY, et al. A comparative study of voiding and sexual function after total mesorectal excision with autonomic nerve preservation for rectal cancer: laparoscopic versus robotic surgery. Ann Surg Oncol. 2012;19:2485–93.

17. Luca F, Valvo M, Ghezzi TL, et al. Impact of robotic surgery on sexual and urinary functions after fully robotic nerve-sparing total mesorectal excision for rectal cancer. Ann Surg. 2013;257(4):672–8.

18. Nagtegaal ID, Van de Velde CJ, Van der Worp E, Cooperative Clinical Investigators of the Dutch Colorectal Cancer Group, et al. Macroscopic evaluation of rectal cancer resection specimen: clinical significance of the pathologist in quality control. J Clin Oncol. 2002;20:1729–34.

19. Baik SH, Kwon HY, Kim JS, et al. Robotic versus laparoscopic low anterior resection of rectal cancer: short-term outcome of a prospective comparative study. Ann Surg Oncol. 2009;16:1480–7.

20. Patriti A, Ceccarelli G, Bartoli A, et al. Short- and medium-term outcome of robot-assisted and traditional laparoscopic rectal resection. JSLS. 2009;13:176–83.

21. Pigazzi A, Luca A, Patriti A, et al. Multicentric study on robotic tumor-specific mesorectal excision for the treatment of rectal cancer. Ann Surg Oncol. 2010;17:1614–20.

22. Hellan M, Stein H, Pigazzi A. Total robotic low anterior resection with total mesorectal excision and splenic flexure mobilization. Surg Endosc. 2009; 23:447–51.

23. Luca F, Cenciarella S, Valvo M, et al. Full robotic left colon and rectal cancer resection: technique and early outcome. Ann Surg Oncol. 2009;16:1274–8.

24. Hussain A, Mahmood H, Singhal T, et al. Long-term study of port-site incisional hernia after laparoscopic procedures. JSLS. 2009;13:346–9.

25. Winslow ER, Fleshman JW, Birnbaum EH, Brunt LM. Wound complications of laparoscopic vs. open colectomy. Surg Endosc. 2002;16:1420–5.

26. Brennan TJ, Zahn PK, Pogatski-Zahn EM. Mechanism of incisional pain. Anesthesiol Clin North America. 2005;23:1–20.

27. Franklin Jr ME, Ramos R, Rosenthal D, Schuessler W. Laparoscopic colonic procedures. World J Surg. 1993;17:51–6.

28. Choi GS, Park IJ, Kang BM, Lim KH, Jun SH. A novel approach of robotic-assisted anterior resection with transanal or transvaginal retrieval of the specimen for colorectal cancer. Surg Endosc. 2009;23:2831–5.

29. Hellan M, Maker JK. Transvaginal excision of a large rectal stromal tumor: an alternative. Am J Surg. 2006;191:121–3.

30. Fu T, Liu B, Zhang S, et al. Transvaginal local excision of rectal carcinoma. Curr Surg. 2003;60:187–97.

31. Sanchez JE, Rasheid SH, Kreiger BR, Frattini JC, Marcet JE. Laparoscopic-assisted transvaginal approach for sigmoidectomy and rectocolpopexy. JSLS. 2009;13:217–20.

32. Diana M, Perretta S, Wall J, et al. Transvaginal specimen extraction in colorectal surgery: current state of the art. Colorectal Dis. 2011;13:e104–11.

33. Franklin ME, Kelley H, Kelley M, et al. Transvaginal extraction of the specimen after total laparoscopic right hemicolectomy with intracorporeal anastomosis. Surg Laparosc Endosc Percutan Tech. 2008;18:294–8.

34. Karahasanoglu T, Hamzaoglu I, Aytac E, Baca B. Transvaginal assisted totally laparoscopic single-port right colectomy. J Laparoendosc Adv Surg Tech A. 2011;21:255–7.

35. Sylla P, Rattner DW, Delgado S, Lacy AM. NOTES transanal rectal cancer resection using transanal endoscopic microsurgery and laparoscopic assistance. Surg Endosc. 2010;24:1205–10.

The Role of a Bedside Assistant

9

Anna Serur, Rebecca Rhee, and Matthew M. Philp

Abstract

Since the introduction of robotic-assisted techniques for colon and rectal surgery in 2002, the role of the first assistant has evolved to include increased responsibility. Typically in conventional laparoscopic surgery, the first assistant provides technical assistance (i.e., camera viewing, suctioning, and retraction). During robotic surgery, the operating surgeon is emerged in the performance of surgery at the console, leaving the bedside assistant responsible for continued support with robotic and laparoscopic instrumentation and more importantly responsible for the patient's safety. We aim to characterize the role of the bedside assistant and how to optimize efficiency during surgery.

Keywords

First assistant • Bedside • Robotic surgery • Laparoscopic assistant • Team

9.1 Introduction

Since the introduction of robotic surgery in a colorectal arena in 2002, more surgeons are becoming interested in performing colorectal surgery using the machine [1]. The use of the robot offers many advantages over conventional laparoscopy but also requires more training not only for the operating surgeon, but for assistants, nurses, and scrub technicians. The role of the assistant is essential in every operation but becomes much more significant in robotic surgery because the assistant is the only human interface between the patient and the robot. The

A. Serur, M.D., F.A.C.S., F.A.S.C.R.S.
Division of Colon and Rectal Surgery, Maimonides Medical Center, Brooklyn, NY, USA
e-mail: ann9002@gmail.com

R. Rhee, M.D. (✉)
Division of Colorectal Surgery, Maimonides Medical Center, 745 64th Street, 2nd Floor, Brooklyn, NY, USA
e-mail: rerhee@maimonidesmed.org

M.M. Philp, M.D.
Division of Colon and Rectal Surgery,
Department of Surgery, Temple University Hospital, Philadelphia, PA, USA

© Springer International Publishing Switzerland 2015
H. Ross et al. (eds.), *Robotic Approaches to Colorectal Surgery*,
DOI 10.1007/978-3-319-09120-4_9

Table 9.1 Clinical application of the bedside assistant

The role of the bedside assistant
• Setup of the room and draping of the robot
• Patient positioning
• Robot docking
• Provide retraction, suction, and irrigation or apply a stapler, energy device, or clip
• Instrument exchange
• Maintain a clean camera and change the angle of the camera as needed
• Assist with adjustment of robot arms
• Perform emergency undocking maneuvers if needed

Table 9.2 Qualities to look for when choosing a bedside assistant

Qualities of a good bedside assistant
• Maintains constant communication with the console surgeon
• Knows the steps of the procedure
• Has knowledge of relevant anatomy
• Understands the instruments and has technical knowledge of the robot system
• Understands the limitations of the robot

surgeon's assistant participates in preoperative setup, patient positioning, operative suite arrangement, trocar placement, intraoperative retraction, and troubleshooting [2–5] as summarized in Table 9.1. Depending on the setting one practices in, the assistant may be another attending surgeon, resident in training, a physician assistant, or an operating room nurse. The robotic assistant should know the steps of a particular operation and be able to aid and facilitate the surgeon in performing a safe and efficient operation as noted in Table 9.2. The role that the assistant takes depends on the kind of surgery performed as well as technical ability of the assistant.

Intuitive has so far came out with three da Vinci robot prototypes, each more advanced than the previous model. With the introduction of robotic suction, energy device, and stapler, the role of the assistant has evolved as well. However, not every hospital has purchased the newer components, and essential parts of surgery can still be done with the older equipment operated by the assistant.

The goal of this chapter is to define the role of the bedside surgeon and to aid surgeons who are starting out on the robot with how to use the bedside assistant more efficiently, facilitating quicker and safer surgery, leading to fewer conversions, and preventing "wear and tear" on the primary surgeon and assistant.

9.2 Preoperative Preparation

The bedside assistant should be involved in preoperative preparation of the patient and the operating suite. We usually check the patient's BMI, other comorbidities, and pre-op status including any dermatologic or neurologic problems. When operating on the elderly or patients with severe arthritis, great care should be taken when positioning them in stir-ups, and more padding should be used for the bony prominences and around the joints. Prior to a patient coming to the operating room, the bedside assistant should check with the OR staff for any concerns with the equipment, draping of the robot, or calibration of the camera.

9.2.1 Patient Positioning

Patient positioning is critical when performing colorectal surgery. A well-defined operative setup and plan can improve efficiency and patient safety when performing robotic colon resection. With robotic surgery, the surgeon is faced with unique challenges. The patient's position cannot be changed after the robot is docked. At times, patient stays in the same position putting pressure on the same places for a long time. Incorrect positioning can lead to pressure ulcers, nerve damage, and other complications. Brachial plexus nerve injuries are discovered after approximately 0.16 % of advanced laparoscopic procedures, and the risk is probably higher for robotic surgery [6].

To minimize the risk of brachial plexus injuries during robotic surgery, the arms should be tucked at the side of the patient whenever possible. Braces should be avoided. Either a moldable beanbag or nonskid mattress should be used. We use The Pink Pad-Pigazzi Positioning System

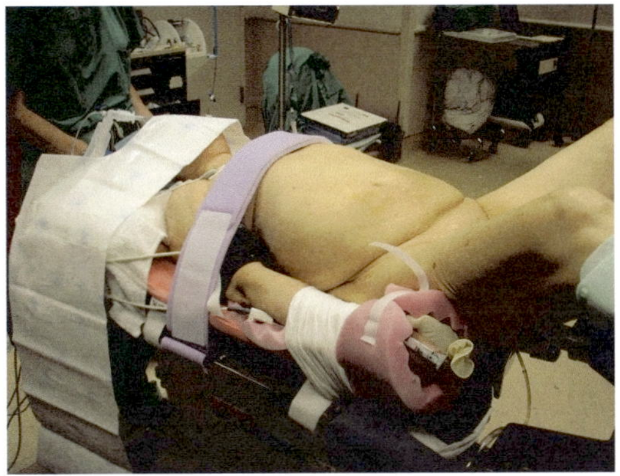

Fig. 9.1 Standard patient lithotomy positioning using The Pink Pad-Pigazzi Positioning System (Xodus Medical Inc.) for left colectomy or pelvic dissection

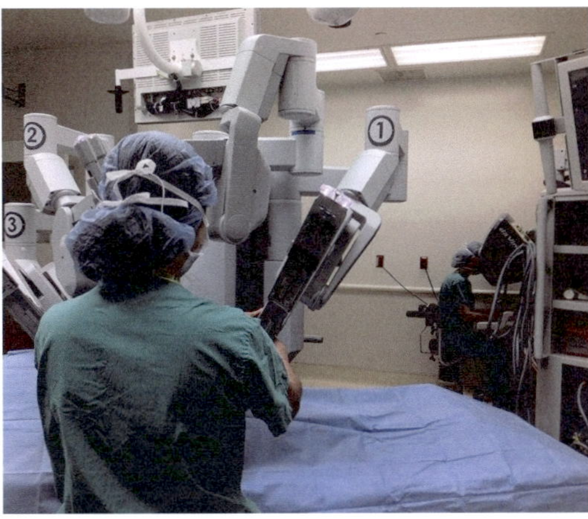

Fig. 9.2 The console surgeon is immersed in the operation, while the bedside surgeon must ensure the safe interaction between the robot and the patient

(Xodus Medical Inc.) to prevent the patient from sliding during surgery and to act as a safeguard to prevent injury by conforming to the patient body and dispersing pressure (see Fig. 9.1). It is primarily the responsibility of the assistant to ensure correct patient positioning, padding, and securing. Once positioned on the Pink Pad, it is very difficult to move the patient. Thus, the position of the mattress should be checked prior to patient's laying down on it, and the patient's positioning should be adjusted when the patient is not anesthetized.

During surgery, the bedside assistant is responsible for checking that the patient has not shifted, and the arms of the robot do not touch the patient to prevent injury. The primary surgeon is neither aware of the positioning of the arms in relation to the patient, since there are no tactile clues, nor has the visual awareness of what is occurring outside the console (see Fig. 9.2).

Once the patient has been optimally positioned and the robot is docked, the bedside assistant takes position by the patient. For a left colon or pelvic procedure, the bedside assistant typically stands on the patient's right side. During a right hemicolectomy, the assistant stands on the patient's left side. We provide the bedside assistant with a sitting stool to maximize comfort and find that the quality of laparoscopic assistance is unaffected (Fig. 9.3).

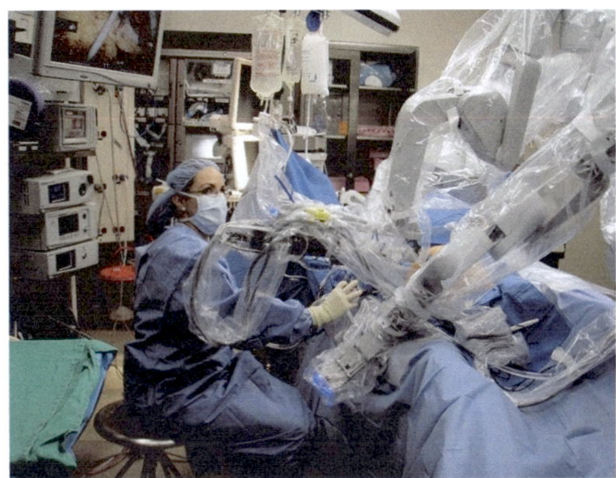

Fig. 9.3 The bedside assistant is sitting comfortably while providing laparoscopic assistance, which promotes endurance throughout the operation. Note the safe distance between the robot and the assistant

9.2.2 Port Placement

Port placement is essential to successful surgery. Each patient has a specific body habitus necessitating port positioning to be individualized. Ports placed too close to each other will hamper movement and cause clash of instruments, whereas ports placed too far from the site of surgery may not allow the instruments to reach the operative site. The bedside assistant is often the one placing the ports (Fig. 9.4).

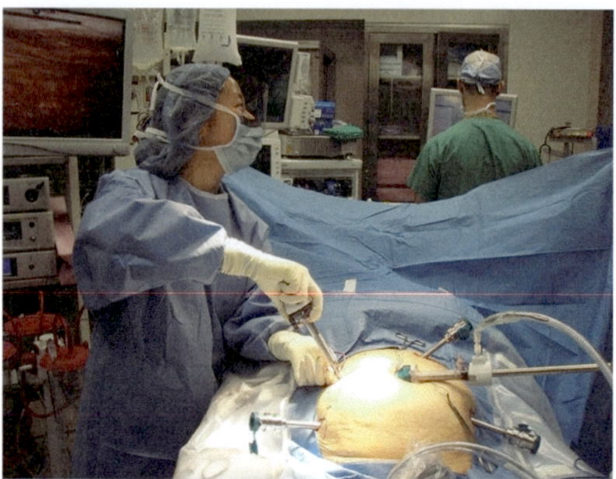

Fig. 9.4 The bedside assistant is often the surgeon who places the robotic and assistant ports

The location of the robotic and assistant ports is specific to the kind of surgery it is. The goal is to allow the bedside assistant to laparoscopically access the area of interest during the surgery while avoiding injury to the patient and assistant and allowing full mobility of the robotic arms. We recommend placing the assistant port no less than 5 cm from the robotic or camera ports.

9.3 Role in Specific Surgeries

9.3.1 Right Hemicolectomy

When performing a robotic-assisted right hemicolectomy, an assistant port is placed in the left lower quadrant. It is used for retraction when getting control of the ileocolic pedicle. If the robotic stapler or energy device is not available, the assistant can divide the pedicle using the energy device, clips, or stapler. When performing an intracorporeal anastomosis, sutures can be passed through the assistant port obviating the need to undock and thus saving time.

9.3.2 Pelvic Dissection

Most colorectal surgeons find the robot to be most useful when performing surgery in the pelvis. For a low anterior resection, abdominoperineal resection, or rectopexy, the assistant port is usually placed in the right upper quadrant. If another port

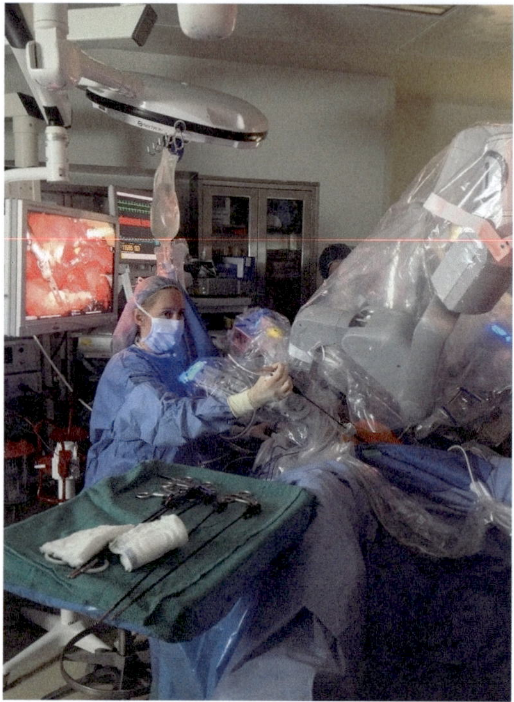

Fig. 9.5 Suprapubic assistant port access during pelvic surgery

becomes necessary, a suprapubic port can be placed approximately 2 cm above the pubic symphysis in the midline (Fig. 9.5). The key is to place the assistant port away from the camera and not in line with other ports. We usually place a 12-mm port approximately 1–2 cm lateral to the midclavicular line and either superior or inferior to the camera port approximately 8 cm superior to the anterior superior iliac spine. This position allows us to use the port for retraction in the initial steps of the operation and for passing a stapler when dividing the rectum, as well as it is very effective in suctioning during the pelvic dissection. The port can be placed at the site of the future diverting ileostomy if it is necessary. However, when placed more medially, it becomes more difficult for the assistant to maneuver the instruments in between robotic arms and occasionally dangerous because of movement of robotic arms in relation to the assistant head or hands. For left hemicolectomy, we usually use three arms only and place an assistant port in a similar location to a pelvic surgery. During surgery, it occasionally becomes necessary to place more ports. The bedside assistant should be able to choose the site and place the ports to facilitate the progression of surgery.

9.4 Robot Installation

Once the patient is placed in position, all the trocars are inserted, and the small bowel is retracted from the site of the surgery, the robot is docked. The camera arm is docked to the central port, while the lateral two or three arms are attached to the respective robotic trocars. The bedside assistant should have knowledge of how to dock and undock the arms quickly and be able to safely place the instruments. If skill level allows, the bedside assistant can receive the robot, while the console surgeon can step back from the patient allowing an overall view of robot to patient alignment to optimize initial setup.

9.5 Change of Robotic Instruments

The bedside assistant should have a thorough understanding of the various robotic instruments. After the robot has been docked, each instrument should be inserted into the robotic port, secured to the arm, and entered under direct visualization with the tip oriented toward the target anatomy. Bipolar or monopolar electrocautery cords should be attached either before or immediately after insertion of the instrument. Throughout the case, the camera will need to be intermittently cleaned, and the angle of visualization may need to be adjusted. The assistant should be adept at manipulating the camera from the port. In order to ease insertion of the camera, we prefer to insert the tip of the camera into the port before securing the hub of the camera to the robotic arm. Additionally, when changing the angle of the camera to view up or down, we prefer to minimize movement by freeing the camera from the robotic arm, rotating the lens, and securing while leaving the tip of the camera in the port (Fig. 9.6). During any operation, instruments need to be exchanged. The da Vinci Surgical System has a built-in instrument position memory to allow for easier instrument insertion throughout the case. It is imperative that the bedside assistant does not

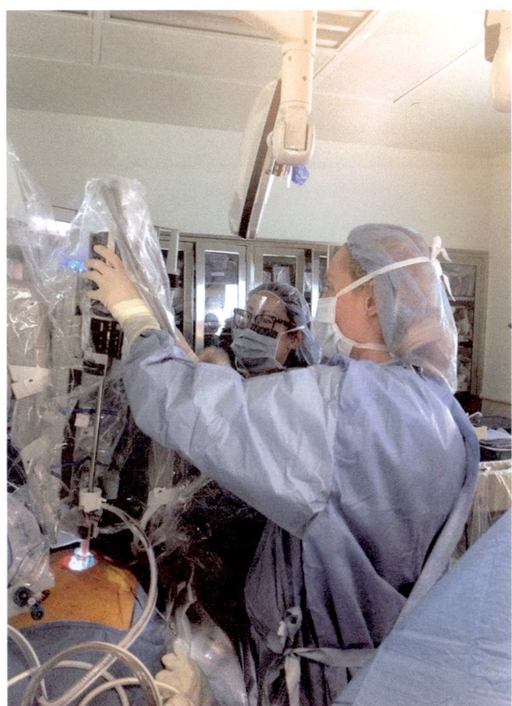

Fig. 9.6 The direction of the camera angle is changed without completely removing the camera from its holster

rely on the position memory of the robotic arm. Caution must always be taken when inserting an instrument to avoid injury to abdominal structures. The bedside assistant has to know the steps of a particular operation and be able to quickly initiate instrument exchanges. Communication between the console surgeon and bedside assistant during instrument insertion or exchange is critical to the safety of the operation. Each movement by the bedside assistant, whether it is removing or inserting an instrument or connecting an electrocautery source, should be clearly communicated to the console surgeon.

9.6 Troubleshooting

9.6.1 Robot Arm Collisions

During the procedure, internal or external collisions may occur necessitating adjustment of the robot arms. We recommend removing the instrument before manipulating the robotic arm to avoid inadvertent intra-abdominal trauma.

9.6.2 Managing Intraoperative Complications

The bedside assistant plays a critical role in maintaining the safety of the patient acting as the human intermediary between the robot and the patient. Complications may arise throughout the case including enterotomy, ureteral injury, and the most urgent of which is intraoperative hemorrhage. In most situations, this can be managed entirely by the console surgeon with the assistant providing proper exposure of the bleeding source by suctioning, providing retraction of tissues, or mobilizing surrounding structures. In other situations, the bedside assistant may obtain hemostasis by application of an energy device, clip, or intracorporeal suture.

Occasionally, a complication requires rapid undocking of the robot in preparation to convert to a laparoscopic or open procedure. The bedside assistant must effectively control the bleeding while concomitantly removing the instruments and disconnecting the arms from the ports. For example, if intraoperative hemorrhage occurs uncontrolled by the robot, the bedside assistant can use a grasper to apply pressure or grasp the bleeding vessel. The console surgeon should release any tissue being held by the instruments. If there is a system fault and the master controller cannot be used to release the tissue, the bedside assistant can use the grip release tool to manually open the grasper. The instruments and endoscope should be rapidly removed, and the arms should be disconnected from the cannulae. As an alternative, once the instruments are removed, the robotic arms can be pulled removing the ports at the same time allowing even faster access to the abdomen from the bedside. However, it is imperative to note that the robot cannot be moved away from the patient until all of the arms are removed from the cannulae unless it is placed in neutral mode. Once the robot is switched from drive to neutral mode, the robot can be pulled away from the bed (Fig. 9.7a, b). The skills of the assistant may be the determining factor if the operation proceeds in the minimally invasive way.

9.6.3 Safety of the Bedside Assistant

A challenge unique to the bedside assistant in robotic surgery is to avoid physical trauma from contact with a moving robotic arms. The operating surgeon is typically immersed in the operative field making him/her unaware of the sudden movement observed of the robotic arms when working throughout the abdomen. The bedside surgeon must be aware of the spatial relationships of the robotic arms to his face, arms, chest, and groin areas. When not engaged laparoscopically in the surgical procedure, the assistant should maintain a safe distance away from the patient.

One way to prevent trauma to the bedside assistant is to maintain constant communication between the bedside and console surgeons. In addition, a bedside assistant will prevent injury by anticipating the steps of the surgery and thus anticipating the movement of the robotic arms. Optimally, the console surgeon should notify the assistant every time the operative field shifts. For instance, after the IMA pedicle is divided and medial to lateral dissection is completed, the surgeon should announce that the lateral attachments are to be divided next. When shifting from the splenic flexure takedown to the pelvic dissection, another warning should be made since the angle of the arms changes completely. In general, sudden movements should be avoided.

9.7 Learning the Procedure

Since more teaching institutions are incorporating robotic surgery into their practice, training on the robot is becoming a part of surgical education. The importance of hands-on training is paramount in developing both laparoscopic and robotic skills. Patient-side assistance is the principal means of acquiring these skills. The bedside assistant is expected to be a safe and efficient assistant but also to acquire necessary skills to graduate to the console surgeon's position. As with laparoscopic surgery, the residents are

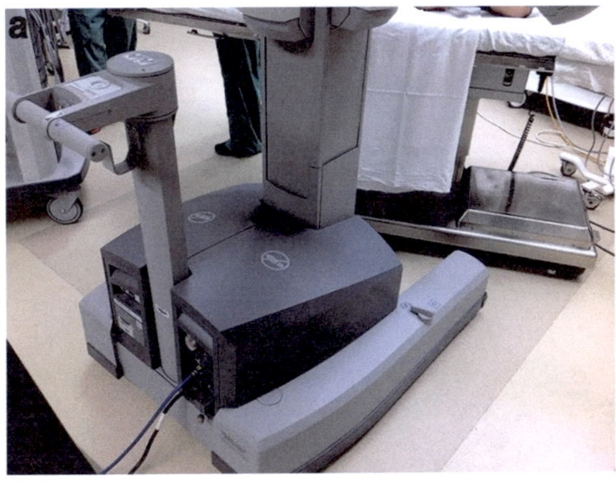
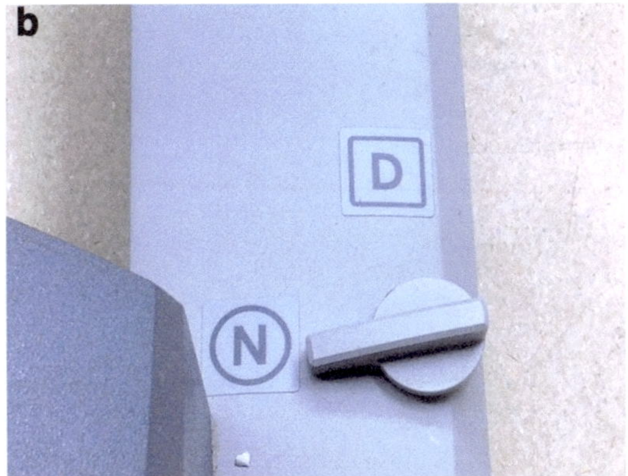

Fig. 9.7 In an emergency conversion to open situation, the bedside assistant can remove the ports attached to the robotic arms, and the robot (**a**) can be moved away from the patient by turning the switch on the bedside cart to neutral (**b**)

expected to participate in pre-, intra-, and postoperative care of the patient [7].

Simulation labs are used in many hospitals to educate the residents and advance their skills. Computer modules and training modules on the actual machine should be used to train the residents in preparation for independent practice.

9.8   Conclusion

In order to perform or to assist in robotic colorectal surgery, one should have the fundamental knowledge of surgical techniques, have familiarity with steps of a particular operation, have detailed knowledge of robotic instruments, and be able to troubleshoot and react quickly. Some centers have presented their experience in having no bedside assistants, facilitating solo surgery [8]. In our opinion, the assistant is a much needed entity in ensuring the safety and efficiency of robotic colorectal surgery, and his role is not going away just yet.

References

1. AlAsari S, Soh Min B. Robotic colorectal surgery: a systematic review. ISRN Surg. 2012;2012:1–12.
2. Smith J, Tewari A. Role of patient side surgeon in robotics. In: Robotics in urologic surgery. Philadelphia: Elsevier Saunders; 2008. p. 31–7.
3. Martin S. The role of the first assistant in robotic assisted surgery. Br J Perioper Nurs. 2004;14(4): 159–63.
4. Yuh B. The bedside assistant in robotic surgery—keys to success. Urol Nurs. 2013;33(1):1–4.
5. Ardilla B, Orvieto M, Patel V. Role of the robotic surgical assistant. In: Robotic urologic surgery. 2nd ed. New York: Springer; 2012. p. 495–505.
6. Shveiky D, Aseff JN, Iglesia CB. Brachial plexus injury after laparoscopic and robotic surgery. J Minim Invasive Gynecol. 2010;17(4):414–20.
7. Chiu A, Browne WB, Sookrai KA, Zenilman ME, Fingerhut A, Ferzli GS. The role of the assistant in laparoscopic surgery: important considerations for the apprentice-in-training. Surg Innov. 2008;15(3): 229–36.
8. Drasin T, Dutson E, Gracia C. Use of a robotic system as a surgical first assistant in advanced laparoscopic surgery. J Am Coll Surg. 2004;199(3):368–73.

Part III

The Procedures: All Appropriate Approaches to Mobilization, Vessel Division, Specimen Extraction, and Anastomosis Will Be Described

Right Colectomy Procedure Guide

10

Kelly Olino, Tushar Samdani, and Julio Garcia-Aguilar

Abstract

This chapter outlines our technique of robotic right hemicolectomy, which we have successfully used in over 100 patients. We generally prefer the three-port technique for extracorporeal right hemicolectomy and the four-port technique for planned intracorporeal anastomosis. There are numerous approaches to dissection of the right colon, but we utilize the medial to lateral approach. This can be modified, based upon surgeon preference. Robotic-assisted right hemicolectomy affords accurate dissection and enhanced visualization and can serve as an alternative platform for the minimally invasive approach.

Keywords

Right hemicolectomy • Intracorporeal right hemicolectomy • Intracorporeal anastomosis • Robotic assisted • Minimally invasive surgery • Instruments • Patient selection • Patient preparation • Patient positioning • Port placement

10.1 Instruments and Accessories

- Basic accessory kit and drapes
- Veress needle
- Laparoscopic 10-mm balloon port trocar (camera port)
- Robotic camera head
- Robotic 0° and 30° endoscopes
- 5-mm laparoscopic camera (in cases where adhesions are anticipated)
- Camera warmer
- Robotic 8-mm trocars (one vented, one non-vented)
- Laparoscopic 5-mm trocar

Electronic supplementary material: This chapter contains video segments that can be found on the following DOI: 10.1007/978-3-319-09120-4_10

K. Olino, M.D. • T. Samdani, M.D.
J. Garcia-Aguilar, M.D., Ph.D. (✉)
Department of Surgery, Memorial Sloan Kettering Cancer Center, 1275 York Avenue, New York, NY 10065, USA
e-mail: garciaaj@mskcc.org

© Springer International Publishing Switzerland 2015
H. Ross et al. (eds.), *Robotic Approaches to Colorectal Surgery*,
DOI 10.1007/978-3-319-09120-4_10

- Smoke evacuator
- 5-mm suction/irrigation device
- Laparoscopic bowel graspers
- Monopolar curved scissors
- Fenestrated bipolar forceps
- Robotic vessel sealer
- Cadiere forceps
- Robotic needle driver (intracorporeal suture)
- Robotic stapler (intracorporeal suture)
- Small Alexis wound protector

10.2 Patient Selection and Preparation

10.2.1 Patient Selection

A number of prospective randomized trials have proven that laparoscopic colectomy reduces postoperative pain, improves short-term outcomes, and provides similar oncologic outcomes compared to open colectomy. The benefits of robotic-assisted colectomy compared to the conventional laparoscopic approach are debatable. Retrospective reviews and a recent meta-analysis indicate that robotic and laparoscopic colectomies are associated with similar complication rates and short-term outcomes. The robotic approach shows trends for lower rates to open conversion and higher rates of intracorporeal anastomosis [1–4]. In the only randomized clinical trial comparing laparoscopic to robotic-assisted right hemicolectomy, surgical and oncologic outcomes were similar [1]. However, time, operating room charges, and overall costs are higher for robotic colectomy.

A right hemicolectomy is an ideal procedure for surgeons beginning to perform robotic-assisted minimally invasive surgery. Patient selection criteria are similar to those of traditional laparoscopic surgery. Due to the enhanced visualization and increased dexterity provided by the robotic platform, this approach is particularly helpful in patients with bulky lymphadenopathy requiring dissection close to the superior mesenteric artery and vein. The robotic platform also facilitates the performance of a total mesocolic excision for tumors located in the vicinity of the hepatic flexure that require dissection of the right gastroepiploic vessels. Contraindications for robotic right colectomy are similar to those for laparoscopic colectomy: patients with locally advanced tumors requiring resection of adjacent organs, patients with peritoneal carcinomatosis, patients with extensive peritoneal adhesions, or those not able to tolerate insufflation.

10.2.2 Patient Preparation

Patients scheduled for robotic-assisted right hemicolectomy undergo oral mechanical bowel preparation with a clear liquid diet and a polyethylene glycol-based agent, in combination with oral antibiotics, on the day prior to surgery. Before induction of anesthesia, a prophylactic dose of low molecular weight heparin and antibiotics are administered. An intravenous dose of a broad-spectrum antibiotic covering gram-negative bacteria and anaerobes is delivered before making the surgical incision.

10.2.3 Operating Room (or) Configuration

The operating room should be spacious enough to allow sufficient room for the surgeon, assistant, scrub nurse, patient cart, robot console, camera tower, and CO_2 insufflation machine. The robot should be positioned on the patient's right side prior to draping, and the robot arms positioned such that arm 1 is positioned toward the head of the patient, the camera arm is centered, and arms 2 and 3 are placed toward the patient's feet. The bedside operating assistant stands on the patient's left side, and the scrub technician and instrument table should be positioned on the left side near the patient's feet. The anesthesia team retains its normal position at the head of the bed. The robot is docked obliquely over the right shoulder, at an almost 45° angle in relation to the axis of the operating table. The video monitors, intravenous fluid poles, equipment booms, and the anesthesia cart should be positioned so as to avoid interference with the cart or robotic arms. Figure 10.1 shows an overhead view of the recommended OR configuration.

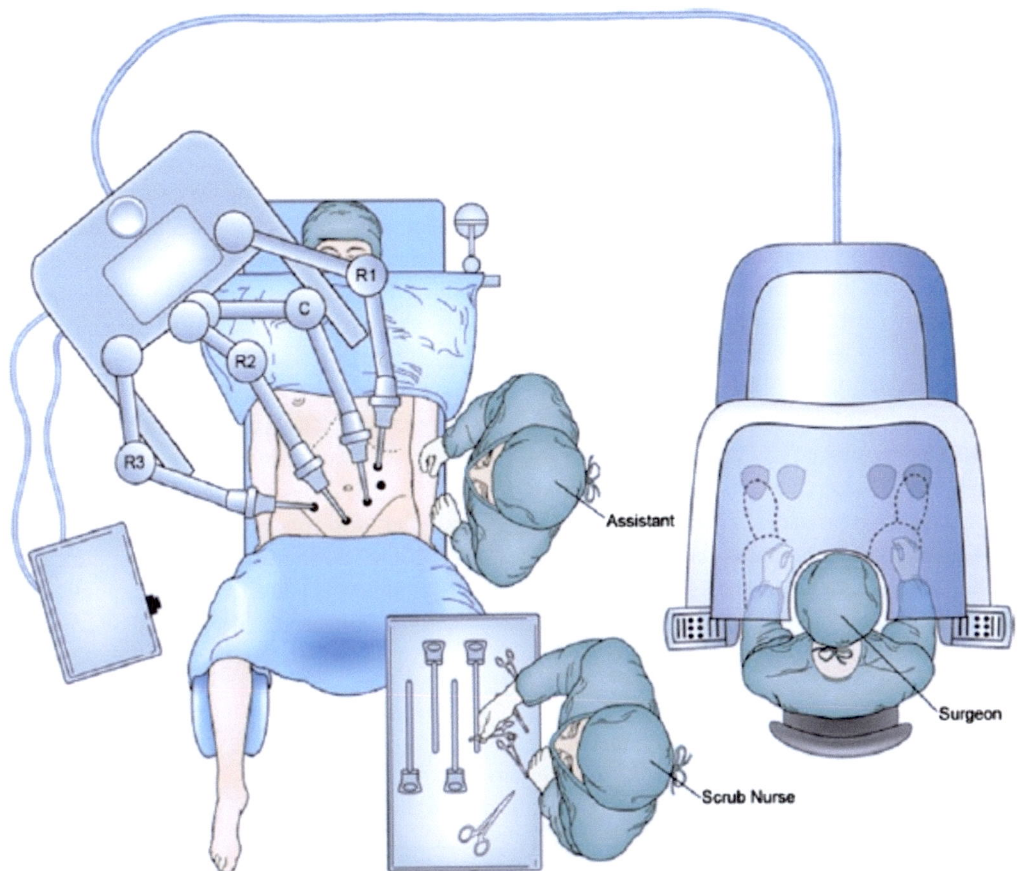

Fig. 10.1 Operating room setup. *With permission from Gossedge G, Jayne D. Robotic Technique for Right Colectomy. In: Kim J, Garcia-Aguilar J, eds. Surgery for* *Cancers of the Gastrointestinal Tract: A Step by Step Approach. Springer, New York 2015; pp. 187–194*

10.3 Positioning, Port Placement, and Docking

10.3.1 Patient Positioning

After intubation and placement of a urinary catheter, orogastric tube, and IV access, the patient is positioned supine with the iliac crest centered over the flexion point joint (break) of the table. The patient's arms are tucked alongside the body and padded to lessen the possibility of brachial plexus injury. This also allows for easier docking of the robot and provides extra space for the assistant at bedside. Pressure points and bony prominences are padded, and the body is secured to the operating table with straps around the legs and shoulders. We also prefer to use antiskid foam cushion in order to avoid the patient sliding with changes in position. Finally, the patient is covered with an upper body warmer to prevent hypothermia. Sequential compression devices are applied to the legs for DVT prophylaxis. (If needed, the table can be flexed 10–15° at the break to lower the patient's legs, in order to prevent external collisions with the robotic arms after docking.) Final table adjustments should be made prior to draping, and an initial safety check performed with the bed rotated in all necessary planes—most importantly in Trendelenburg and left-sided tilt position.

10.3.2 Port Placement

When performing robotic-assisted right hemicolectomy, thought must be given prior to port placement and decisions made based upon the patient's size and body habitus, extent of the dissection of the transverse colon, and whether an intra- or extracorporeal anastomosis is planned. In general, we recommend a 4-trocar approach (camera, two robotic trocars, and an auxiliary laparoscopic trocar) when an extracorporeal anastomosis is planned. In this case, the specimen is extracted by extending the incision used for the camera trocar. The intracorporeal anastomosis requires one additional robotic or laparoscopic large-bore trocar (12–15 mm) to introduce the stapler. Basic principles for port placement dictate that the camera port be 15–18 cm from the site of dissection, and the distance between ports, following insufflation, should be around 8 cm to prevent collisions.

10.3.2.1 Camera Port, 12 mm

Pneumoperitoneum is established either with a Veress needle placed in Palmer's point so as to achieve insufflation of 12–15 mmHg. A 10–12-mm balloon port for the camera is placed either supraumbilically or to the left of the umbilicus, 2–3 cm medial to the midclavicular line (MCL), depending upon body habitus and site of the lesion. (The spino-umbilical line is drawn from the anterior superior iliac spine to the umbilicus.) Alternatively, the open Hasson technique can be used. The camera is then introduced, and inspection for metastatic disease is performed.

10.3.2.2 Four-Port Robotic Right Hemicolectomy with Planned Extracorporeal Anastomosis

The position of the robotic and laparoscopic trocars is only decided after pneumoperitoneum has been created:

- *Instrument Arm 1, Vented Robotic Port, 8 mm*: Place the port approximately two fingerbreadths below the left costal margin along the left MCL. The distance to the camera port should be at least 8–10 cm. This port should be vented to connect the smoke evacuator.

- *Instrument Arm 2, Robotic Port, 8 mm*: This port is placed in the vicinity of the intersection of the left MCL with the SUL and always more than two fingerbreadths medial to left anterior superior iliac spine. However, it is important to take into consideration the fact that the instrument introduced through this trocar should reach the hepatic flexure and may need to be moved medially in large patients. The distance to other instrument ports and the camera port should be at least 8–10 cm.

- *Assistant Port (5 mm)*: Place a 5-mm laparoscopic port lateral to the left MCL, at least 8–10 cm away from both instrument arms.

- *Instrument Arm 3*: Some surgeons prefer to use the third robotic arm to obtain additional exposure during the dissection. An 8- or 12-mm port is placed in the suprapubic area at least two fingerbreadths above the pubic bone.

10.3.2.3 Five-Port Robotic Right Hemicolectomy with Intracorporeal Anastomosis (Fig. 10.1)

- When an intracorporeal anastomosis is planned, some surgeons prefer to place the camera port to the left of the umbilicus and at least 2–3 fingerbreadths from the MCL.

- *Instrument Arm 1 and 2 ports and a laparoscopic auxiliary port* are placed for an extracorporeal anastomosis.

- *For Instrument Arm 3*, a 12-mm trocar (either robotic or laparoscopic, depending on the stapling device used) is placed in the suprapubic area, 2–3 fingerbreadths above the pubic bone and to the right of the midline. The incision for this trocar should be in transverse orientation, so that it can be enlarged to create a small Pfannenstiel incision in order to remove the specimen.

10.3.2.4 Exposing the Area of Dissection

Prior to docking the robot, the bed is tilted left side down with slight Trendelenburg positioning. When an intracorporeal anastomosis is planned, the operating room table can be flexed slightly at the hips (kidney bend) to gain additional range of motion for instrument arm 3 and avoid collision with the patient's legs. After inspecting the peritoneal cavity, the omentum and the transverse colon are pushed cephalad over the stomach using laparoscopic instruments. The small intestine is gently moved to the left to expose the ileocolic pedicle and duodenum.

10.3.3 Robotic Cart Docking and Instrument Placement

A clear path for the patient cart free of all cords and other equipment should be made prior to driving the draped patient cart. The cart should approach the OR table from the right, at a 45° degree angle over the right shoulder.

When docking the arms, it is important to ensure that the camera port, target anatomy, and robotic cart center column are aligned. Port and arm clutch maneuvers should be used to dock the remaining instrument arms. Once the cart is docked, the position of the bed cannot be changed without undocking. While docking, the camera arm should be in the "sweet spot" to maximize range of motion for the camera and instrument arms. The blue arrow should align with the blue marker on the second joint or create a 90° angle between the first and third joint on the camera arm. When using all three instrument arms, it is useful to place the arm joints as lateral as possible away from the field, to avoid collision.

10.3.3.1 Loading the Robotic Arms with Instruments

Four-Port Robotic Right Hemicolectomy with Extracorporeal Anastomosis (Fig. 10.2)

- Camera Arm: After weight balancing, a warmed robotic 0° endoscope is inserted into the camera port. The entire procedure can usually be performed with a 0° endoscope, but a 30° endoscope may be required for optimal exposure in obese patients with a deep hepatic flexure.
- Instrument Arm 1 Port, 8 mm: Monopolar curved scissors and the robotic vessel sealer are used most often in this port.
- Instrument Arm 2 Port, 8 mm: A bipolar grasper or a Cadiere grasper is used to hold the bowel and provides exposure for dissection.
- Assistant Port (5 mm): The suction irrigator and laparoscopic bowel grasper are commonly used by the assistant during the procedure.

Five-Port Robotic Right Hemicolectomy with Intracorporeal Anastomosis

- Instrument Arm 3: A Cadiere grasper can be used for additional tissue exposure during the dissection. However, this instrument arm will be used mainly for the introduction of the stapler and/or the robotic needle driver during the anastomosis.

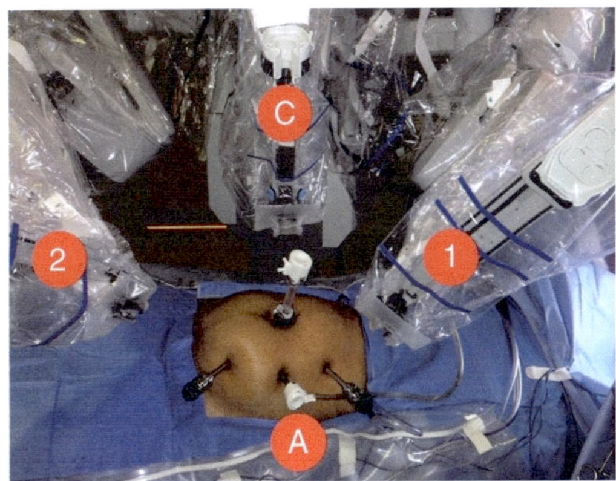
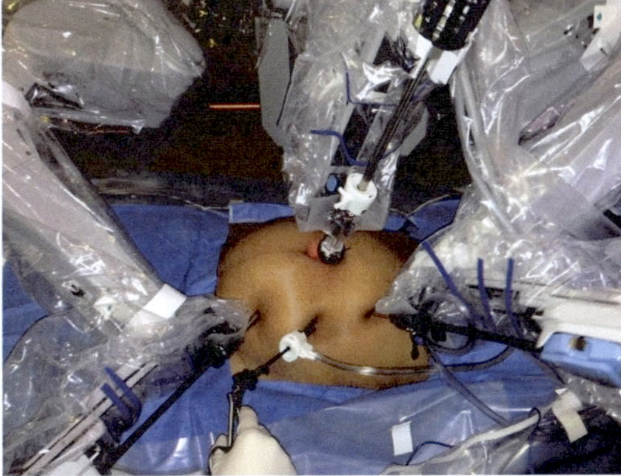

Fig. 10.2 Robotic docking and instrument position

10.4 Procedure Steps

10.4.1 Right Hemicolectomy

10.4.1.1 Initial Exposure

We prefer to use a medial to lateral approach. However, the procedure can be performed with a lateral to medial approach. If not performed previously, the omentum is retraced cephalad, and the small bowel to the patient's left, in order to expose the colonic mesentery. The assistant may have to continue to hold appropriate retraction, particularly in obese patients with sizeable omentum (see Video 10.1).

10.4.1.2 Vascular Control

High Ligation of Ileocolic Vessels
The course of the ileocolic vessels is demonstrated by grasping the mesentery at the ileocolic junction and pulling gently toward the left lower quadrant. Once identified, the fenestrated bipolar grasper (arm 2) is used to hold up the ileocolic vessel about 5 cm from its takeoff from the SMA (Fig. 10.3). A robotic monopolar scissor (arm 1) is used to score the peritoneum on the medial side of the ileocolic vessels and enter the retroperitoneum (Fig. 10.3). A small cave is created underneath the mesentery by posteriorly sweeping the retroperitoneal structures and the duodenum. The dissection is continued until the origin of the ileocolic vessels in the superior mesenteric vessels is reached.

The peritoneum around the origin of the ileocolic vessels is scored to expose the origin of the superior mesenteric vessels and the duodenum. Once the anatomy is defined, the ileocolic vessels are skeletonized near the origin leaving the mesenteric nodes in the specimen side (Fig. 10.3). The vessels are then divided either between Hem-o-lok® clips or with the vessel sealer® (Fig. 10.3).

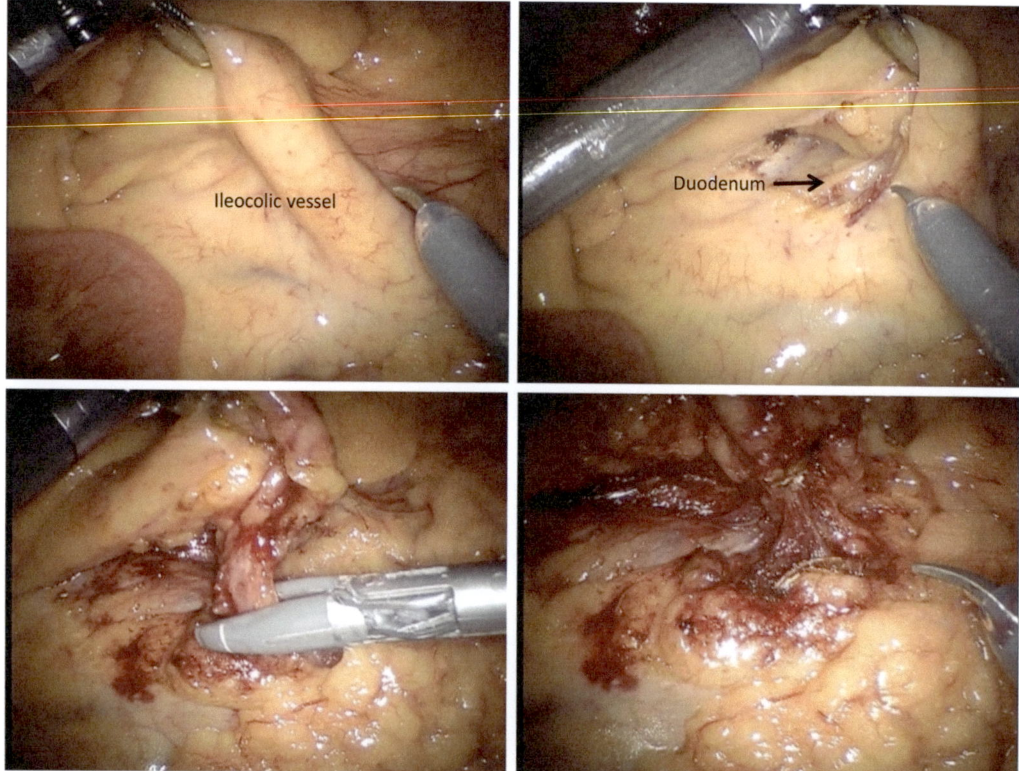

Fig. 10.3 Dissection and division of ileocolic pedicle

10.4.1.3 Medial to Lateral Dissection

The mesocolon is lifted from Toldt's fascia and the retroperitoneal structures bluntly and sharply, with the monopolar scissors reintroduced through arm 1 (Fig. 10.4). The dissection continues laterally, using the bipolar forceps to provide counter-tension until the abdominal wall is reached. The dissection continues along this plane superiorly and medially over the duodenum and the head of the pancreas. This avascular plane should be easily identified, as the pancreas has a different color and texture than the mesocolic fat (Fig. 10.4). The dissection is then continued at the root of the mesentery along the superior mesenteric vessels, until the origin of the right colic vessels is encountered. The vascular anatomy in this area is variable, and some patients do not have a right colic artery (Fig. 10.4). In these patients, the next vessels encountered are the middle colic vessels. Again, after carefully inspecting the anatomy, the vessel is dissected clearly down to the origin and divided with the vessel sealer. The right branch of the middle colic is also routinely divided (Fig. 10.4).

For tumors located on the right side of the transverse colon, an extended right colectomy may be required. In those cases, the trunk of the middle colic vessels is divided close to the origin. In the presence of bulky lymphadenopathy at the origin of the middle colic vessels, this portion of the dissection can be particularly challenging, as the lymph nodes may adhere to both the pancreas and the root of the mesentery. For these tumors, we recommend removing the lymph nodes along with the right gastroepiploic vessels, which can be dissected and divided near the head of the pancreas from beneath the mesocolon (Fig. 10.5).

Once the vascular pedicles have been divided and the right side of the transverse mesocolon separated from the pancreas and retroperitoneum, we then turn our attention to the greater omentum and the gastroepiploic arcade. The colon and mesentery are pulled toward the pelvis.

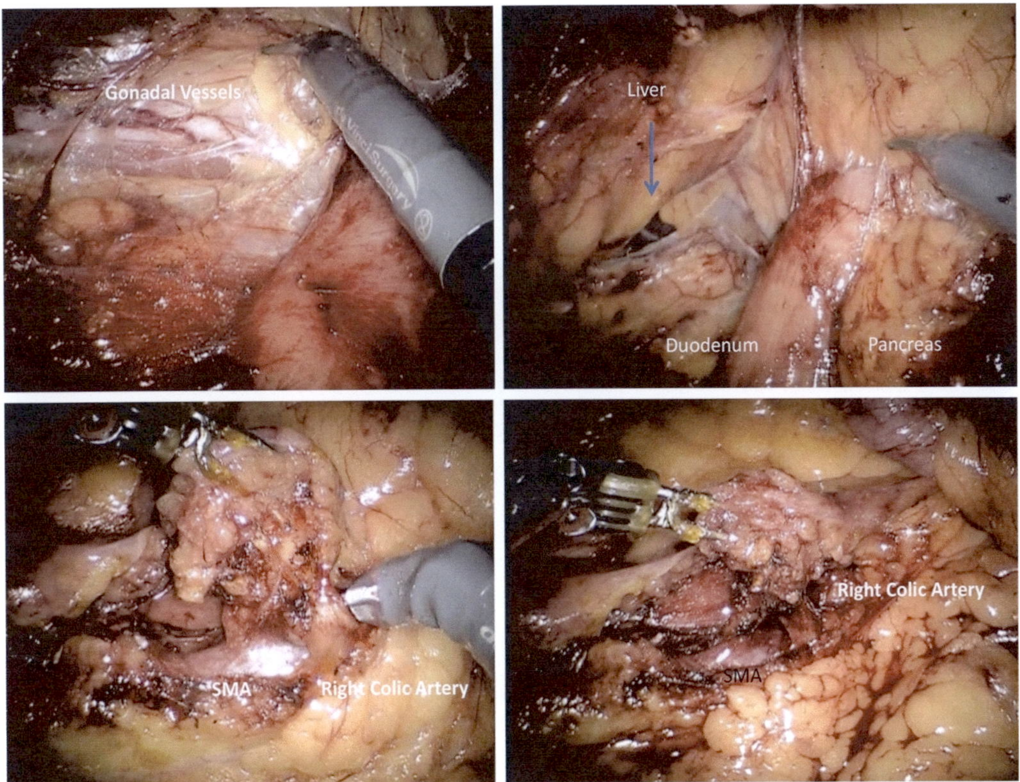

Fig. 10.4 Medial to lateral dissection and division right colic artery

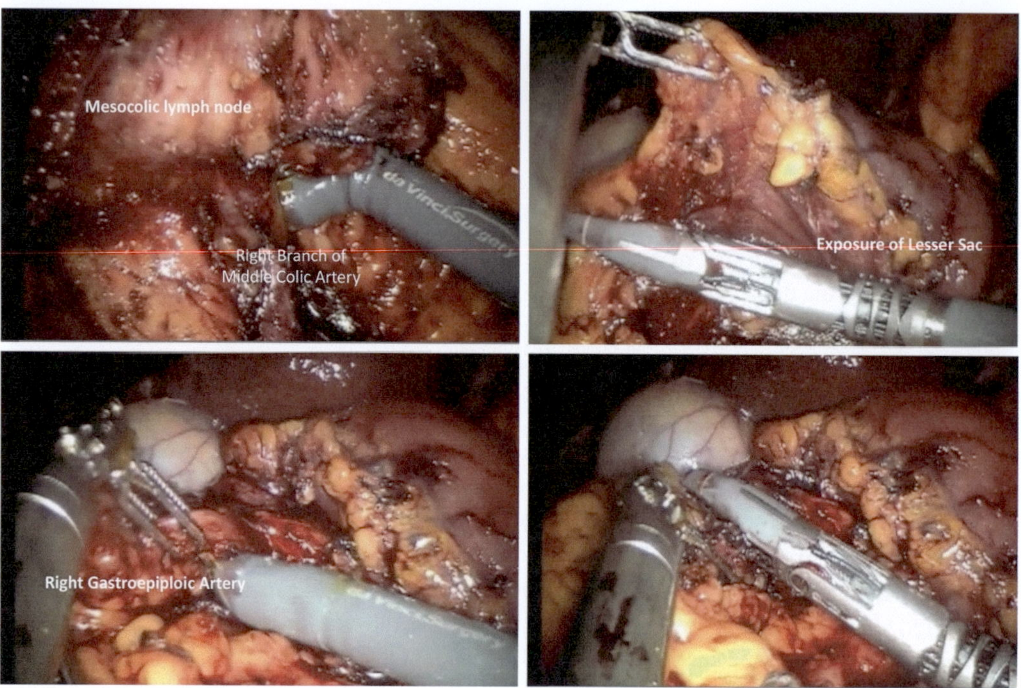

Fig. 10.5 Dissection of right colic with bulky lymphadenopathy, entrance into lesser sac, and division of right gastro-epiploic pedicle

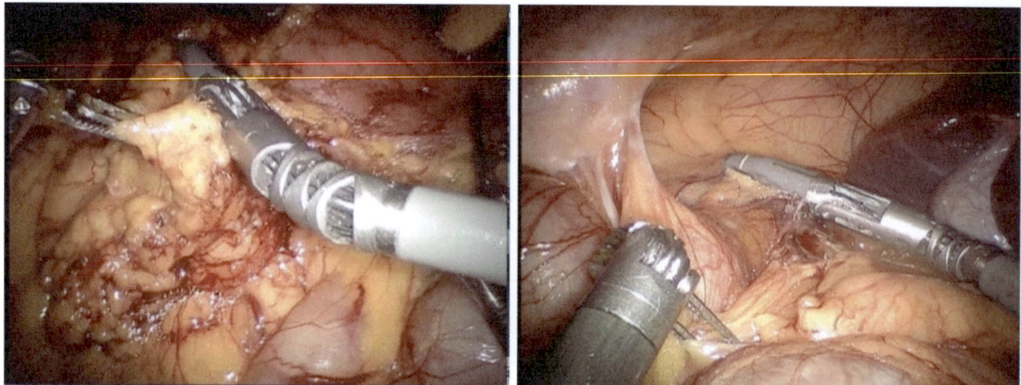

Fig. 10.6 Standard entrance into lesser sac with sparing of the right gastroepiploic pedicle with mobilization of lateral colon attachments

For a standard right colectomy, the omental vessels are divided outside the gastroepiploic, using the vessel sealer. At this point, it is important to enter the lesser sac, which is often partially obliterated by adhesions. Once the lesser sac is exposed, the surgeon encounters the plane of dissection already developed from beneath the transverse mesocolon. The attachments of the omentum and the colon are sequentially divided from medial to lateral, around the hepatic flexure, and toward the ascending colon. Finally, the cecum, appendix, and terminal ileum are mobilized by dividing the peritoneal attachments in the right lower quadrant. Care should be taken to avoid injuring the gonadal vessels or the right ureter (Fig. 10.6).

10.4.1.4 Division of the Mesentery and Omentum

Ample mobilization of the terminal ileum is recommended, particularly when an extracorporeal anastomosis is anticipated. The mesentery of the terminal ileum is divided with the vessel sealer approximately 5–6 cm away from the ileocolic vessels (Fig. 10.7).

Attention is turned to the transverse mesocolon held in place by the bipolar grasper (arm 2) and the laparoscopic assistant grasper. The marginal arteries are sealed with a vessel sealer, and the mesentery is divided parallel to the vasa recta all the way to the bowel wall. The omentum is then divided at the same level as the transverse mesocolon. The portions of the transverse colon and mesocolon distal to the point of transection should be mobile to allow a tension-free anastomosis, particularly when an extracorporeal anastomosis is anticipated.

10.4.1.5 Anastomosis and Specimen Removal

Extracorporeal Anastomosis

Once the entire right colon is mobilized and hemostasis is confirmed, the appendix is held with a laparoscopic bowel grasper through the assistant port. The robot is then undocked, releasing the robotic arms but leaving the trocars in place. The robotic cart is carefully backed away from the patient. One must make certain to raise the level of the arms to avoid trauma to the patient. The camera port incision is extended up to 4 cm, and a wound protector is placed. The appendix is delivered into the incision site and the specimen delivered outside the body for extracorporeal anastomosis. We prefer to perform a stapled side-to-side functional end-to-end anastomosis, after carefully ensuring proper alignment of the mesentery. After the anastomosis is performed, we do not close the mesenteric defect. The fascia from the specimen retrieval site is irrigated, and figure-of-8 sutures are used to close the fascia with reabsorbable monofilament sutures. We prefer to close the skin of the midline incision with vertical mattress nylon stitches and the port sites with subcuticular monofilament reabsorbable sutures (Fig. 10.8).

Intracorporeal Anastomosis

The terminal ileum and the transverse colon are divided with a laparoscopic or robotic stapler. We prefer a functional end-to-end anastomosis. The ends of the terminal ileum and the transverse colon are aligned side to side with interrupted stitches for at least 8 or 10 cm in length, ensuring contact with the antimesenteric borders. The sutures are kept long to facilitate orientation of the bowel while the stapler is fired. The sutures holding the bowel together are placed by arms 1 and 3. Arm 2 is used to create enterotomies with a monopolar scissor in the transverse colon, about 2 cm proximal to the stapled ends. The openings should be large enough to accommodate the stapler. The sutures are then held with arms 1 and 2,

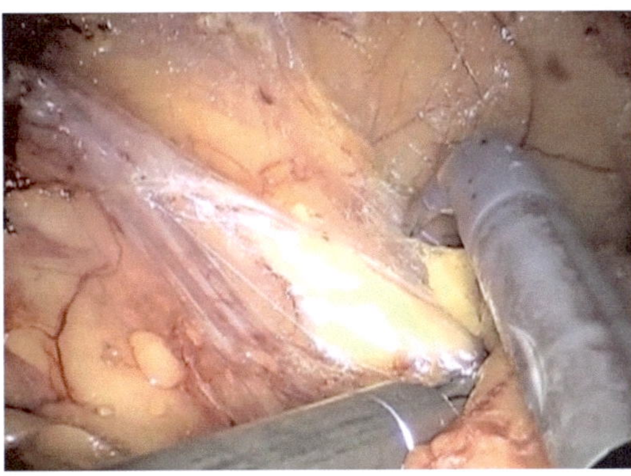
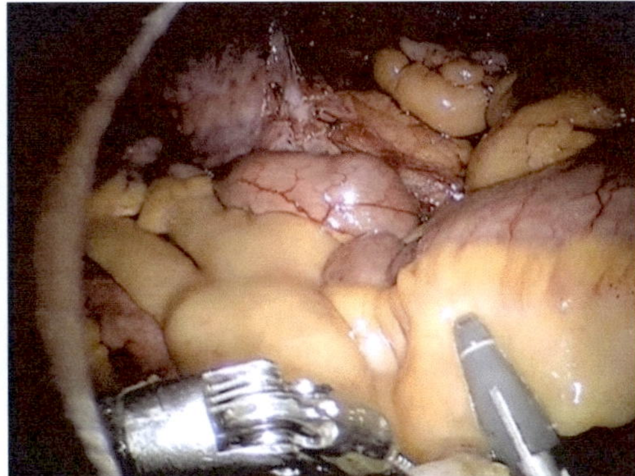

Fig. 10.7 Mobilization of the terminal ileum with division of the mesentery

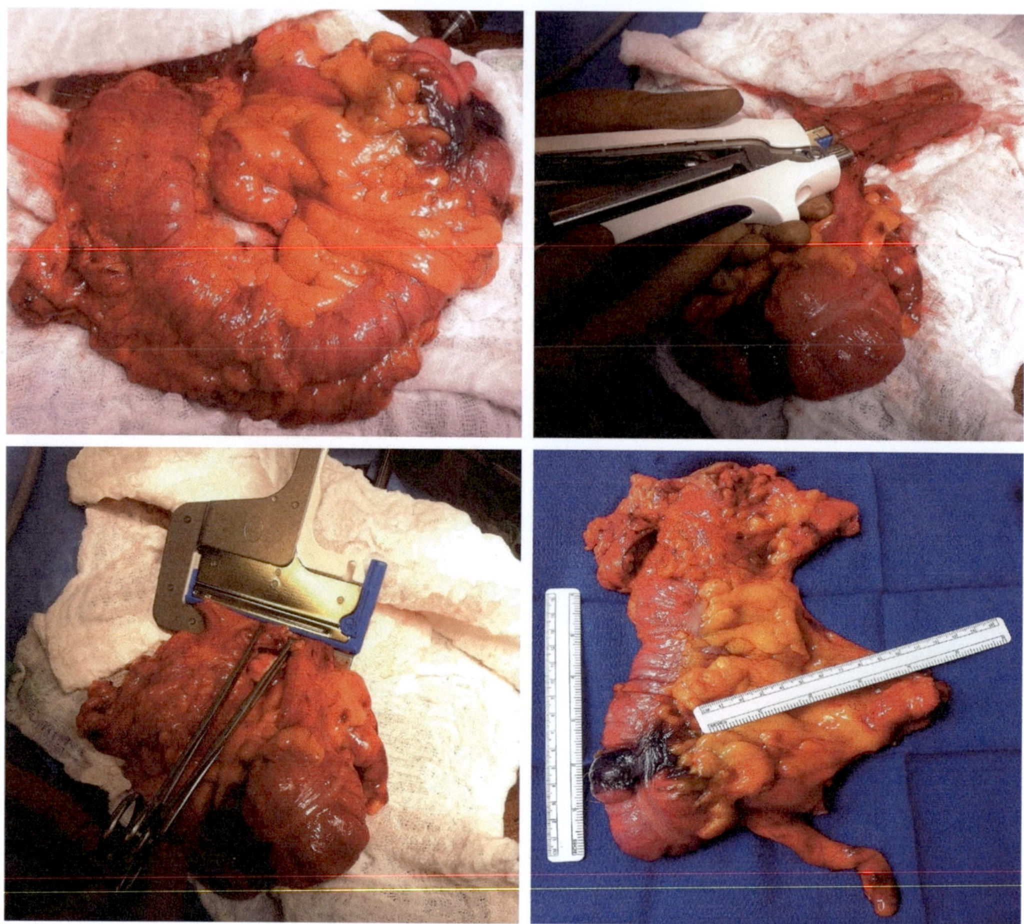

Fig. 10.8 Extracorporeal ileocolonic anastomosis

and a 45-mm robotic stapler with a blue load (3.5 mm staples) is now introduced through the 15-mm port and directed toward the bowel opening. The stapler is oriented so that the broader jaw is placed into the enterotomy in the transverse colon and the smaller jaw in the ileum. The stay sutures are used to advance the tissue onto the stapler. The assistant can help align the bowel so that the stapler fires along the antimesenteric borders. The common enterotomy is closed with interrupted absorbable sutures. The staple lines are inspected for excessive bleeding, malformed staples, or tissue gaps, and the peritoneal cavity is inspected for any bleeding and to ensure proper orientation of the bowel. Once hemostasis is confirmed, the specimen is held with laparoscopic bowel grasper, while the robotic arms are undocked, and the robotic cart is moved away from the bed. The incision of the port for arm 3 is extended to deliver the specimen, and a wound protector is placed. Once the specimen is removed, this incision and the camera port are closed with PDS suture. The skin is then closed.

10.5 Postoperative Care

Postoperative pain management is minimal, with patients requiring IV narcotics through the first postoperative day. Diet can be advanced as tolerated. Most patients have return of bowel function by postoperative day 2–3. We have had patients discharged as early as postoperative day 2, but the time of average discharge is day 3.

10.6   Key Points

- To avoid intraoperative complications, create adequate exposure, and use proper traction and countertraction. As there is no tactile feedback, great attention must be given to the retracting hand. Injuries involving tearing of the mesentery are common when first using this platform. Avoid, whenever possible, prolonged periods of holding the bowel directly, as tears or traction injury can occur.
- Develop the correct planes to avoid bleeding and inadvertent damage to neighboring viscera.
- Standardize the assistant's role, and create a team with whom you will operate.
- Study any available preoperative imaging to ascertain variations of the vasculature or anatomy.
- Port position varies based on patient size. In obese patients, ports should be placed medially to the usually described position, as the instrument may not reach the hepatic flexure. Use bariatric instruments when needed. In thin patients, ports should be placed laterally to described positions to prevent overcrowding of arms.

This chapter outlines our technique of robotic right hemicolectomy, which we have successfully used in over 100 patients. We generally prefer the three-port technique for extracorporeal right hemicolectomy and the four-port technique for planned intracorporeal anastomosis. There are numerous approaches to dissection of the right colon, but we utilize the medial to lateral approach. This can be modified, based upon surgeon preference. Robotic-assisted right hemicolectomy affords accurate dissection and enhanced visualization and can serve as an alternative platform for the minimally invasive approach.

References

1. Park JS, Choi GS, Park SY, Kim HJ, Ryuk JP. Randomized clinical trial of robot-assisted versus standard laparoscopic right colectomy. Br J Surg. 2012;99:1219–26.
2. deSouza AL, Prasad LM, Park JJ, Marecik SJ, Blumetti J, Abcarian H. Robotic assistance in right hemicolectomy: is there a role? Dis Colon Rectum. 2010;53:1000–6.
3. Juo YY, Hyder O, Haider AH, Camp M, Lidor A, Ahuja N. Is minimally invasive colon resection better than traditional approaches?: first comprehensive national examination with propensity score matching. JAMA Surg. 2014;149:177–84.
4. Liao G, Zhao Z, Lin S, et al. Robotic-assisted versus laparoscopic colorectal surgery: a meta-analysis of four randomized controlled trials. World J Surg Oncol. 2014;12:122.

Robotic Left Hemicolectomy and Sigmoidectomy

Carrie Y. Peterson, Doaa Alsaleh, Sang W. Lee, and Govind Nandakumar

Abstract

A robotic approach to left hemicolectomy and sigmoidectomy is becoming a more widely utilized minimally invasive technique. In early reports, there appeared to be no difference in short-term outcomes when compared to laparoscopy. Currently, the benefit of robotic dissections remains unclear due to a lack of randomized controlled trials, yet anecdotal experience and several series suggest the benefits of robotic approaches elsewhere translate to colorectal surgery. In this chapter, we will provide a step-by-step technique to perform robotic left hemicolectomy and sigmoid resection, including things to consider in patient selection, room arrangement, and what to do in an emergency. We will also briefly review the literature on robotic left hemicolectomy and sigmoidectomy and evaluate the reported short-term and oncologic outcomes.

Keywords

Robotic • Left • Hemicolectomy • Sigmoidectomy

11.1 Introduction to Robotic Colectomy

The application of a robotic platform to colorectal surgery is an evolving area. Robotic colon resection, first described in 2001, is beginning to grow in both acceptability and applicability [1]. The technologic advantages of the robotic platform—three-dimensional, high-definition cameras, wrExisted instruments, motion stabilizing, and tireless retraction —may offer an advantage over laparoscopic surgery. Yet, it is currently unclear what

C.Y. Peterson, M.D. • D. Alsaleh, M.D.
S.W. Lee, M.D., F.A.C.S., F.A.S.C.R.S. (✉)
G. Nandakumar, M.D. (✉)
Division of Colorectal Surgery, New York-
Presbyterian Hospital, Weill Cornell Medical Center,
525 East 68th Street, Box 172, New York, NY 10021,
USA
e-mail: sal2013@med.cornell.edu;
doctorgovind@gmail.com

© Springer International Publishing Switzerland 2015
H. Ross et al. (eds.), *Robotic Approaches to Colorectal Surgery*,
DOI 10.1007/978-3-319-09120-4_11

this advantage may be and at what economic cost. Current hypotheses propose the largest benefit from robotic colorectal surgery comes from the use of the robotic platform during pelvic operations, where the precise dissection resulting from the improved visualization and wristed instruments may have an advantage over open and laparoscopic techniques in the small, confined space of the pelvis. As such, the majority of the literature to date has examined the impact and outcomes of robotic techniques for proctectomy, as is discussed in detail in Chap. 13 [2–4]. The focus of this chapter is to provide step-by-step procedural instructions for completing a left hemicolectomy or sigmoidectomy, as well as to discuss a variety of important topics to consider when planning your robotic segmental colectomy.

11.2 Indications for Robotic Segmental Colectomy

The indications for use of the robotic platform for left colon and sigmoid resections are similar to the indications for laparoscopic left and sigmoid colectomy. First and foremost, the patient must have appropriate physiologic reserve to undergo general anesthesia and pneumoperitoneum. Early in the surgeon's experience with robotic techniques, many reports demonstrate significantly longer operative times [5]. Patients should also have minimal adhesions or at least be amenable to laparoscopic adhesiolysis prior to the robotic portion of the procedure. The robotic arms are designed specifically for movement around a focal target and are not suited for large movements into many quadrants of the abdomen. Because the robotic platform lacks tactile feedback, procedures that depend on distinguishing the correct operative plane by palpation, such as inflammation from acute or chronic diverticulitis or locally invasive recurrent malignancies, are not ideal for robotic techniques (at least not initially), as the danger of positive margins and inadvertent damage to surrounding organs

outweighs the potential benefit. These caveats considered, robotic resection of left hemicolectomy and sigmoidectomy has been described with excellent outcomes for both benign diseases and colonic malignancies [6–8].

11.3 Procedure for Robotic Left Hemicolectomy or Sigmoidectomy

11.3.1 Room Set-up

- A number of viable arrangements for room set-up are possible depending on your institution's space and resource utilization.
  - It is helpful to start with the patient-side cart on the patient's left side to minimize the distance the cart must travel during docking.
  - Angling the patient bed can further reduce the distance traveled and give the assistant more room (see Fig. 11.1).
- The bedside assistant is on the patient's right side, next to the scrub table.

11.3.2 Patient Positioning

- Modified lithotomy position is ideal. Due to concerns of prolonged operative time and the risk of venous thromboembolic disease and extremity complications, a split-leg table might also be used.
- Secure the patient to the table, as incidents of sliding off the operating table during steep Trendelenburg have been reported [9].
  - Our preferred technique is to use curved pink pads on each shoulder with elastic tape wrapped circumferentially around the upper torso and across the shoulders securing the patient to the bed (see Fig. 11.2).
  - Perform a "tilt test" prior to prepping and draping the patient with maximal Trendelenburg and right side down tilt to ensure minimal movement on the table.

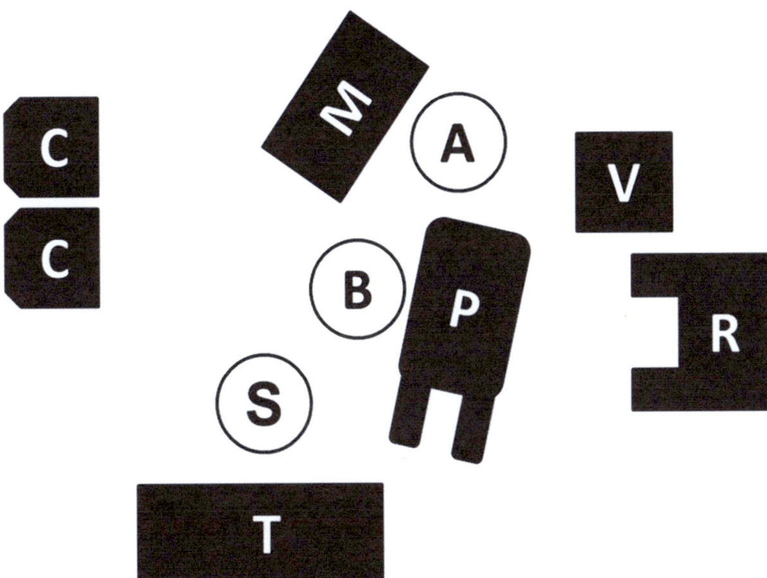

Fig. 11.1 Diagram of possible operating room layout and positioning of equipment and personnel

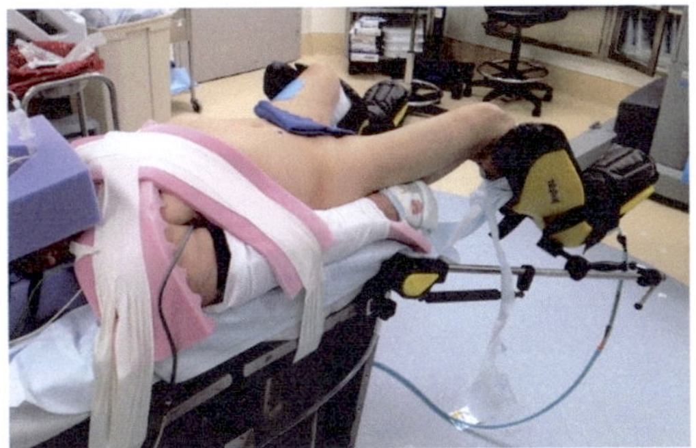

Fig. 11.2 Photograph of patient undergoing robotic sigmoid colectomy demonstrating our technique for securing the patient to the bed using foam pads and circumferential tape across the shoulders and upper torso

11.3.3 Port Placement

- Begin by inserting a 12 mm balloon port in the supraumbilical position via an open technique for use as the camera port. A balloon port is ideal as it is long enough for the camera to fit through and allows for the least amount of "extra" trocar to be in the abdomen.
  - The robotic camera is held by the assistant and inserted into the abdomen.
- For lesions in the distal descending and sigmoid colon that require splenic flexure mobilization, use a set-up similar to that of a low anterior resection with the ports arrayed around a vector pointing at the target lesion in the left lower quadrant (LLQ) (see Fig. 11.3a).
  - Draw a line on the skin from the ASIS to the camera port—placing ports below this line can cause crowding during any pelvic dissection and can limit the reach to the splenic flexure.
  - An 8 mm robotic port is placed in the right upper quadrant (RUQ) on the mid-clavicular line.
  - An 8 mm robotic port is also placed in the right lower quadrant (RLQ) port 8 cm from the camera port and usually 1–2 cm above the marked line. Alternatively, a 10–12 mm laparoscopic port with an 8 mm robotic port placed through it can be placed here to allow for intracorporeal stapling.
  - Another 8 mm robotic port in the LLQ is placed on the opposite side.
  - For procedures where retraction in the pelvis is important, we will also place a fourth 8 mm robotic port laterally in the left flank, 8 cm lateral to the LLQ port and 1–2 cm superior to allow for third-arm retraction during pelvic dissection.

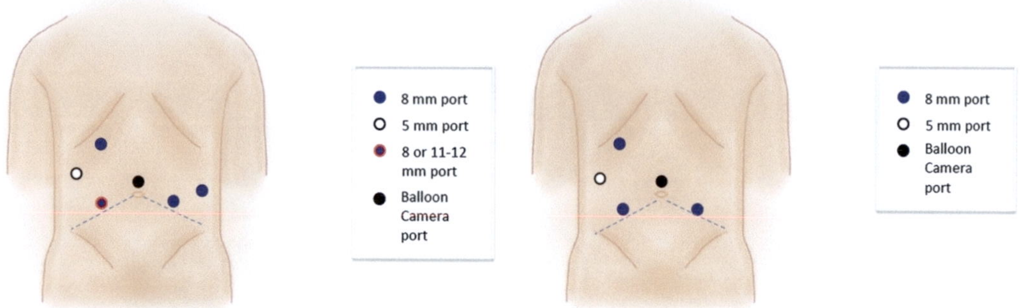

Fig. 11.3 Port placement for (**a**) distal descending and sigmoid colon lesions and (**b**) distal transverse and proximal descending colon target lesions

- A 5 mm laparoscopic port is placed in the right mid-abdomen between the RUQ and RLQ ports for use by the bedside assistant.
- For target lesions proximal to the mid-descending colon, use an amphitheater approach to port placement surrounding a vector directed at the target lesion in the left upper quadrant (LUQ) (see Fig. 11.3b).
  - An 8 mm robotic port in the right upper quadrant (RUQ) and another in the right lower quadrant (RLQ) are placed along the midclavicular line.
  - A third 8 mm robotic port is placed in the left lower quadrant (LLQ) for the third arm, but may not be necessary for a left colectomy and can interfere with other working arms causing collisions. This can be minimized if the RLQ and LLQ ports are not in the same sagittal plane.
  - Each port should be at least 8 cm away to avoid arm collisions. In addition, ports should not be placed directly in front or behind the camera port, as visualization will be limited.
  - A 5 mm laparoscopic port placed in the right mid-abdomen is very useful and allows your bedside assistant to help with retraction and suction as needed.

11.3.4 Docking the Patient-Side Cart

11.3.4.1 Exposing the Left Colon

- Use laparoscopic graspers in the RUQ and RLQ ports and the robotic camera held by the assistant.
  - Tilt the patient to approximately 30° Trendelenburg and 15° left side-up.
  - Reflect the transverse colon & omentum superiorly above the liver and arrange the small bowel into the right side of the abdomen, exposing the Ligament of Treitz, Inferior Mesenteric Vein (IMV) and the vascular pedicle of the sigmoid.
- Take note of the specific location of the target lesion and any anatomical variances, such as redundancy.

11.3.4.2 Angled Docking

- This configuration is ideal for most distal left colectomies and sigmoid resections as it gives reach to the splenic flexure, yet allows for pelvic dissection without re-docking.
- Position the patient-side cart at a 45° angle to the pedestal of the operating bed on the lower left side, resulting in the patient-side cart approaching over the left hip (see Fig. 11.4).

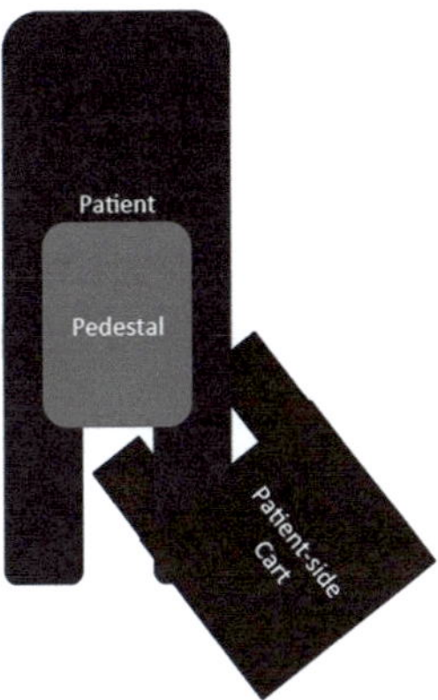

Fig. 11.4 Diagram of angle docking used for left hemicolectomy and sigmoidectomy. The patient-side cart straddles the pedestal of the operating table at approximately a 45° angle

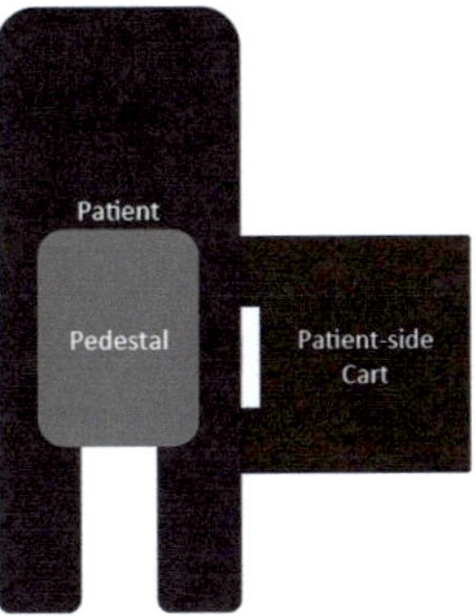

Fig. 11.6 Diagram of side docking for proximal left colon lesions. The patient-side cart approaches the left side of the patient and table perpendicularly

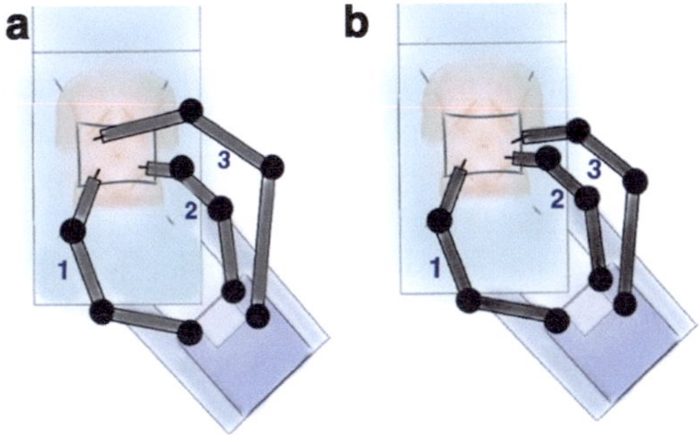

Fig. 11.5 Diagram of the arm arrangement for angle docking. (**a**) This arrangement is best suited for the splenic flexure portion. Arm 3 must be locked at the base of the patient-side cart to maximize its reach. (**b**) For the sigmoid or pelvic portions, move Arm 3 to the lateral left port and unlock it from its base

- The third arm of the patient-side cart may change ports during the procedure.
  - During pedicle dissection, ligation and splenic flexure mobilization, Arm 3 is over the patients' LUQ and inserted into the RUQ port. Arm 1 is placed in the RLQ port (see Fig. 11.5a). Arm 2 is usually not used, but can be placed in the LLQ port for some limited retraction if needed. The hinge of Arm 3 closest to the patient-side cart should be locked during this part of the operation to maximize the reach.
  - For pelvic dissection, Arm 3 is unlocked and moved to the left lateral port. Arm 2 is placed in the LLQ port while Arm 1 remains in the RLQ port (see Fig. 11.5b).

11.3.4.3 Side Docking

- This position is ideal for target lesions in the proximal descending, splenic flexure or distal transverse.
- The patient-side cart is positioned perpendicular to the pedestal of the operating bed over the patient's left flank (see Fig. 11.6).
  - Arm 2 is placed in the RUQ port and Arm 1 in the RLQ port.
  - Arm 3 is left unlocked and placed extending over the patient's left hip into the LLQ port with a grasping instrument.

11.3.4.4 Instrument Selection

- The monopolar scissors or the vessel sealer should be used in the surgeon's right hand, Arm 1.
- The surgeon's left hand (Arm 2 or 3) should have a bipolar grasper, either the Chaudière or the Prograsp.
- The retracting arm not in active use by the surgeon should have another grasper, such as the double fenestrated grasper.

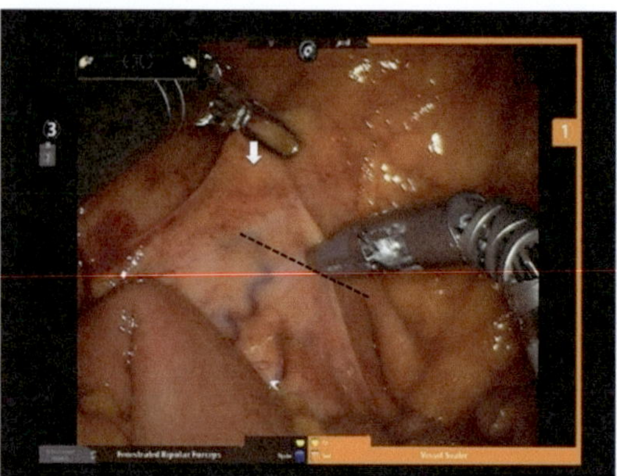

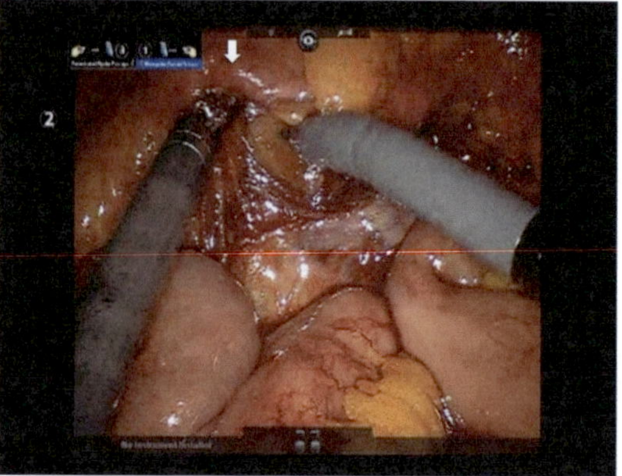

Fig. 11.7 Intraoperative photograph of the appearance of the vascular pedicle when placed on tension during robotic dissection. During this exposure, the surgeon's left hand lifts up on the sigmoid mesentery (*white arrow*) exposing the Inferior Mesenteric Artery (IMA) pedicle. The assistant can help by retracting the sigmoid colon to the left pelvis. The vessel sealer or monopolar scissors are used to incise the peritoneum and begin the dissection along the *dashed line* indicated

Fig. 11.8 Dissect posterior to the Inferior Mesenteric Artery by lifting up on the artery (*white arrow*) with the surgeon's left hand to visualize the tension and define the correct plane for dissection laterally. Blunt dissection of the avascular plane laterally can be performed with the right hand

11.3.5 Vascular Dissection

- Using the retracting third arm or the bedside assistant, the sigmoid mesentery is placed on slight tension to identify the vascular pedicle of the Inferior Mesenteric Artery (IMA).
- Divide the peritoneum just to the right of the base of the pedicle at the level of the sacral promontory; using soft sweeping motions expose the IMA and dissect posterior to the vessel (see Fig. 11.7).
  - The correct plane is avascular and generally bloodless.
  - Protect the hypogastric nerves in this area as dissection proceeds toward the origin of the IMA.
  - Continue the dissection superiorly around the base of the IMA and identify the bifurcation of the Left Colic Artery (see Fig. 11.8).
  - Creating a wide window behind the IMA facilitates identification of the retroperitoneal strictures.
  - Division of the vascular pedicle can be performed at this time if the left ureter can be identified and protected.

- For maximal splenic flexure mobilization, extend the peritoneal incision superiorly to the IMV, dividing any adhesions to the Ligament of Trietz (see Fig. 11.9a).
  - The mesentery of the left colon is gently lifted up near the IMV and the peritoneum is incised. The IMV is dissected from surrounding structures, including the retroperitoneum and can be divided at this time to prevent avulsion (see Fig. 11.9b).

11.3.6 Medial-to-Lateral Mesocolic Dissection and Mobilization

- The plane developed when dissecting posterior to the IMV or the superior hemorrhoidal artery is extended laterally and will guide you into the proper plane for dissecting the mesocolon from the retroperitoneum.
  - Gently place one operating arm under the mesocolon and lift up, opening the plane and showing the tension. Gentle blunt dissection will separate the mesocolon from the retroperitoneum (see Fig. 11.10a).
  - Using a blunt bipolar grasper in the left hand and another blunt instrument, such as the vessel sealer, in the right hand is

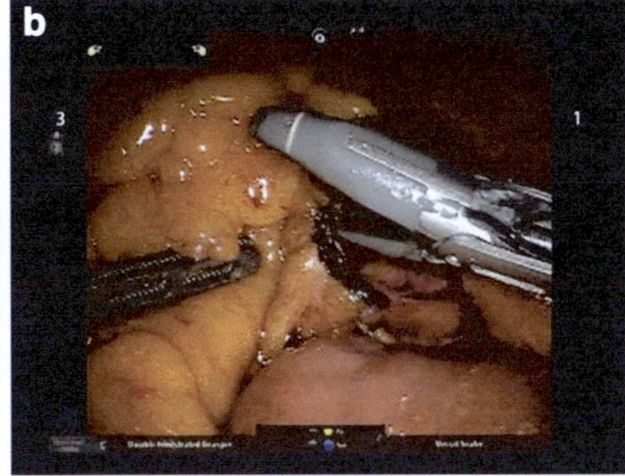

Fig. 11.9 Taking the Inferior Mesentery Vein (IMV) proximally allows for greater mobilization of the left colon. In addition, it is easy to identify as can be seen here. (**a**) The left hand lifts up on the mesentery just lateral to the IMV, which can be seen clearly in the retroperitoneum. (**b**) After incising the peritoneum and dissecting posterior to the IMV, the vessel can be divided using the vessel sealer

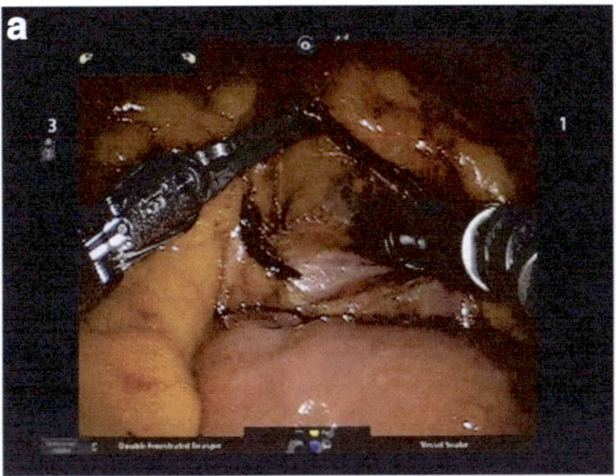

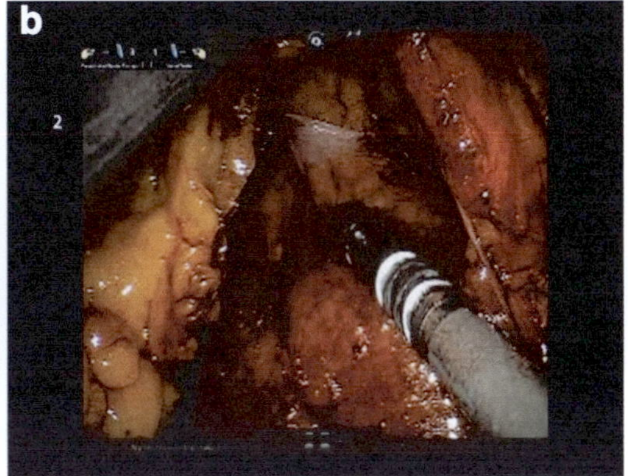

Fig. 11.10 The proper plane for medial-to-lateral dissection can be entered in several locations, including posterior to the IMA and the IMV. (**a**) Demonstrates the dissection posterior to the IMV. (**b**) As the dissection is carried laterally, a *white line* is identified that is the retroperitoneal fascia, which should be preserved

preferred. Pointed instruments such as Maryland graspers or scissors can make this dissection difficult and more traumatic.
- Again, the correct plane is avascular and nearly bloodless.
- Often you will notice a "white line" of thin filmy fascia—this is the retroperitoneal fascia and should be dissected down to stay on the retroperitoneum (see Fig. 11.10b).
- Continue laterally and inferiorly to develop the dissection extending from the transverse colon to the sigmoid.
- Once the plane lateral to the IMA pedicle is dissected and the Left Colic Artery is located, it is time to identify the left ureter, which is usually located in the retroperitoneum just to the left of the IMA pedicle (Fig. 11.11).
- Using the left grasper or the assistant, come under the IMA, tenting this up and exposing the view to the retroperitoneum.
- Using the right hand and possibly the third arm, gently dissect the retroperitoneum to expose the left ureter, looking for the characteristic vascular pattern and vermiculation to identify the structure.
- Ureteral stents are of little help in these cases as there is no tactile feedback to help locate the ureter. Because of the improved visualization of the robotic camera, we have seldom had difficulty in identifying the ureter.

- If the mesocolic dissection is too deep or the ureter is not found quickly, look for the structure on the posterior surface of the mesocolon, which is now tented up.
- After identification of the left ureter, it is safe to divide the vascular pedicle (see Fig. 11.12a).
  - The robotic vessel sealer can be used for pedicle ligation. If it is not yet available in your area, the RLQ robotic arm can be removed and another bipolar sealing and cutting device can be inserted through the same port and operated by the assistant (see Fig. 11.12b).

- In cases of severe atherosclerosis, changing the RLQ port to an 11–12 mm port and using a laparoscopic stapling device to divide the pedicle is recommended. Alternatively, an ENDOLOOP™ (Ethicon, Cincinnati, OH) may be used after division of the pedicle with an energy device. Following this, the 8 mm robotic port can be placed through the larger laparoscopic port (a "port-in-port" technique) to return to using the robotic arm.
- The avascular plane between the mesocolon and the retroperitoneal fascia can now be dissected further in the lateral, superior and inferior directions (see Fig. 11.13).
  - The lateral boundary of the mesocolic dissection is the abdominal wall, which will be noted as the dissection plane takes a sharp turn anteriorly.
  - During the dissection superiorly, the surgeon must be wary around the pancreas; the proper plane is anterior. It is easy to dissect posterior to the pancreas and cause moderate bleeding that may be difficult to control.
  - Once the superior edge of the pancreas is identified, the dissection has extended sufficiently.
  - Extending this dissection laterally, being conscious of the close proximity of the spleen, can make the splenic flexure mobilization much easier, particularly when it is very high.

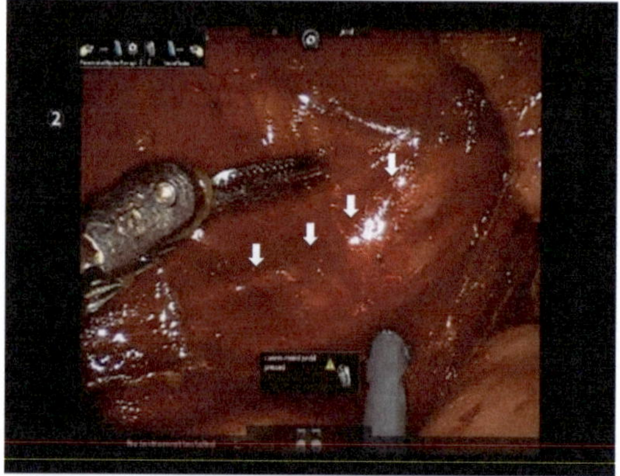

Fig. 11.11 Identification of the left ureter (*white arrows*) is a key step in the procedure, performed before vascular pedicle ligation. Is this photograph, the surgeon is retracting the IMA superiorly out of view using the right hand. The assistant is helping to clear the view using suction to expose the ureter

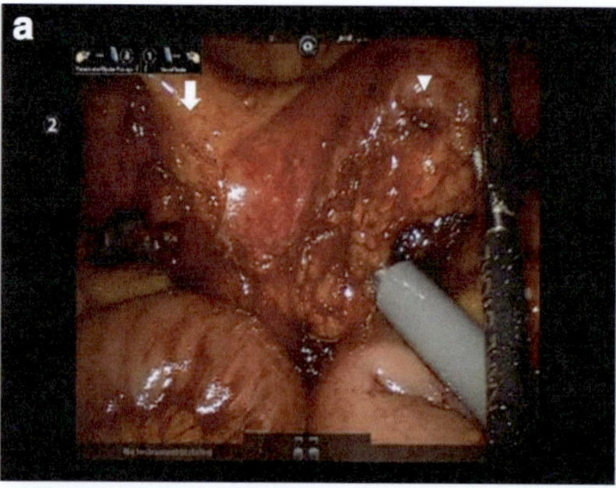
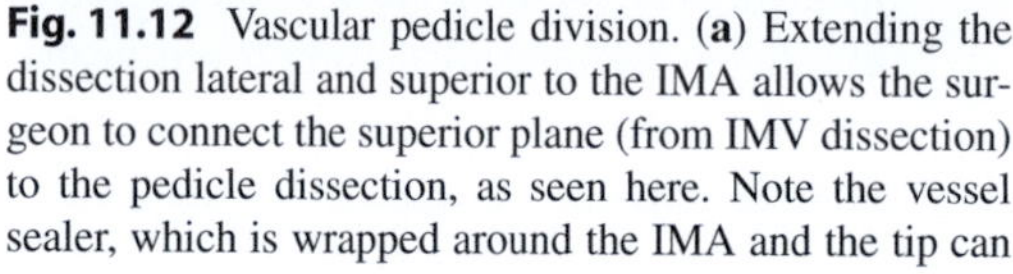
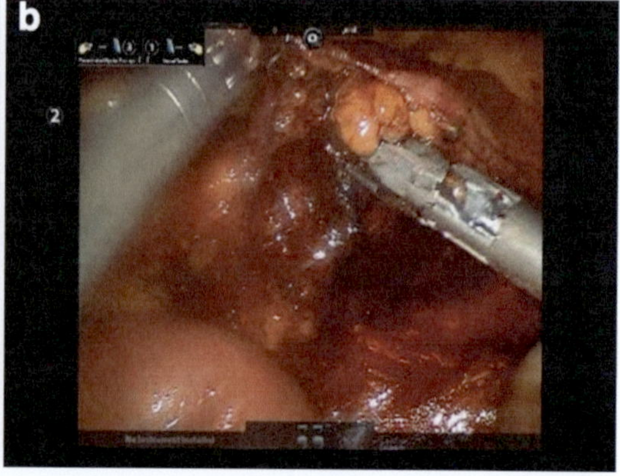

Fig. 11.12 Vascular pedicle division. (**a**) Extending the dissection lateral and superior to the IMA allows the surgeon to connect the superior plane (from IMV dissection) to the pedicle dissection, as seen here. Note the vessel sealer, which is wrapped around the IMA and the tip can be seen superior in the left of the screen. The Left Colic Artery is identified by the *white arrow* and the IMA by the *white arrowhead*. (**b**) The IMA (as seen here) or the Left Colic Artery can be divided using the EndoWrist® One™ Vessel Sealer (Intuitive Surgical Inc., Sunnyvale, CA)

11.3.7 Splenic Flexure Mobilization

- The assistant provides retraction and counter-tension using an atraumatic laparoscopic grasper inserted through the 5 mm port in the right lateral abdomen.
- Beginning at the mid-transverse colon, identify the plane and dissect the transverse colon from the omentum in the standard fashion (see Fig. 11.14).
  - Carry the dissection in the direction of the splenic flexure as far as possible.

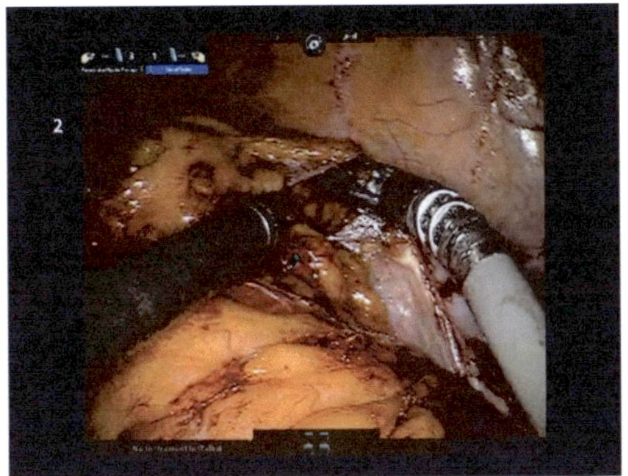

Fig. 11.15 Incise the lateral attachments of the descending and sigmoid colon. The plane from the mesocolic dissection should be clear and easy to identify if taken far enough laterally. Is this photograph, the right hand has just entered the plane created during the medial-to-lateral dissection

11.3.8 Lateral Mobilization

- Because of the extensive medial-to-lateral mesocolic dissection that has already been performed, the plane is easy to identify.
  - The assistant grasps the sigmoid and descending colon retracting medially and the peritoneum at the White Line of Toldt is incised (see Fig. 11.15).
  - Begin with the lateral attachments of the sigmoid colon inferiorly and continue to the splenic flexure.
  - Monopolar scissors or the robotic vessel sealer can be used for this portion of the dissection.
- Stay anterior and adjacent to the bowel wall when dissecting near the left kidney as dissecting posteriorly can send you into the retroperitoneum.
  - We use a technique of "rolling the colon over" toward the midline by grasping the descending colon on the lateral edge and rolling it medially to expose the posterior mesocolon (see Fig. 11.16a).
  - If you were able to dissect to the splenic flexure from the transverse colon previously, your dissection planes will connect, allowing excellent exposure from both directions to divide the splenocolic ligaments (see Fig. 11.16b).

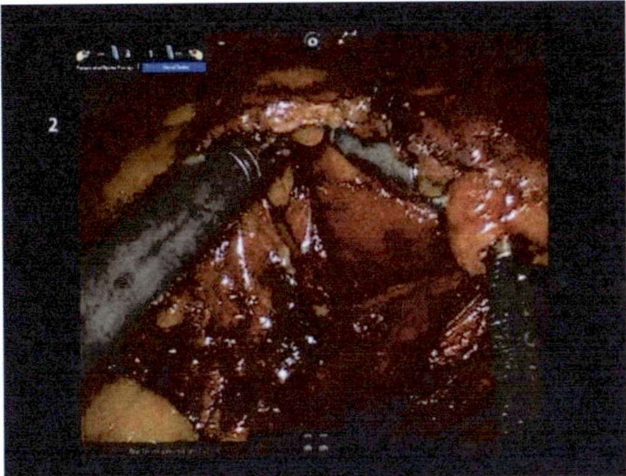

Fig. 11.13 After pedicle ligation, the mesocolic dissection is extended laterally and superiorly in a similar fashion, by lifting with the left hand and gently, bluntly dissecting with the right hand

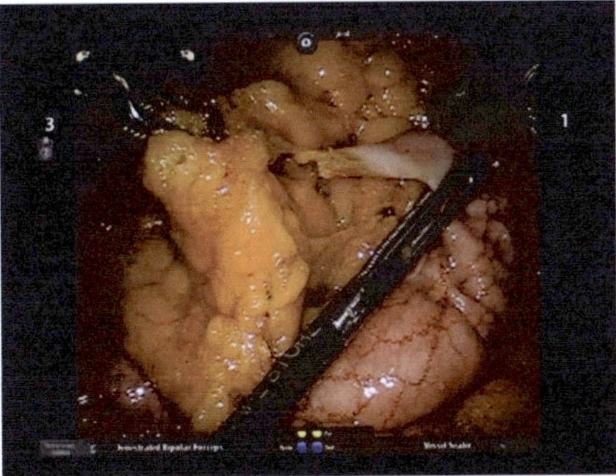

Fig. 11.14 Divide the omental attachments to the transverse colon in the usual fashion. The assistant can be particularly helpful here to retract the transverse colon inferiorly

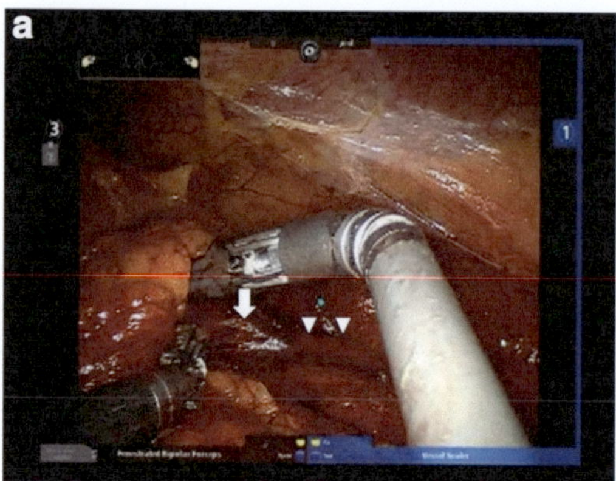

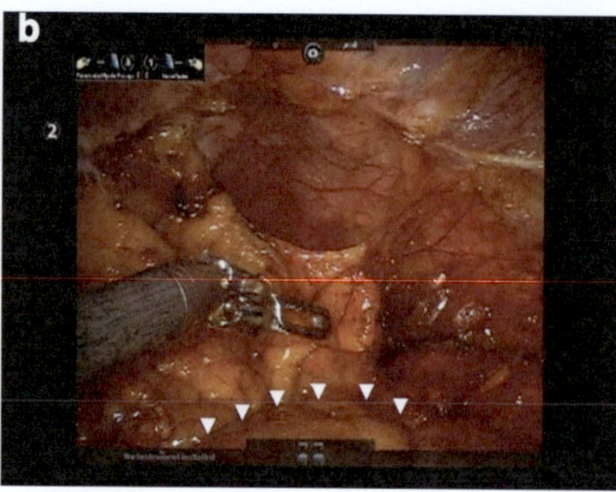

Fig. 11.16 Splenic flexure mobilization. (**a**) Demonstration of the "rolling over" of the descending colon. Here, the surgeon's left hand is hooking and retracting the descending colon medially and the right hand vessel sealer is ligating a band tethering it. Other bands identifying the proper plane of dissection are noted at the *white arrow*. The *white arrowheads* identify the incorrect plane when the dissection is taken to far laterally into the retroperitoneum. (**b**) When the transverse and lateral descending colon mobilization is thorough, the planes of dissection will meet at the splenic flexure as demonstrated here (*white arrowheads* outline the retracted splenic flexure of the colon)

- Rotate the transverse and descending colon toward the midline and even to the right side and expose the extent of the dissection to ensure appropriate mobilization has been completed.

11.3.9 Pelvic Dissection

- This setup can be used when further pelvic and upper rectal dissection is needed.
  - With the patient-side cart in an angled docking position, Arm 1 remains in the RLQ port with a monopolar scissors.
  - Arm 2 is moved to the LLQ port with a bipolar grasper, and Arm 3 is moved to the left lateral port with another grasper.
- Using Arm 3, lift up the sigmoid colon slightly toward to the left side, sometimes by performing a "hooking" maneuver under the mesocolon with the third arm.
  - This maneuver exposes the plane for a total mesorectal excision and dissection of the upper rectum in this avascular plane can be performed to the extent needed (see Fig. 11.17).
  - When rectal mobilization is complete, the mesorectum can be divided to the bowel wall using either the robotic vessel sealer or another bipolar sealing device.

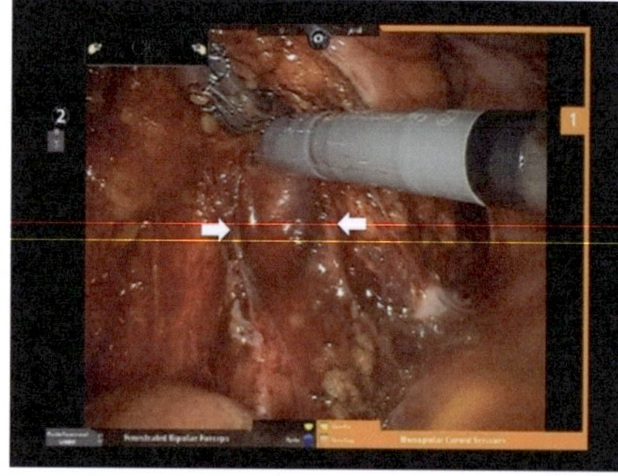

Fig. 11.17 Retract the sigmoid colon anteriorly to expose the correct plane for pelvic dissection. The left hand can lift up on the posterior aspect of the distal sigmoid/upper rectum to expose the mesorectal plane, which can be divided using monopolar scissors, as in this photograph. Note the bilateral hypogastric plexi (*white arrows*), which are easily identified and protected

11.3.10 Resection, Extraction and Anastomosis

- For most distal descending and sigmoid lesions, intracorporeal distal resection and an end-to-end anastomosis using a circular stapler is preferred.
  - Begin by performing the distal resection first. This can be done using either the

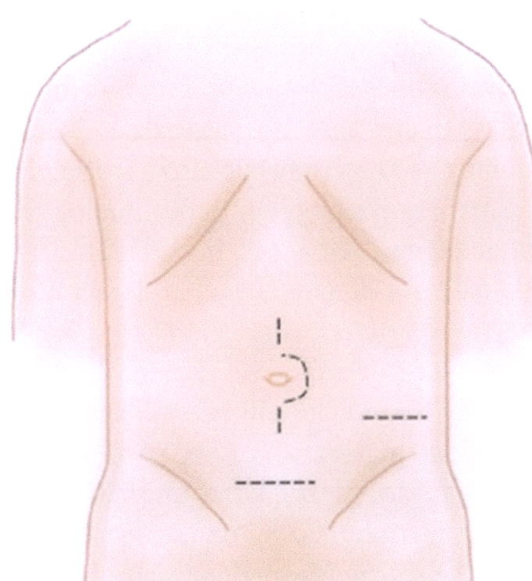

Fig. 11.18 Possible locations of incision for extracting the specimen include periumbilical, Pfannenstiel or left transverse

robotic stapling device or a laparoscopic stapler using a port-in-port technique, as described above.

- Once this is completed, remove the robotic arms and undock the patient-side cart.
- Identify the extraction incision site, either periumbilical or Pfannenstiel depending on the location of the tumor and patient body habitus (see Fig. 11.18).
- Eviscerate the colon and perform the proximal resection using a laparoscopic stapler. If you have the capability of robotic stapling, the proximal resection can be completed prior to creating the extraction incision.
- The end-to-end circular stapling is performed in the usual fashion with insertion of the anvil and closure of the proximal bowel prior to reintroducing it into the abdomen.
- The periumbilical extraction incision is closed by twisting the wound protecting device around the camera port (for periumbilical incisions), covering with abdominal pads to protect the plastic, and using two large clamps to secure the air-tight seal. Alternatively, fascial sutures can be placed and tightened with Rummel tourniquets to close the fascia around the balloon port.

- The abdomen is reinsufflated and the robotic camera is held in place by the assistant and reinserted as in the beginning of the procedure. The circular anastomosis is completed, after which an air-leak test is performed. If there are no bubbles and no diverting ostomy is necessary, the abdomen is desufflated, the ports removed, and in the incisions closed in the standard fashion.
- For those patients with very redundant colons and more proximal lesions, extracorporeal resections and anastomoses may be optimal.
  - Perform the extraction incision after completing the mobilization. Most often, this is in the periumbilical location, but could also be a transverse left incision if needed, as shown in Fig. 11.18.
  - After inserting a wound protector and eviscerating the colon, the resection and anastomosis is performed in the standard fashion.
  - The anastomosis is inspected, tested if possible, and replaced in the abdomen and the incision closed.

11.4 Planning Your Robotic Operative Approach

The pre-operative planning for robotic colonic resections is important to consider closely. Because the da Vinci system (Intuitive Surgical® Inc., Sunnyvale, CA) is less mobile and maneuverable compared to laparoscopy, it is imperative to have considered a number of options before the start of the procedure. We will address a number of considerations specific to operations on the left and sigmoid colon and for more information, please see Chaps. 4 and 5 for a detailed analysis of other pre-operative considerations.

11.4.1 Disease Location Matters

The arms and camera of the da Vinci® Surgical System are designed to function best in a focused area surrounding a central point or target. For left colon resections, this focal point could range from a splenic flexure mass to diverticulitis in the distal sigmoid colon and cover a relatively large area. Understanding the precise location of the target anatomy is crucial to making several important decisions early in the operative procedure. It is highly recommended to review imaging and procedure reports closely to precisely determine disease location and the target area of anatomy.

If the target lesion is located proximal to the mid-descending colon, an amphitheater approach with a focal point in the left upper quadrant, similar to that used for left colectomy as described by Spignolio et al. [10], works very well. These tumors are also often ideal for docking the patient-side cart perpendicular to the patient on the left side. If the diseased area is located in the sigmoid colon, port placement is slightly altered allowing for changing of the arms to reach splenic flexure mobilization and sigmoid dissection, which is facilitated by angled-docking of the robotic cart similar to the procedure described by Luca et al. [11] Our practice and preference for port placement and robotic cart docking is described below in more detail, but a general guideline is to use side docking for proximal descending colon or higher tumors and angled-docking for those in the distal descending and lower.

11.4.2 Patient Characteristics to Consider

Unlike in robotic rectal resections, where obese patients and those with ultra-low tumors were shown to have low rates of conversion to open operations, there is currently no data indicating favorable or challenging patient characteristics for robotic left colectomies [12, 13]. It is the authors' experience that the extremes of weight are most challenging. Those patients who are underweight and very thin have very thin colonic mesenteries, and the dissection can be quite challenging, especially when tactile feedback is limited. Conversely, obese patients with a heavy, thick omentum and mesentery can be equally

challenging. In these cases, the robotic graspers may tear the tissue because of the weight, and prolonged retraction by holding up omentum or mesentery can lead to increased bleeding. Positioning and exposure can also be difficult and may require undocking and repositioning to get an optimal view.

The patient's height is another aspect of their habitus to consider when planning your port placement and docking site. For those patients with a long torso who will need splenic flexure mobilization, placement of the working ports along a line drawn from the umbilicus to the Anterior Superior Iliac Spine (ASIS) can make reaching the splenic flexure and transverse colon challenging. Our practice is to keep the ports at least 1 cm above this line or even higher in a patient with a very long torso. Anticipating this in advance can help avoid re-docking or even conversion to laparoscopy.

Lastly, understanding the patient's individual colonic anatomy can help you plan your operation. Reviewing any cross-sectional imaging for redundancy in the transverse or sigmoid colon as well as the colonic vasculature may allow you to limit your splenic flexure mobilization and pedicle dissection.

11.4.3 Hybrid vs. Totally Robotic Approach

The hybrid technique, where part of the operation is completed with laparoscopic cameras and instruments, can be useful during sigmoidectomy and can also help reduce the operating time for surgeons new to robotics. Some surgeons advocate the hybrid approach as a way to increase resident and fellow involvement in the cases as well. If you choose to incorporate this into your practice, we recommend placing your ports in an optimal location for completion of the robotic portion of the case and take advantage of the flexibility of laparoscopy. For more detail information regarding hybrid techniques, we refer the reader to Chap. 8.

11.4.4 Robotic Accessories

The da Vinci® Surgical System *Si*-model, the most advanced on the market today, has a number of optional accessories and tools that are useful for left colectomies. The EndoWrist® One™ Vessel Sealer (Intuitive Surgical Inc., Sunnyvale, CA) is a useful device that performs independent bipolar sealing and cutting for vessels up to 7 mm in diameter, as well as grasping and blunt dissection. Our experience with this device has been quite favorable and we have found reduced operating times resulting from fewer instrument changes. The EndoWrist® One Stapler 45, newly FDA-approved and currently available only in select areas, is a wristed endoscopic stapling device that deploys a 45 mm double-row of 1.5 or 2.0 mm (closed height) staples with cutting capabilities. Having the stapler in the control of the operating surgeon during transection of the bowel is a much-needed advancement in the technology. Additionally, Firefly™ (Intuitive Surgical Inc., Sunnyvale, CA) is a near-infrared fluorescence imaging technique using injectable indocyanine green to highlight vascular structures and perfusion in real time. Its use has been reported in case series with good results and may help in identifying vascular pedicles and bowel perfusion [14, 15]. Lastly, the EndoWrist® One Suction/Irrigator is a 45° wristed device with dual control capabilities, either the surgeon console or the bedside assistant, and may be helpful in the third arm for maintaining a clear surgical field. If you are considering increasing your robotic practice, it may be warranted to consider adding some of these accessories to facilitate your operations.

11.4.5 Other Tips and Tricks for Success

As is true for many things, having a committed team of surgical technicians, nurses, assistants and anesthesiologists that assist you can make the operations much more efficient and pleasurable. Establishing a "Robotic Team" that will work with you frequently on the same cases every time, helps your assistants to learn your preferences, understand the flow of the procedure and anticipate your needs.

We generally perform our procedures in the same sequence and using the same equipment, changing only if significant outstanding needs exist. Many variations for robotic procedures exist and no "Standard Technique" has been defined, which can be confusing. In addition, having a clear plan of each step of the operation (i.e., port placement, docking position, extraction technique, resection strategy, etc.), and communicating these with your team early in the case will also help to improve the flow of the operation and the ease in which the case progresses. All of the above will ultimately result in decreased operative times, which will reduce cost by improving operative efficiency.

11.4.6 In an Emergency…

Although rare, emergency situations can and do arise during robotic procedures. Whether as a result of the operation or not, a procedure to address the emergent needs of the patient must be in place. We suggest adding a special "Time Out" or having an algorithm on view in the operating room where several key steps for emergent undocking are reviewed (Table 11.1). This may help to reduce confusion and improve response times when critical situations emerge. Another way to reduce response times for assembling supplies and tools is to have a "Robotic Conversion Tray" with necessary basic tools used during conversion.

Table 11.1 Key points to review prior to a robotic emergency and examples of personnel who can be responsible for various tasks

Task	Person responsible
Tamponade bleeding vessels	Patient-side Assistant/surgeon
Remove robotic arms	Surgical technician
Undock robot from patient	Circulating RN
Open emergency surgical tray	Circulating RN
Call for anesthesia assistance, call for blood	Anesthesia MD/CRNA
Call for surgical assistance	Surgeon

This way, opening large laparotomy trays can be avoided, but needed basic equipment is rapidly available. Also, reviewing with operating staff where the key for a hard reset of the robot is located is useful; this can often derail an otherwise smooth operation. In short, robotic procedures are complex and any way in which the procedure can be simplified and each person's roles clarified will go a long way to improving operative efficiency.

11.5 The Evidence for Robotic Left Hemicolectomy and Sigmoidectomy

Because of the early interest in the application of robotics for pelvic surgery, an abundance of literature is available exploring outcomes for robotic low anterior resection. When considering colon resections, either right, left or sigmoidectomy, the data is much more sparse and often heterogeneous. Indeed, early in the experience all colectomies and rectal resections were reported together in larger case series and differentiating the outcomes for each type of operation is difficult. Delaney et al. [8] reported in their initial experience, which included three robotic sigmoid resections, an average operating time of 300 min compared to 140 min for matched laparoscopic cases. This is supported by Rawlings et al. [16] in a series of 13 robotic sigmoid colectomies and 12 laparoscopic resections performed in the same time period; the average case time was nearly 26 min longer in the robotic group (225.2 vs. 199.4 min), though this was not statistically significant. In a review of the literature specifically addressing robotic colectomy, Antoniou et al. [17] reported that the average operative time for robotic left and sigmoid colectomies was 185 min, a time much improved from the earlier series [8, 11, 16].

These operative times are difficult to generalize to a larger population for a number of reasons. As has been reported in the robotic proctectomy literature, the impact of a learning curve on operative time is not insignificant; and improvements in docking time, console time and overall operative time are seen in the first 15–35 cases until mastery is achieved [18–20]. The surgeons performing these first cases and who currently comprise the majority of actively publishing robotic surgeons, are those with extensive training in laparoscopy and other minimally invasive techniques. Furthermore, the time reported for laparoscopic cases in many series does not reflect the surgeon's initial experience with laparoscopy and the comparisons may not be equivalent. If we extrapolate from what we know about robotic rectal resections, we can expect significant improvements in operative time after the learning curve has been reached and more surgeons gain experience.

Antoniou et al. [17] also evaluated the rate of conversions in robotic left colectomy and sigmoidectomy and noted there were significantly fewer conversions to either laparoscopic or open operations (7.6 % on average) compared to the early laparoscopic colectomy experience (ranging from 14 to 41 %). A variety of reasons were reported for conversion from robotic, ranging from technical problems to ischemia [17]. Interestingly, the inability to reach and mobilize the splenic flexure was only reported in one case out of 105 and does not seem to be a frequent occurrence, despite the perceived inherent limitations in multi-quadrant mobility. The previous experience with rectal resections, where we have learned a number of techniques to achieve the needed reach, has most likely influenced the experience in colectomy [11, 17, 21].

Initial reports indicate that the operative and short-term outcomes may not be significantly different in robotic surgery when compared to laparoscopy. This is somewhat difficult to interpret as series of robotic colectomies are often reported together and include such disparate operations as right, left and transverse colectomies; however, several studies report no differences in estimated blood loss, return of bowel function, hospital stay and complication rates [8, 10, 22]. Two series report the outcomes specifically for robotic left and sigmoid resections separate and found no difference in blood loss, return of bowel function or hospital stay when compared to laparoscopic cases [16, 23]. In one nonrandomized series of

180 consecutive patients who underwent robotic or laparoscopic sigmoid resections, there were no mortalities in either group and no differences in the number of complications or readmissions. Of note, the authors did report a statistically significant shorter return of bowel function and hospital stay in the robotic group, both by less than 1 day, though the clinical significance of this is likely small [6].

In patients with malignancy, robotic techniques may offer an oncologic improvement over laparoscopy. In reviewing the literature on robotic colectomy, Fung and Aly [24] found that the median lymph node harvest for robotic colectomies was 22.2, a yield significantly higher than 14.8 reported in reviews of multiport laparoscopic colectomy. The authors opine that this is related to the increased visualization and enhanced mobility of the wristed instruments, which allow more complete and extensive lymphadenectomy. Whether this results in improvements in survival or leads to stage-shifting has yet to be determined. To date, only one study has reported on longer-term follow-up with 3-year overall and disease-free survival and found no difference between robotic and laparoscopic sigmoidectomy for colon cancer [6]. Clearly, the literature addressing robotic colonic resections is limited and our understanding of the results is likewise incomplete. Future randomized comparative studies will need to be performed to clearly understand these risks and the potential benefit robotic techniques offer.

11.6 Summary

In our chapter we discussed a stepwise approach to performing robotic left hemicolectomy and sigmoid resections, including such considerations as port placement, docking technique, and splenic flexure mobilization, along with reviewing various options for intracorporeal versus extracorporeal resection and anastomoses. Patient body habitus and target lesion location is important to note preoperatively, as it may impact both the setup as well as the procedure. Lastly, we reviewed the limited evidence for robotic

left hemicolectomy and sigmoidectomy, which demonstrates patient benefit may be due to the minimally invasive nature of the operation by having faster return of bowel function and shorter recovery times; but has yet to demonstrate a clear benefit of robotic techniques over laparoscopy. In it, our hope that by providing you with further information about performing robotic surgery, more surgeons will become facile with the technology and the beneficial outcomes of robotic colorectal surgery will become clear.

11.7 Key Points

- The steps of the operation and technique for left/sigmoid colectomy using a robotic approach are similar to laparoscopy—just different equipment, setup, and learning curve.
- Port placement and robotic positioning are keys to being efficient and avoiding collisions with the robotic arms.
- Your bedside assistant is much more valuable than you may think. Ensure they have a thorough understanding of the procedure.
- Both the hybrid and multi-docking approach may be required for successful completion of a multiple quadrant surgery such as a left/sigmoid colectomy and splenic flexure mobilization.
- Have a plan for what you are going to do in case of an emergency.

References

1. Weber PA, Merola S, Wasielewski A, Ballantyne GH. Telerobotic-assisted laparoscopic right and sigmoid colectomies for benign disease. Dis Colon Rectum. 2002;45(12):1689–94; discussion 95–6.
2. Peterson CY, Weiser MR. Robotic colorectal surgery. J Gastrointest Surg. 2014;18(2):398–403.
3. Baek SK, Carmichael JC, Pigazzi A. Robotic surgery: colon and rectum. Cancer J. 2013;19(2):140–6.
4. Yang Y, Wang F, Zhang P, Shi C, Zou Y, Qin H, et al. Robot-assisted versus conventional laparoscopic surgery for colorectal disease, focusing on rectal cancer: a meta-analysis. Ann Surg Oncol. 2012;19(12): 3727–36.
5. Parra-Davila E, Ramamoorthy S. Lap colectomy and robotics for colon cancer. Surg Oncol Clin N Am. 2013;22(1):143–51, vii.

6. Lim DR, Min BS, Kim MS, Alasari S, Kim G, Hur H, et al. Robotic versus laparoscopic anterior resection of sigmoid colon cancer: comparative study of long-term oncologic outcomes. Surg Endosc. 2013;27(4):1379–85.

7. Neme RM, Schraibman V, Okazaki S, Maccapani G, Chen WJ, Domit CD, et al. Deep infiltrating colorectal endometriosis treated with robotic-assisted rectosigmoidectomy. JSLS. 2013;17(2):227–34.

8. Delaney CP, Lynch AC, Senagore AJ, Fazio VW. Comparison of robotically performed and traditional laparoscopic colorectal surgery. Dis Colon Rectum. 2003;46(12):1633–9.

9. Huettner F, Pacheco PE, Doubet JL, Ryan MJ, Dynda DI, Crawford DL. One hundred and two consecutive robotic-assisted minimally invasive colectomies—an outcome and technical update. J Gastrointest Surg. 2011;15(7):1195–204.

10. Spinoglio G, Summa M, Priora F, Quarati R, Testa S. Robotic colorectal surgery: first 50 cases experience. Dis Colon Rectum. 2008;51(11):1627–32.

11. Luca F, Cenciarelli S, Valvo M, Pozzi S, Faso FL, Ravizza D, et al. Full robotic left colon and rectal cancer resection: technique and early outcome. Ann Surg Oncol. 2009;16(5):1274–8.

12. deSouza AL, Prasad LM, Marecik SJ, Blumetti J, Park JJ, Zimmern A, et al. Total mesorectal excision for rectal cancer: the potential advantage of robotic assistance. Dis Colon Rectum. 2010;53(12):1611–7.

13. Scarpinata R, Aly EH. Does robotic rectal cancer surgery offer improved early postoperative outcomes? Dis Colon Rectum. 2013;56(2):253–62.

14. Bae SU, Baek SJ, Hur H, Kim NK, Min BS. Intraoperative near infrared fluorescence imaging in robotic low anterior resection: Three case reports. Yonsei Med J. 2013;54(4):1066–9.

15. Jafari MD, Lee KH, Halabi WJ, Mills SD, Carmichael JC, Stamos MJ, et al. The use of indocyanine green fluorescence to assess anastomotic perfusion during robotic assisted laparoscopic rectal surgery. Surg Endosc. 2013;27(8):3003–8.

16. Rawlings AL, Woodland JH, Vegunta RK, Crawford DL. Robotic versus laparoscopic colectomy. Surg Endosc. 2007;21(10):1701–8.

17. Antoniou SA, Antoniou GA, Koch OO, Pointner R, Granderath FA. Robot-assisted laparoscopic surgery of the colon and rectum. Surg Endosc. 2012;26(1):1–11.

18. Bokhari MB, Patel CB, Ramos-Valadez DI, Ragupathi M, Haas EM. Learning curve for robotic-assisted laparoscopic colorectal surgery. Surg Endosc. 2011;25(3):855–60.

19. Sng KK, Hara M, Shin JW, Yoo BE, Yang KS, Kim SH. The multiphasic learning curve for robot-assisted rectal surgery. Surg Endosc. 2013;27(9):3297–307.

20. Jimenez-Rodriguez RM, Diaz-Pavon JM, de la Portilla de Juan F, Prendes-Sillero E, Dussort HC, Padillo J. Learning curve for robotic-assisted laparoscopic rectal cancer surgery. Int J Colorectal Dis. 2013;28(6):815–21.

21. Obias V, Sanchez C, Nam A, Montenegro G, Makhoul R. Totally robotic single-position 'flip' arm technique for splenic flexure mobilizations and low anterior resections. Int J Med Robot. 2011;7(2):123–6.

22. D'Annibale A, Morpurgo E, Fiscon V, Trevisan P, Sovernigo G, Orsini C, et al. Robotic and laparoscopic surgery for treatment of colorectal diseases. Dis Colon Rectum. 2004;47(12):2162–8.

23. Deutsch GB, Sathyanarayana SA, Gunabushanam V, Mishra N, Rubach E, Zemon H, et al. Robotic vs laparoscopic colorectal surgery: an institutional experience. Surg Endosc. 2012;26(4):956–63.

24. Fung AK, Aly EH. Robotic colonic surgery: is it advisable to commence a new learning curve? Dis Colon Rectum. 2013;56(6):786–96.

Robotic-Assisted Total Abdominal Colectomy

12

Cristina R. Harnsberger, Luis Carlos Cajas-Monson, Seung Yeop Oh, and Sonia Ramamoorthy

Abstract

Robotic-assisted total abdominal colectomy (TAC) has been demonstrated to be safe and effective in patients suitable for minimally invasive surgery. Most surgical techniques described to date report a multi-dock approach. However, a single-dock approach utilizing three robotic arms, a robotic camera, and one assistant port is technically feasible without the need for a change in patient positioning. We have found that the single-dock technique improves efficiency while performing a robotic-assisted TAC.

Keywords

Robotic assisted • Total abdominal colectomy • Minimally invasive surgery • Robotic surgery • Single-dock technique

12.1 Introduction

Minimally invasive approaches to colorectal surgery have become increasingly popular. The reported advantages compared to open surgery have been well described and include decreased postoperative pain, shorter hospital stay, reduced intra-abdominal adhesions, etc. Outcomes have been shown to be similar to those of open technique in terms of estimated blood loss, extent of resection, leak rates, and number of lymph nodes removed [1–8]. Despite the advantages, widespread adoption of this technique remains limited. National databases report that 30–40 % of colectomies are performed laparoscopically. Technical limitations with laparoscopic surgery have been cited as one of the most common causes for limited adoption. These include

Electronic supplementary material: This chapter contains video segments that can be found on the following DOI: 10.1007/978-3-319-09120-4_12

C.R. Harnsberger, M.D.
Department of Surgery, University of California, San Diego, CA, USA

L.C. Cajas-Monson, M.D., M.P.H. • S. Ramamoorthy, M.D., F.A.C.S., F.A.S.C.R.S. (✉)
Department of General Surgery, UC San Diego Health System, San Diego, CA, USA
e-mail: sramamoorthy@mail.ucsd.edu

S.Y. Oh, M.D.
Department of Surgery, Ajou University School of Medicine, Suwon, South Korea

two-dimensional imaging with loss of depth perception, long instruments that often invert the surgeon's movement and do not allow for the same degrees of freedom as a surgeon usually has during open procedures, lack of advanced camera movements, multiquadrant inaccessibility, and limitations in tight spaces such as the pelvis.

Robotic approaches for colorectal disease were first described in 2001. The reported advantages of robotic surgery over traditional approaches is the ability of robotics to overcome many of the technical limitations of laparoscopic surgery. Those include three-dimensional imaging, third arm for fixed retraction, fine motion scaling, and articulated instruments, which provide superior dexterity and degrees of freedom of movement, master control over the camera and robotic arms, single incision, energy, and stapling capability within a single platform [9, 10]. The degrees of freedom provided by the robot are in/out movement, pitch (up/down), yaw (left/right), rotation, grasp, internal pitch, and internal yaw of instrument tip [11].

Since the first robotic operation, multiple studies have been performed to evaluate its performance against laparoscopic surgery [10]. Despite the reported advantages, multiple studies have not found a significant difference in outcomes over conventional laparoscopic surgery. Several studies have shown a statistically significant difference in cost and length of surgery when comparing robotic surgery and laparoscopic surgery [1–8].

One study found statistically significant differences in postoperative ileus and length of hospital stay between robotic surgery and laparoscopic surgery. The results were favorable toward robotic surgery [9]. It is possible that with more experience, operating times and outcomes in robotic surgery will improve and that current studies are reflective of the learning curve [6]. Additionally, the costs of robotic surgery may decrease over time, as is the typical pattern following release of a new technology.

In this chapter, we will describe a total abdominal colectomy (TAC) using robotic surgery. One of the approaches involves changing the robot's position in order to complete dissection in multiple quadrants of the abdomen, termed a multi-dock technique. The second approach, which we use at our institution, is a single-dock technique in which the robot does not need to be undocked and repositioned.

12.2 Indications for Robotic-Assisted Total Abdominal Colectomy

The indications for TAC can be broadly categorized into two groups: those conditions resulting from a primary lesion and those due to secondary lesions [12]. Diffuse adenomatosis of the colon falls into the former category and is most commonly seen in the form of the inherited syndrome, familial adenomatous polyposis (FAP), which is managed by TAC as the lifetime risk of carcinoma development is nearly 100 %. Additionally, hereditary nonpolyposis colorectal cancer (HNPCC), or Lynch syndrome, is a primary lesion that can also be managed with total colectomy, as the risk of metachronous colon cancer is high if segmental colectomy is performed [13].

Secondary lesions that may warrant total colectomy include inflammatory bowel disease (IBD), pseudomembranous colitis, and motility disorders. Ulcerative colitis with bloody stool that is refractory to medical management and chronic ulcerative colitis with complications or dysplasia are indications for total colectomy. Additionally, Crohn's disease that has failed medical management and has multi-segment colonic involvement or short skip lesions can be managed with total colectomy, although the indications for colonic preservation are not clearly defined [14, 15]. Pseudomembranous colitis resulting from Clostridium difficile infection that is not responsive to medical management or causes toxic megacolon is treated with TAC. The motility disorder characterized by weak muscular activity of the colon such as the case of colonic inertia that is refractory to medical management should be managed with TAC as well [16].

In the case of any of the above indications for TAC, the patient should be a suitable candidate for minimally invasive surgery. Cases in which surgery is emergent secondary to colonic perforation and gross contamination are not appropriate for minimally invasive surgery. Obesity, however, is not a contraindication to minimally invasive surgery, though conversion rates are higher than in the nonobese [17].

12.3   Multi-Dock Technique

12.3.1   Background

One of the early limitations of robotic surgery was the time it took to dock the robot. With experience, many robotic teams have reduced "docking time," but in cases of dedocking and redocking for repositioning, prolonged operative times are a consideration. If surgical dissection must be accomplished in different sectors of the abdomen, the task of undocking and redocking the robot can seem daunting. In order to successfully complete a TAC, it is necessary to work in all quadrants of the abdomen and pelvis. The following summarizes a multi-dock technique, which takes advantage of each position of the patient and robot in order to minimize the number of times the robot must be redocked.

12.3.2   Patient Preparation and Initial Positioning

Patients undergo standard colectomy preparation including consultation with ostomy nurses if ileostomy is planned. Patients are prepped in the usual fashion as if a laparoscopic colectomy was to be performed. The patient can be in a modified lithotomy position with the thighs at the level of the abdomen or in a split-leg position in order to minimize interference with the arms of the robot. Initially, the patient is positioned in slight Trendelenburg with the right side up.

12.3.3   Port Placement

A 12 mm port is placed at the umbilicus and a laparoscope is inserted to confirm that there are no contraindications to proceeding with a robotic-assisted TAC. Subsequently, four additional 8–12 mm trocars are placed for the robotic arms, which will be rotated throughout the case. Additionally, if extra assistance is required, 5 mm ports can be placed at the level of the umbilicus in the left or right flank or in the suprapubic region. Initially, the robot is docked over the right upper quadrant of the patient, the camera is inserted at the umbilicus, and robotic arms 1 and 2 are placed in right lower quadrant (RLQ) and left upper quadrant (LUQ) ports.

12.3.4   Surgical Technique

Dissection is started with the ascending colon. The LLQ port is utilized by the assistant for retraction of the terminal ileum, thereby extending the ileocolic vascular pedicle. Once isolated, the ileocolic vascular pedicle is divided with a laparoscopic linear stapler where it crosses the duodenum. The transected pedicle can be used to retract the colon as the other two instruments bluntly dissect Gerota's fascia from the mesocolon. At this stage, care must be taken to identify the right ureter and gonadal vessels and preserve them. This dissection is continued in a medial to lateral (MtL) manner caudally until the cecum and terminal ileum are mobilized. The terminal ileum is then divided with a linear stapler. Next, the dissection proceeds cranially, through the hepatic flexure. At this point, the lateral attachments of the ascending colon are left in place to keep the colon from falling into the field of vision. The omentum can be taken off the proximal portion of transverse colon using the robotic vessel sealer or an energy device through the assistant port. The lateral fascia of Toldt is then divided to finish the right-sided portion of the procedure. At this point, the robot is undocked.

The patient is now positioned for the left-sided dissection. Slight Trendelenburg position is maintained, but the bed is tilted with the left side up. The robot is redocked to the left side of the patient to the cart over the left hip at a 30–40° angle to the bed. The camera is inserted through the umbilical port, and now the first robotic arm is placed through the RLQ port, and the second and third arms through the LUQ and RUQ ports. The curved monopolar scissors and Maryland bipolar grasping forceps are placed in the first arm of the robot and a Cadiere grasper in the second and third arms. The inferior mesenteric artery (IMA) pedicle is identified and retracted anteriorly using the Cadiere grasper, allowing development of the plane between the IMA and the aorta. The IMA is divided with the robotic vessel sealer or an energy device through the assistant port. Next, the inferior mesenteric vein (IMV) is identified and divided near the inferior border of the pancreas. A (MtL) dissection is performed in a similar fashion to the right-sided portion of the TAC, from the sigmoid colon proceeding cranially, lifting the mesocolon off of Gerota's fascia taking care not to injure the ureter or gonadal vessels. Next, dissection continues through the splenic flexure and to the midportion of the transverse colon using the robotic vessel sealer or an energy device through the assistant port to divide the gastrocolic ligament. At this point, the colon should be mobilized with the exception of the rectum.

The final change in robot positioning involves moving the robotic arms only, while leaving the patient-side cart in place. The first robotic arm is maintained in the RLQ port, and the second and third robotic arms are moved to the LLQ and LUQ ports, allowing better retraction and dissection of the rectum. The dissection will proceed with standard total mesorectal excision principles. Start the dissection inferiorly, then laterally, and finally anteriorly. Once the appropriate level of dissection has been reached, the rectum is transected using a robotic stapler.

12.4 Single-Dock Technique

12.4.1 Background

Literature on technique for robotic TAC is limited. All current reports describe a multi-dock approach, as was summarized above. Due to the utility of different patient positions, different ideal camera angles, and different robotic arm configurations for the various aspects of a TAC, a single-dock approach may seem like a technical impossibility. However, below we describe a robotic-assisted TAC via a single-dock technique with an accompanying video (Video 12.1).

12.4.2 Patient Preparation and Positioning

All patients undergo a mechanical bowel preparation prior to surgery and have an ileostomy site marked. The patient is positioned supine in slight Trendelenburg and in a split-leg configuration with both arms tucked. The suction, electrocautery, energy devices, and all lines are connected toward the head of the patient.

12.4.3 Port Placement and Robot Docking

Pneumoperitoneum is obtained via Veress needle insufflation in the right upper quadrant. Port placement is illustrated below (Fig. 12.1). Initially, an 8 mm incision is made in the left subcostal position in the mid-clavicular line, and a Visiport® optical trocar is placed (this is later replaced with an 8 mm robotic trocar used for the surgeon's second robotic arm). Under laparoscopic visualization, another 8 mm robotic port is placed in a left lateral position, approximately parallel or just inferior to the umbilicus (this port will later be used for the surgeon's third robotic arm). The falciform ligament is then taken down laparoscopically to facilitate placement of the robotic camera port in the subxiphoid position, as superiorly as possible.

Following placement of the robotic camera port, the remaining 8 mm port is placed in the right subcostal position, lateral to the mid-clavicular line, and will initially be used for the surgeon's first robotic arm. Finally, the 12 mm assistant port is placed in the RLQ, as lateral as possible and just inferior to the anterior superior iliac spine. Typically, the assistant port is unable to be placed at the previously marked ileostomy site, which is usually more medial and superior to an optimally placed assistant port.

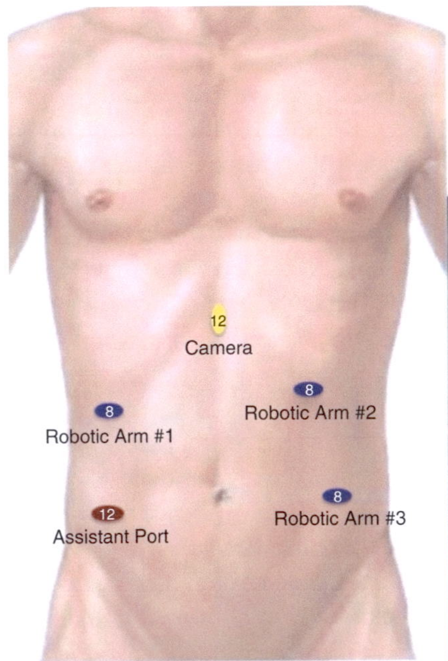
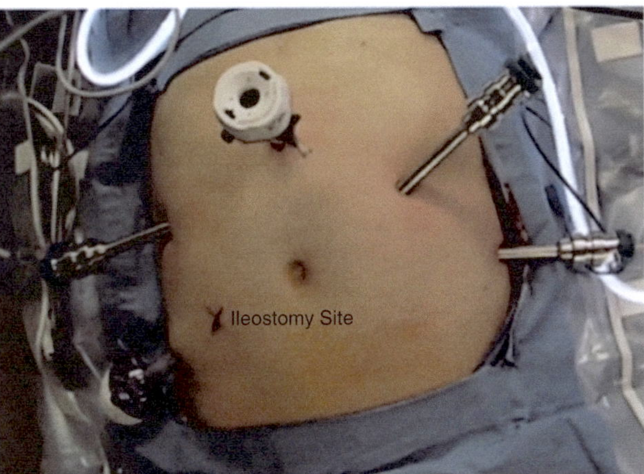

Fig. 12.1 Single-dock port placement

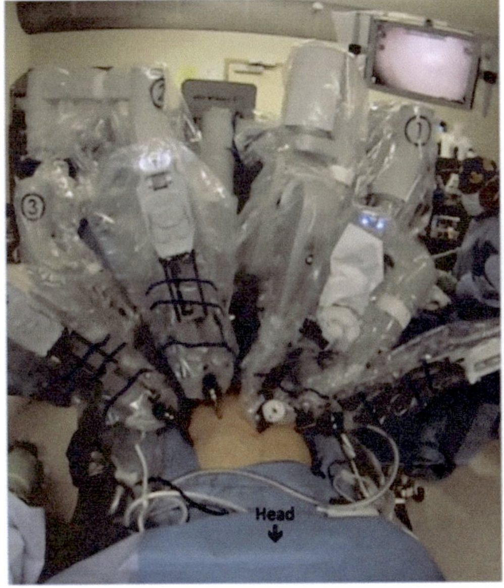

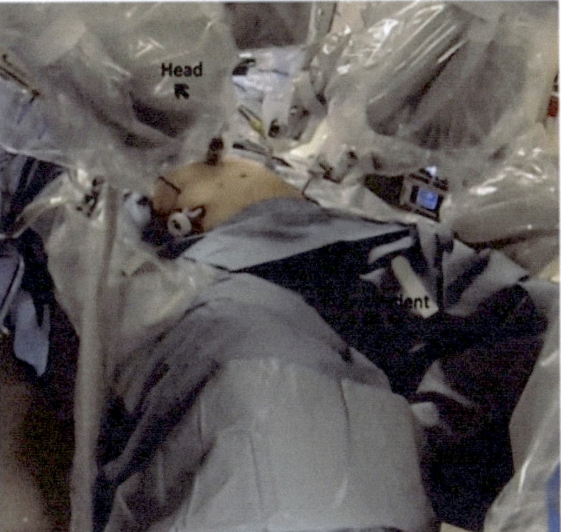

Fig. 12.2 Robotic docking in single-dock technique

The da Vinci® robot is then docked from between the patient's legs, in-line with the bed. The arm for the robotic camera is docked in the subxiphoid position; the first, second, and third robotic arms are docked in the right subcostal, left subcostal, and left lateral ports, respectively (Fig. 12.2).

12.4.4 Surgical Technique

The robotic vessel sealer and hook cautery are alternated in the surgeon's first robotic arm, the Cadiere forceps in the second robotic arm, and a fenestrated grasper in the third robotic arm. In a female patient, the uterus can be retracted and fixed anteriorly using temporarily placed transabdominal sutures. The sigmoid colon is mobilized until the rectosigmoid junction is identified. At this point, the rectosigmoid junction is dissected and divided using a laparoscopic linear stapler via the assistant port.

The left colon is then mobilized, and left colic artery (or IMA) is divided with the robotic vessel sealer, or alternatively, by an energy device introduced through the assistant port. Dissection proceeds toward the splenic flexure, and the assistant retracts the left colon inferomedially. Once the splenic flexure is mobilized, the dissection continues up to the mid-transverse colon. Often this is accomplished by retracting the flexure and transverse colon inferiorly toward the pelvis and taking the mesentery of the colon from the side closest to the stomach within lesser sac.

Following mobilization of the splenic flexure, the dissection can continue along the transverse colon mesentery if visualization is optimal and or turn toward the terminal ileum. The ileocolic artery is identified and divided with the robotic vessel sealer or energy device via the assistant port. The assistant retracts the right colon medially and cephalad as the terminal ileum and ascending colon mobilized. The terminal ileum is then divided with a linear stapler through the assistant port.

The last part of the dissection is the mobilization of the hepatic flexure and completion of dissection of the transverse colon. This can be challenging as the camera is often placed off-center toward the right, so having the TI mobilized and the transverse colon mobilized allows the inferior retraction of the colon leftward and toward the pelvis to better visualize the flexure. The middle colic artery is identified and divided with the robotic vessel sealer or energy device through the assistant port. Additionally, the IMV or branches thereof are divided.

12.4.4.1 Anastomosis and Specimen Extraction

If an end-to-end ileorectal anastomosis is planned, the proximal end of the divided terminal ileum is grasped and brought out through the 12 mm assistant trocar site. The anvil is introduced, and a standard purse-string suture is used to secure the anvil in place prior to replacing the ileal stump into the abdomen. This can also be performed intracorporeally.

The specimen can be extracted via a Pfannenstiel incision, through an enlarged incision at an ileostomy site, or transrectally. In the former, an extracorporeal anastomosis can be performed. If an ileostomy is performed, an incision can be made at that site large enough for the specimen to be extracted. Alternatively, the specimen can be removed in a transrectal fashion. Our technique for transrectal extraction is to irrigate the rectal stump prior to proctotomy. A proctotomy is made along the staple line with robotic scissors through which a flexible endoscope is introduced into the peritoneal cavity. A looped snare is used to grasp the distal end of the specimen (usually the stapled TI), which is then extracted through the proctotomy under robotic visualization, taking care to minimize tension on the specimen and rectal stump during extraction. The robotic arms are used to hold the rectum open to facilitate extraction. The proctotomy is closed with a linear stapler, and an end-to-end ileorectal anastomosis is performed in the standard fashion using an EEA stapler.

The anastomosis is then evaluated endoscopically and a leak test is performed. The final step of the procedure is creation of a diverting loop ileostomy, if indicated. A pelvic drain can be placed through the left lateral port site.

12.5 Conclusion

Robotic-assisted TAC has been demonstrated to be safe and effective in patients suitable for minimally invasive surgery. Most surgical techniques described to date report a multi-dock approach. However, a single-dock approach utilizing three robotic arms, a robotic camera, and one assistant port is technically feasible without need for change in patient positioning. We have found that the single-dock technique improves efficiency while performing a robotic-assisted TAC.

References

1. Buchs NC, et al. Totally robotic right colectomy: a preliminary case series and an overview of the literature. Int J Med Robot. 2011;7(3):348–52.
2. Caputo D, et al. Conversion in mini-invasive colorectal surgery: the effect of timing on short term outcome. Int J Surg. 2014;12(8):805–9.
3. Davis BR, et al. Robotic-assisted versus laparoscopic colectomy: cost and clinical outcomes. JSLS. 2014;18(2):211–24.
4. Park JS, et al. Randomized clinical trial of robot-assisted versus standard laparoscopic right colectomy. Br J Surg. 2012;99(9):1219–26.
5. Shin JY. Comparison of short-term surgical outcomes between a robotic colectomy and a laparoscopic colectomy during early experience. J Korean Soc Coloproctol. 2012;28(1):19–26.
6. Juo YY, et al. Is minimally invasive colon resection better than traditional approaches?: first comprehensive national examination with propensity score matching. JAMA Surg. 2014;149(2):177–84.
7. Kim CW, Kim CH, Baik SH. Outcomes of robotic-assisted colorectal surgery compared with laparoscopic and open surgery: a systematic review. J Gastrointest Surg. 2014;18(4):816–30.
8. Zeng WG, Zhou ZX. Mini-invasive surgery for colorectal cancer. Chin J Cancer. 2014;33(6):277–84.
9. Casillas Jr MA, et al. Improved perioperative and short-term outcomes of robotic versus conventional laparoscopic colorectal operations. Am J Surg. 2014;208(1):33–40.
10. Rawlings AL, et al. Robotic versus laparoscopic colectomy. Surg Endosc. 2007;21(10):1701–8.
11. Huettner F, et al. One hundred and two consecutive robotic-assisted minimally invasive colectomies—an outcome and technical update. J Gastrointest Surg. 2011;15(7):1195–204.
12. Rankin FW. Total colectomy: its indications and technique. Ann Surg. 1931;94(4):677–704.
13. Stupart DA, et al. Surgery for colonic cancer in HNPCC: total vs segmental colectomy. Colorectal Dis. 2011;13(12):1395–9.
14. Guy TS, Williams NN, Rosato EF. Crohn's disease of the colon. Surg Clin North Am. 2001;81(1):159–68, ix.
15. Tekkis PP, et al. A comparison of segmental vs subtotal/total colectomy for colonic Crohn's disease: a meta-analysis. Colorectal Dis. 2006;8(2):82–90.
16. Pinedo G, et al. Laparoscopic total colectomy for colonic inertia: surgical and functional results. Surg Endosc. 2009;23(1):62–5.
17. Delaney CP, et al. Is laparoscopic colectomy applicable to patients with body mass index >30? A case-matched comparative study with open colectomy. Dis Colon Rectum. 2005;48(5):975–81.

Low Anterior Resection/Proctectomy

Amit Merchea and David W. Larson

Abstract

Robotic use in rectal resection is increasing in utility and popularity. Reported benefits of the robotics over traditional laparoscopy are varied. Robotic pelvic dissection is a technically demanding operation. A surgeon who is competent with pelvic laparoscopy may be at an advantage to benefit from the opportunities robotics may offer.

In general the robot improves operative ergonomics and three-dimensional high-definition visualization of the pelvis, which may translate into technical and functional benefits. This chapter reviews the technical aspects of both a hybrid and totally robotic approach to proctectomy (low anterior, coloanal, and abdominoperineal resection).

Keywords

Robotic • Proctectomy • Low anterior resection • Coloanal • Abdominoperineal resection

Electronic supplementary material: This chapter contains video segments that can be found on the following DOI: 10.1007/978-3-319-09120-4_13.

A. Merchea, M.D.
Section of Colon and Rectal Surgery, Mayo Clinic, Jacksonville, FL, USA

D.W. Larson, M.D., M.B.A. (✉)
Division of Colon and Rectal Surgery, Mayo Clinic, 200 First Street SW, Rochester, MN 55905, USA
e-mail: larson.david2@mayo.edu

13.1 Introduction

The benefits of robotic surgery are many and follow the national trend of increasing minimally invasive surgery for complex operations. Patient selection is a key component to assuring outstanding outcomes when undertaking robotic surgery. This is particularly important for the novice robotic surgeon. The learning curve is both steep and long for complex pelvic surgery and one may shorten this curve if they are facile with more traditional laparoscopic techniques prior to attempting their first robotic resection [1]. Robotic techniques may have lower rates of conversion to open in cancer when compared with laparoscopy without a difference in margin positivity [2]. However, recent studies have demonstrated no clinical or oncologic benefit to robotics over laparoscopy [3].

The robotic platform may be used to treat both benign and malignant pelvic diseases. The overall process that we use in our practice combines this minimally invasive approach with best practice processes by incorporating enhanced recovery pathway (ERP) principles with robotic surgery. As is consistent with ERP, the use of oral mechanical bowel preparation is avoided due to the limited data to support their use [4]. Enhanced recovery pathways include multimodal pre-, intra-, and postoperative elements in an attempt to operate in a physiologically normal state, optimize postoperative pain control, manage postoperative nausea, limit fluids, and allow for institution of a general diet [5–7].

13.2 Operative Technique (Video 13.1)

13.2.1 Patient and Robot Positioning

The ultimate docking position of the robot is dependent upon the surgical approach being undertaken. For a patient undergoing rectal resection, a modified lithotomy position is chosen to provide access to the perineum. Furthermore, the robot model itself may determine the flexibility, or lack thereof, in such positioning. The new da Vinci Xi is more forgiving than the older S and Si platforms, allowing for the ability to operate in all quadrants without repositioning (Fig. 13.1a, b).

The technical approaches may include either a fully robotic or a hybrid operation. In the hybrid technique, the colorectal vasculature is ligated and the colon mobilized prior to docking the robot. In a completely robotic approach, ligation of vasculature, colonic, and rectal mobilization is completed entirely with the robot.

In the hybrid technique, the patient position may be easily changed to aid the dissection prior to robot docking. Once the laparoscopic mobilization is completed, the patient is placed in steep Trendelenburg and leveled in the horizontal plane or a slight right-side-down tilt. The robot can be docked either between the patient legs for the pelvic dissection in a non-reconstructive operation or over the left hip for a reconstructive operation in which access to the perineum is required. When performing a totally robotic dissection, the robot is docked over the patient's left hip after the patient is placed in Trendelenburg with the right side tilted downward. It is helpful to have adequate exposure of the colon, splenic flexure, and pelvis simultaneously as the patient bed may not be repositioned with the robot docked. Too steep Trendelenburg will make visualizing the splenic flexure and transverse colon difficult and too steep right-side tilt may inhibit visualization of the pelvis. In such situations, the robotic arms may be disengaged, the bed appropriately adjusted, and the arms re-engaged.

13.2.2 Trocar Placement

Abdominal access can be obtained by a variety of methods. We prefer the use of a modified open technique, utilizing an OPTIVIEW® trocar (Ethicon Endo-Surgery, Inc.) placed under direct visualization in the midline just superior to the umbilicus. The OPTIVIEW® trocar has particular benefit in an obese patient in which a traditional open technique is difficult secondary to poor visualization. Ideally, the 30-degree camera is positioned roughly 15 cm from the target anatomy and is positioned at a 30-degree down angle. It is critical with older S and Si models that the working arms are positioned outside this camera cone area, which is the visual field of the camera based on the target anatomy. Additional trocars are placed once insufflation is achieved to ensure the appropriate 8–10 cm distances between ports for S and Si system and 6–8 cm for the Xi system to avoid external or internal collisions.

In the hybrid technique we generally place 4 additional trocars (Fig. 13.2a). Robotic trocars are placed in the right and left lower quadrants (arms 1 and 2, respectively), approximately at the midclavicular lines. Another robotic trocar (arm 3) is placed in the left lateral abdomen, cranial to both the anterior superior iliac spine and arm 2. An additional 5-mm trocar (assistant port) is placed in right upper quadrant.

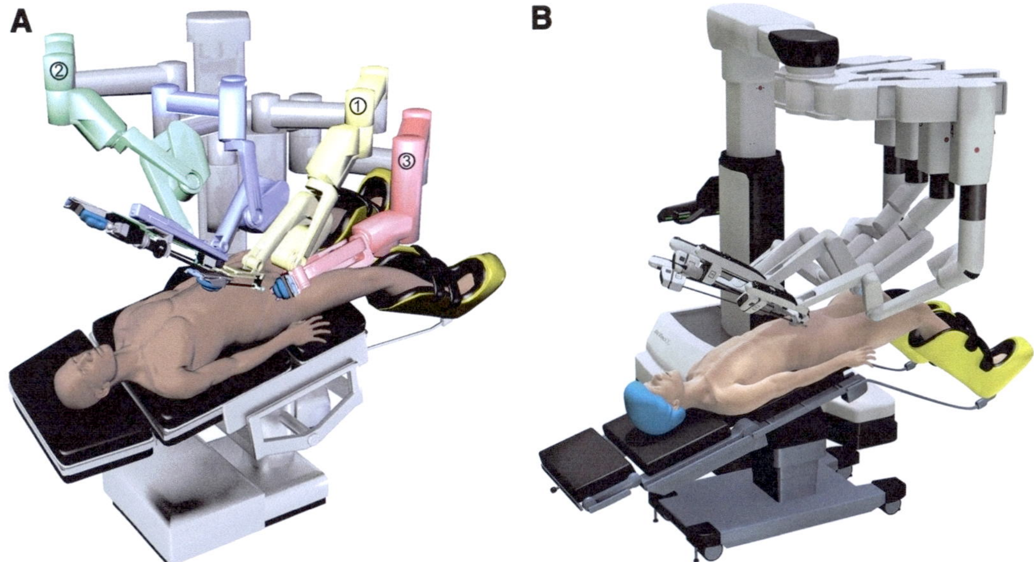

Fig. 13.1 The newer da Vinci Xi (**a**) and previous generation (**b**), systems are seen here. The Xi offers greater flexibility with overhead instrument arm location and the ability to operate in all abdominal quadrants without repositioning the robot. *With permission from Intuitive Surgical, Sunnyvale, CA*

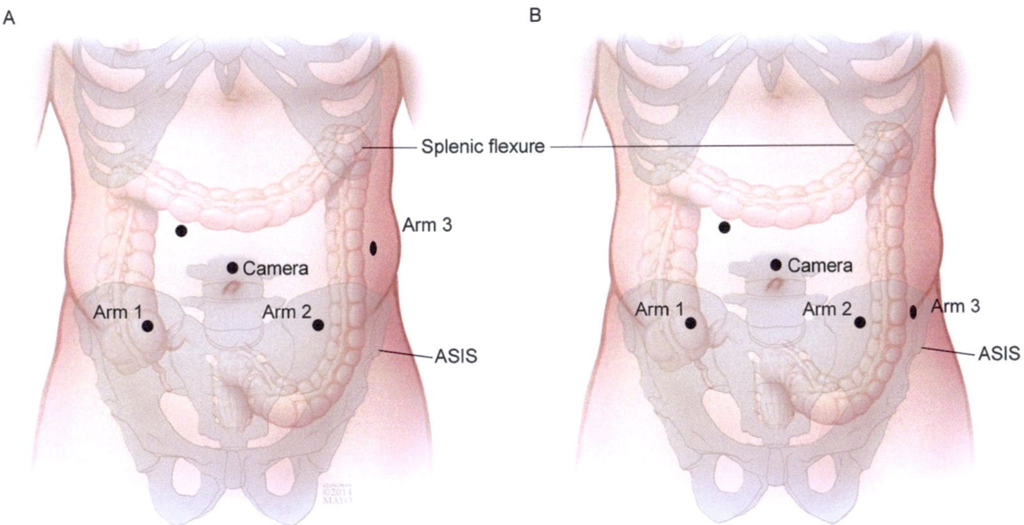

Fig. 13.2 (**a**) Trocar positions for a hybrid robotic approach and (**b**) trocar positions for a completely robotic approach. *With permission from Intuitive Surgical, Sunnyvale, CA*

Port placement differs slightly in the completely robotic technique. Abdominal access is obtained in the same position and manner as previously described. Robotic instrument ports (arms 1 and 2) are placed in similar positions. A robotic trocar (arm 3) is placed in the left lateral abdomen, just superior to anterior iliac spine. A similar trocar is placed for the third arm in the right upper quadrant just to the right of midline—this position is used for the splenic flexure. The robot should be positioned over the left hip such that a straight line drawn from the midpoint of the camera arm attachment crosses the anterior superior iliac spine. The most distal aspect of the camera arm and port should be in line with the patient's spine. It is critical that the alignment of arm 1 and the camera is not in the identical vector toward the left colon and splenic flexure, as this position would impede mobilization and dissection (Fig. 13.2b).

Issues that are critical to consider include the distance to the target anatomy and the potential for the boney aspects of the pelvic sidewall and sacral promontory to impede surgical dissection. For example, the monopolar scissors is 57 cm in length with a working length of 27 cm from the remote center to tip. Trocars placed too far cephalad in a patient with a long torso will make the presacral dissection toward the pelvic floor difficult secondary to reach. Likewise, the sacral promontory acting as a fulcrum can lead to a poor angle of dissection into the presacral space. Finally, trocars placed too far laterally (particularly in a male patient) will make the low pelvic dissection difficult secondary to collisions with the lateral pelvic sidewall.

13.2.3 Operative Technique

13.2.3.1 Step 1: Initial Exposure

The greater omentum should be reflected over the transverse colon toward the liver and the small bowel retracted out of the pelvis into the right upper quadrant. In a female patient, it may be necessary to suspend the uterus to obtain an unobstructed view into the deep pelvis. We place a suture transabdominally around the round ligaments to suspend the uterus anteriorly or directly through the fundus of the uterus. Alternatively, a uterine manipulator may be placed transvaginally to suspend the uterus and vagina away from the rectum to allow easier dissection in the rectovaginal septum.

13.2.3.2 Step 2: Control of the Inferior Mesenteric Artery and Inferior Mesenteric Vein

Depending on the length of colon needed, vessel ligation may include any combination of inferior mesenteric artery (IMA), proximal or distal to the left colic artery, as well as inferior mesenteric vein (IMV) ligation. Whether this particular portion of the operation is done with traditional laparoscopic techniques or robotic techniques, the principles remain the same. If being completed laparoscopically, the patient is placed in steep Trendelenburg; the assistant grasps the rectosigmoid junction and retracts the rectum superiorly out of the pelvis. Robotically, a monopolar-curved scissors is initially used in arm 1 (right lower quadrant) and a fenestrated bipolar forceps used in arm 2 (left lower quadrant); a double-fenestrated atraumatic bowel grasper is placed in arm 3 (left lateral abdomen). Using arm 3, the rectosigmoid junction is grasped and the rectum is placed on tension proximally, pulling it out of the pelvis. Alternatively, an assistant may grasp this area, allowing arm 3 to grasp more distally on the rectum to provide additional traction, placing the rectosigmoid mesocolon and mesorectum on tension. It is critical that the upper rectum be elevated in such a way as to stretch the peritoneum overlying the right pelvic gutter, as well as the superior rectal artery to help separate the vessels from the sacral promontory. Electrocautery is then utilized to incise the peritoneum along the right side of the rectum, caudal to the sacral promontory. This exposes and opens the presacral space (Fig. 13.3a, b).

Dissection is carried cephalad along the posterior aspect of the mesorectum toward the IMA (Fig. 13.4a), taking care not to breach the fascia propria of the rectum and avoiding injury to the superior hypogastric nerves. Injury to the nervous structures around the IMA may result in retrograde ejaculation and/or bladder dysfunction. As one dissects directly below the superior rectal artery and above the retroperitoneal fascial planes, the left ureter and gonadal vessels should be identified just above the pelvic brim.

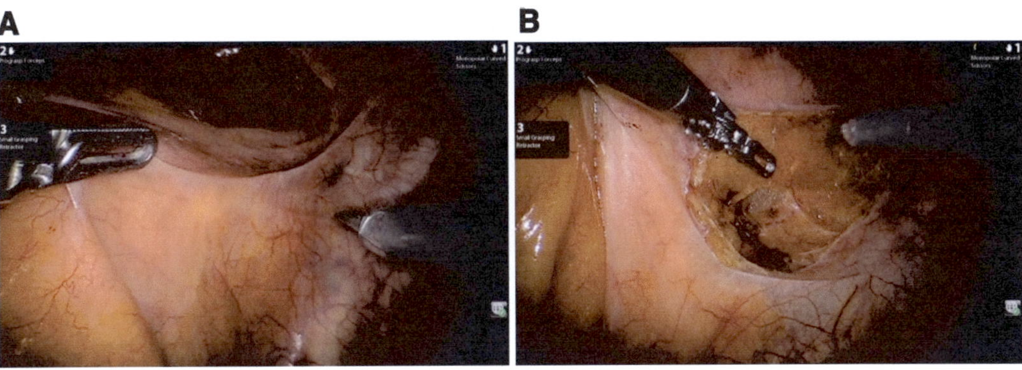

Fig. 13.3 (**a**, **b**) An unobstructed view of the pelvis is obtained. The rectum is retracted cephalad and to the left using arm 3. The rectum must be elevated to stretch the peritoneum and raise the superior rectal artery anteriorly to separate the vessels from the sacral promontory. Electrocautery is then used to incise the peritoneum along the right side of the rectum, caudal to the sacral promontory

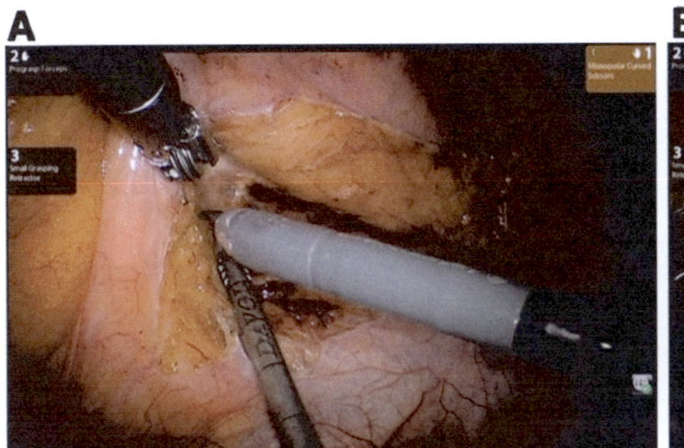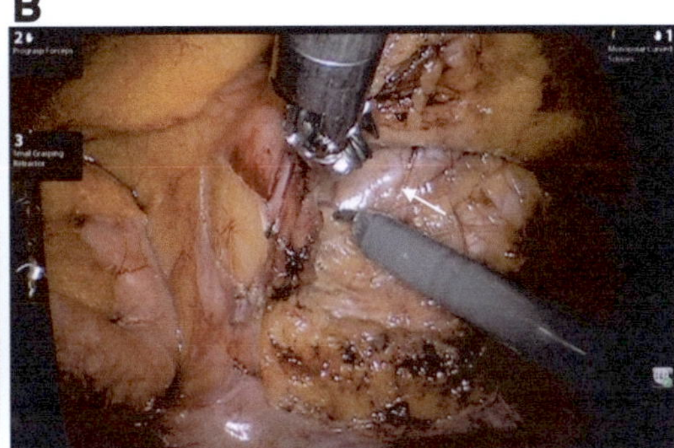

Fig. 13.4 (**a**, **b**) Identifying and isolating the inferior mesenteric artery—dissection is carried cephalad along the posterior aspect of the mesorectum toward the IMA. Arm 2 (LLQ) is placed posterior to the vascular bundle and mesorectum and retracted anteriorly. The assistant may place countertraction using either a laparoscopic grasper or suction device to aid the dissection. The vessel is elevated from the retroperitoneum, and the gonadal vessels and ureter (white arrow) should be identified within the retroperitoneum, just above the pelvic brim, posterior and lateral to the IMA

As this dissection continues in this plane, the vessel is elevated from the retroperitoneum and the ureter and gonadal vessels can be easily swept bluntly posteriorly to maintain their position within the retroperitoneum, posterior and lateral to the IMA (Fig. 13.4b).

While there is no oncologic benefit to high versus low ligation of the IMA, we prefer to ligate this vessel at its origin to obtain maximal length for a potential low pelvic anastomosis and to minimize tension [8]. Once the IMA is isolated at its origin, we ligate this using either a 5-mm blunt tip LigaSure (*Covidien Surgical Solutions, Mansfield, MA*) vessel sealer or the da Vinci® EndoWrist® One™ vessel sealer (*Intuitive Surgical Inc., Sunnyvale, CA*) (Fig. 13.5). Other methods of vascular control include the use of endoscopic staplers, clips, or sutures. The colonic mesentery can now be elevated off the retroperitoneum proximally and laterally. If in the correct plane, much of this dissection can be carried out bluntly. The extent of dissection is superior to the inferior border of the pancreas and laterally overlying the Gerota's fascia. The cut edge of the colonic mesentery can continue to be transected superiorly, lateral to the duodenum to include the IMV. If the IMV cannot be reached in this manner, it may be transected prior to releasing the splenic flexure.

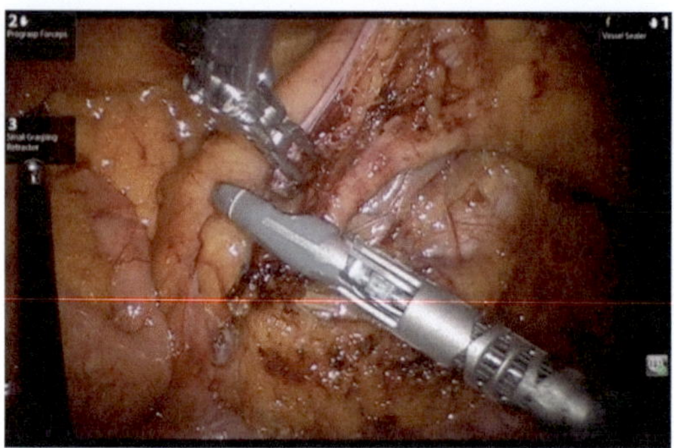

Fig. 13.5 Ligation of the IMA is shown. One must take care to not inadvertently include the retroperitoneum in the vessel sealer. Prior to ligation, this retroperitoneal plane should be developed such that the empty space between the IMA and left colic artery in the colonic mesentery is visualized. Arm 3 continues to retract the rectum out of the pelvis and places the IMA on a near-vertical orientation. Arm 2 can be used to grasp the peritoneum overlying the vessel (as shown) or the vessel itself, distal to the transection point. Care must be taken to not put the vessel on excess tension while ligating it

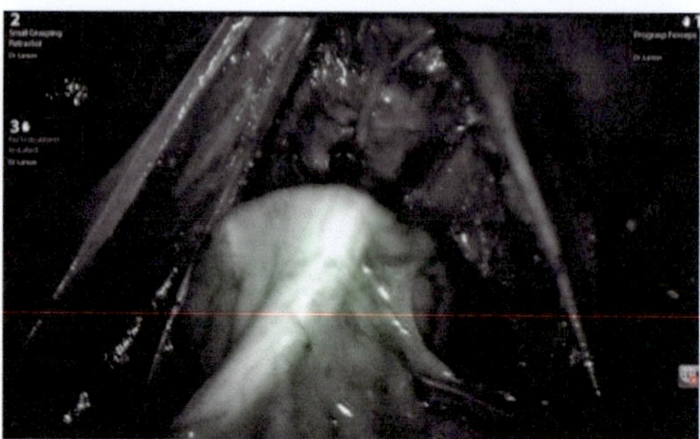

Fig. 13.6 Fluorescence angiographic imaging evaluates the blood supply of the bowel prior to performing an anastomosis

An alternative method to IMV ligation with the hybrid technique involves placing the patient into reverse Trendelenburg position, with the left side elevated. The greater omentum is reflected superiorly and the transverse colon is retracted anteriorly and superiorly. The ligament of Treitz is identified, and the IMV can usually be seen coursing within the colonic mesentery just lateral to the fourth portion of the duodenum. To enter the lesser sac through the transverse mesocolon, the peritoneum of the transverse mesocolon, just superior to the IMV and lateral to the duodenum, is incised. Dissection is carried through the mesocolon and into the lesser sac. The pancreas should be identified posteriorly. To achieve enough length for any coloanal anastomosis, the IMV generally needs to be divided at the inferior boarder of the pancreas. This medial approach to the vein flows into the lesser sac dissection and facilitates complete mobilization of the splenic flexure. Any remaining colonic mesentery between the region of dissection of the IMA and IMV is then also transected with the vessel sealer.

Our typical approach at this point includes taking the colonic mesentery from the primary feeding vessel of the rectum to the edge of the sigmoid or descending colon. This allows for complete vascular isolation of the target anatomy

and provides an estimate as to the proximal area for anastomosis. Near-infrared perfusion angiography (PINPOINT System, *Novadaq, Canada*) and fluorescence angiographic imaging (FIREFLY, *Novadaq,* Canada) to evaluate the blood supply of the bowel to be used for the anastomosis may be evaluated either at this time or after construction of the anastomosis (Fig. 13.6) [9–11]. In general, we prefer to use the more compliant descending colon for any low anterior resection. Once the mesentery has been divided, we do not divide the bowel as it provides a fantastic opportunity for retraction during the pelvic dissection.

13.2.3.3 Step 3: Medial-to-Lateral and Splenic Flexure Mobilization

The mesentery and lateral attachments of the descending and sigmoid colon are all that remain to be divided. From the medial side, the appropriate avascular plane can be quickly and easily separated in a blunt manner. It is imperative to ensure that the Toldt's fascia is preserved and the retroperitoneum is not violated—doing so places the retroperitoneal structures (kidney, ureter, and gonadal vessels) at risk of injury. This dissection is complete when all that remains of the colonic attachments are the lateral peritoneal attachments and filmy attachments to the splenic flexure. Without changing position these attachments can be cut with electrocautery. Alternatively, one may prepare the robot for the pelvic portion of the dissection and place the patient in Trendelenburg position and the left side slightly elevated. Prior to engaging the pelvis, one can quickly detach the lateral peritoneal attachments

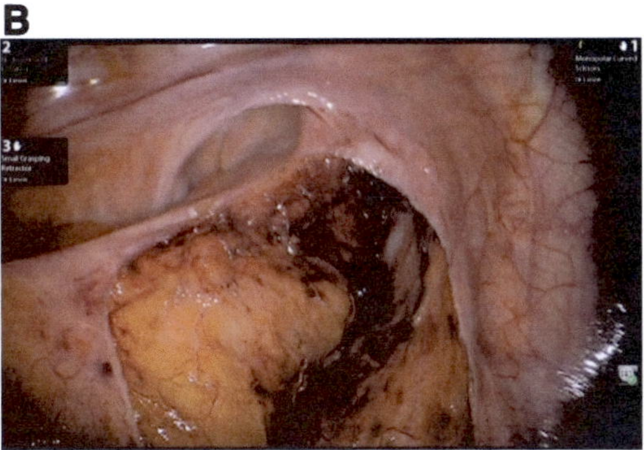

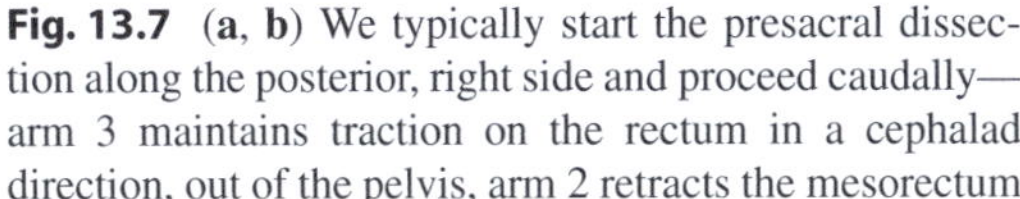

Fig. 13.7 (**a, b**) We typically start the presacral dissection along the posterior, right side and proceed caudally—arm 3 maintains traction on the rectum in a cephalad direction, out of the pelvis, arm 2 retracts the mesorectum toward the patient's left side, and arm 1 is used to perform the dissection. This dissection is carried as far to the left pelvic sidewall as possible to decrease the amount of dissection necessary from the patient's left side

to the left colon and sigmoid by starting at the pelvic brim and continued proximally toward the splenic flexure. This is then taken down completely with a combination of a medial-to-lateral and lateral-to-medial dissection.

When releasing the splenic flexure robotically, the right and left lower quadrant robotic ports (arms 1 and 2) and the right upper quadrant port (arm 3) are utilized. A double-fenestrated atraumatic bowel grasper can be placed in arm 1, and the monopolar-curved scissors and a bipolar fenestrated grasper can be exchanged between arms 2 and 3 to help facilitate the splenic flexure dissection in a medial-to-lateral or lateral-to-medial approach.

If an abdominoperineal resection (APR) is to be performed, it is not necessary to ligate the IMV highly and the splenic flexure is not mobilized. The colonic mesentery is instead transected with the vessel sealer to the border of the sigmoid colon and the colon is divided with an endoscopic stapler.

13.2.3.4 Step 4: Rectal Dissection

In the hybrid approach, the robot is docked between the legs for a non-reconstructive operation. If reconstruction is considered, the robot may be docked over the left hip. Arm 3 (left lateral abdomen—graptor) or an instrument through the accessory port directed by the first assistant is used to grasp the rectum and retract it out of the pelvis anteriorly. Arms 1 (monopolar-curved scissors) and 2 (fenestrated bipolar forceps) then begin the dissection in the avascular mesorectal plane. We typically start this dissection along the

posterior, right side and proceed caudally—in this case, arm 2 retracts the rectum toward the patient's left side and arm 1 is used to perform the dissection. This dissection is carried as far to the left pelvic sidewall as possible to decrease the amount of dissection necessary from the patient's left side (Fig. 13.7). The instrumentation in arms 1 and 2 may always be exchanged in order to complete the dissection along the left side of the rectum. The posterior dissection is continued distally, including the lateral stalks, which are taken with monopolar cautery. If a middle rectal vessel is present within the lateral stalks and not controlled with cautery, this may be controlled with either the bipolar or the robotic vessel sealer. Dissection that is too lateral in the region of the lateral stalks places the nervi erigentes at risk for injury, which can lead to erectile dysfunction.

The anterior dissection is then undertaken. Arm 3 is used to pull down and out of the pelvis to provide proper tension on the anterior structures. The assistant aids the dissection by placing a suction device or grasper anterior at the level of the seminal vesicle or posterior vagina and lifting anteriorly. This countertraction anterior to the rectum allows the dissection to progress to the level of the pelvic floor (Fig. 13.8). In patients with an anterior tumor, our dissection plane is always anterior to the Denonvilliers' fascia. With posterior-based tumors, our dissection plane is just posterior. The periprostatic nerve plexus carries mixed sympathetic and parasympathetic fibers and may be injured during this phase of the dissection.

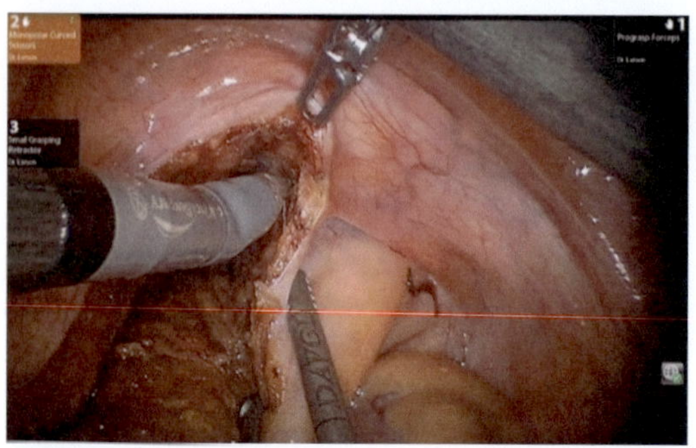

Fig. 13.8 The anterior dissection, either anterior or posterior to the Denonvilliers' fascia (dependent upon tumor location), is performed by placing the rectum on tension in a posterior and cephalad direction (arm 3). Arm 1 retracts anteriorly and arm 2 is performing the direction (these may be interchanged). Additional countertraction can be obtained by having the assistant either retract posteriorly (as shown) or anteriorly

In the completely robotic approach, the technique for rectal dissection is similar, as is the instrumentation. This position is still instrumented with an atraumatic bowel grasper for retraction of the rectum out of the pelvis.

A total mesorectal excision is completed circumferentially to the pelvic floor for patients undergoing coloanal anastomosis. For more proximal tumors, the dissection proceeds to a level that includes a 5-cm distal mesorectal margin. In this case, the mesorectum at the distal transection point is ligated using either a handheld vessel sealer or the robotic vessel sealer in order to isolate the rectum and prepare it for transection in a proper tumor-specific mesorectal excision.

13.2.3.5 Step 6: Anastomotic Technique

In patients undergoing APR, the rectal dissection proceeds robotically to the pelvic floor in a cylindrical manner. The bare area of the rectum distal to the mesorectum must not be unroofed. In this scenario, the pelvic floor musculature can even be incised from the pelvis and the ischioanal space entered, exposing the ischioanal fat. The perineal portion of the resection is then conducted in the usual open fashion and the rectum is extracted through the perineum. Finally, the abdomen is insufflated after closure of the perineal incision

and the end colostomy is identified and matured usually in the left lower quadrant.

For those patients with a low rectal tumor and undergoing a coloanal anastomosis, a mucosectomy is completed just proximal to the dentate line. Placement of a Lone Star retractor (*Cooper Surgical, Trumbull, CT*) generally provides adequate visualization. The mucosectomy is carried proximally to just above the anorectal ring. The pelvis is then entered from the perineal side just anterior to the coccyx. A finger placed into the pelvis, transanally, is then utilized to identify the correct plane of dissection to free the rectum circumferentially with electrocautery. When performing this dissection anteriorly, one must take care not to injure the urethra in males or the vagina in females. Once completely mobilized, the rectum may be extracted transanally and divided at the previously identified proximal transection point on the descending colon. A single-layer hand-sewn coloanal anastomosis is then fashioned with interrupted absorbable sutures placed circumferentially.

Patients undergoing low anterior resection can have the rectum transected, once the mesorectum has been cleared with the vessel sealer, either intracorporeally using the robotic stapling device (Fig. 13.9) or transabdominally, through a small Pfannenstiel incision. An end-to-end stapled anastomosis is then fashioned. An alternative to a straight colorectostomy, a colonic J-pouch, or a transverse coloplasty may be fashioned to increase the reservoir capacity of the colon [12, 13].

A diverting loop ileostomy is routinely used in patients with low (below the anterior peritoneal reflection) anastomoses or those patients who received preoperative radiation therapy. Consideration for ileostomy reversal occurs 3 months after the index operation or once any potential adjuvant therapy is completed.

13.3 Summary

Robotic rectal resection is both safe and feasible. With appropriate surgeon experience and patient selection, either a hybrid laparoscopic-robotic or

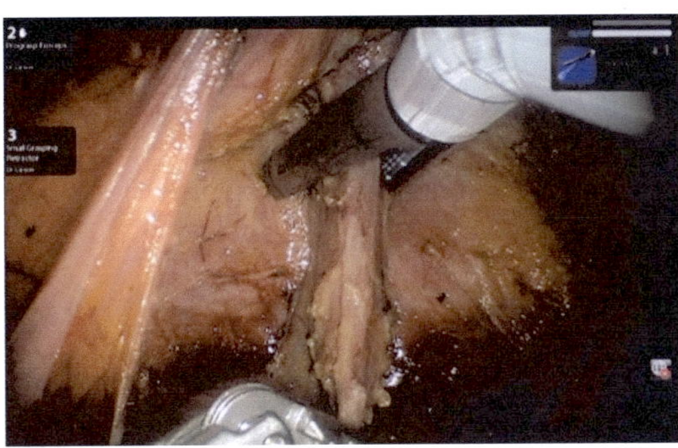

Fig. 13.9 The robotic stapler is utilized to transect the rectum (here for an LAR). The mesorectum has already been cleared with the robotic vessel sealer

completely robotic approach may be used. As newer robotic technologies become available (da Vinci Xi system), additional complex pathology and or multi-quadrant operations may be amenable to such minimal techniques.

13.4 Key Points

- Robotic rectal resection is complex and has a steep learning curve.
- To optimize success, the operating surgeon should initially be facile with laparoscopic techniques.
- Hybrid or totally robotic approaches may be used. For proctectomy, a single docking position is all that is generally necessary.
- Appropriate trocar placement is vital to ensure adequate visualization, limitation of external and internal collisions, and effective and efficient dissection.
- The robot provides improved three-dimensional and high-definition visualization of the pelvis.

References

1. Park EJ, Kim CW, Cho MS, Baik SH, Kim DW, Min BS, et al. Multidimensional analyses of the learning curve of robotic low anterior resection for rectal cancer: 3-phase learning process comparison. Surg Endosc. 2014;28(10):2821–31.
2. Memon S, Heriot AG, Murphy DG, Bressel M, Lynch AC. Robotic versus laparoscopic proctectomy for rectal cancer: a meta-analysis. Ann Surg Oncol. 2012;19(7):2095–101.
3. Park EJ, Cho MS, Baek SJ, Hur H, Min BS, Baik SH, et al. Long-term oncologic outcomes of robotic low anterior resection for rectal cancer: a comparative study with laparoscopic surgery. Ann Surg. 2014; 261(1):129–37.
4. Guenaga KF, Matos D, Wille-Jorgensen P. Mechanical bowel preparation for elective colorectal surgery. Cochrane Database Syst Rev. 2011;(9):CD001544.
5. Khreiss W, Huebner M, Cima RR, Dozois ER, Chua HK, Pemberton JH, et al. Improving conventional recovery with enhanced recovery in minimally invasive surgery for rectal cancer. Dis Colon rectum. 2014;57(5):557–63.
6. Lovely JK, Maxson PM, Jacob AK, Cima RR, Horlocker TT, Hebl JR, et al. Case-matched series of enhanced versus standard recovery pathway in minimally invasive colorectal surgery. Br J Surg. 2012;99(1):120–6.
7. Hubner M, Lovely JK, Huebner M, Slettedahl SW, Jacob AK, Larson DW. Intrathecal analgesia and restrictive perioperative fluid management within enhanced recovery pathway: hemodynamic implications. J Am Coll Surg. 2013;216(6):1124–34.
8. Bonnet S, Berger A, Hentati N, Abid B, Chevallier JM, Wind P, et al. High tie versus low tie vascular ligation of the inferior mesenteric artery in colorectal cancer surgery: impact on the gain in colon length and implications on the feasibility of anastomoses. Dis Colon Rectum. 2012;55(5):515–21.
9. Sherwinter DA. Transanal near-infrared imaging of colorectal anastomotic perfusion. Surg Laparosc Endosc Percutan Techn. 2012;22(5):433–6.
10. Sherwinter DA, Gallagher J, Donkar T. Intra-operative transanal near infrared imaging of colorectal anastomotic perfusion: a feasibility study. Colorectal Dis. 2013;15(1):91–6.
11. Jafari MD, Lee KH, Halabi WJ, Mills SD, Carmichael JC, Stamos MJ, et al. The use of indocyanine green fluorescence to assess anastomotic perfusion during robotic assisted laparoscopic rectal surgery. Surg Endosc. 2013;27(8):3003–8.
12. Biondo S, Frago R, Codina Cazador A, Farres R, Olivet F, Golda T, et al. Long-term functional results from a randomized clinical study of transverse coloplasty compared with colon J-pouch after low anterior resection for rectal cancer. Surgery. 2013;153(3): 383–92.
13. Heriot AG, Tekkis PP, Constantinides V, Paraskevas P, Nicholls RJ, Darzi A, et al. Meta-analysis of colonic reservoirs versus straight coloanal anastomosis after anterior resection. Br J Surg. 2006;93(1):19–32.

Robotic Abdominoperineal Resection

14

Jorge A. Lagares-Garcia, Anthony Firilas,
Carlos Martinez Parra, Mary Arnold Long,
and Raquel Gonzalez Heredia

Abstract

Robotic utilization in rectal cancer has several distinct advantages. The clear benefits of the magnification and visualization, combined with the improved dexterity in confined places such the true pelvis, make robotic-assisted surgery optimal for distal rectal cancers. Current literature shows short-term outcomes comparable with laparoscopic approach. Large prospective international studies are underway to provide an answer about the short-and long-term oncologic and functional outcomes with this technique. In this chapter, we provide the reader with detailed description of how to perform robotic APR. Attention to patient selection, the importance of preoperative stoma marking, positioning, room arrangement, and troubleshooting in an emergency situation are illustrated. Literature review and outcomes are described with the most up-to-date short-term and oncologic outcomes.

Keywords

Robotic • Distal rectal cancer • Abdominoperineal resection

J.A. Lagares-Garcia, M.D., F.A.C.S.,
F.A.S.C.R.S. (✉)
Division of Colon and Rectal Surgery,
Department of Surgery, Charleston Colorectal
Surgery, Roper Hospital, 125 Doughty Street Suite
280, Charleston, SC, USA
e-mail: Jorge.lagares-garcia@rsfh.com

A. Firilas, M.D.
Roper St Francis Physicians Partners,
Charleston, SC 29403, USA

C.M. Parra, M.D.
Division of General and Transplant Surgery,
University of Illinois at Chicago, Chicago, IL, USA

M.A. Long, A.P.R.N.
Department of Nursing, Roper Hospital,
Charleston, SC, USA

R.G. Heredia, M.D., Ph.D.
Division of General, Minimally Invasive and Robotic
Surgery, University of Illinois at Chicago,
Chicago, IL, USA

© Springer International Publishing Switzerland 2015
H. Ross et al. (eds.), *Robotic Approaches to Colorectal Surgery*,
DOI 10.1007/978-3-319-09120-4_14

"

14.1 Introduction to Robotic Proctectomy

Robotic technology is currently undergoing a significant expansion in the field of colorectal surgery. Although it was originally seen as more appropriate to be used in a single quadrant area, the introduction of the new platform da Vinci Xi™ (Intuitive Surgical Inc., Sunnyvale, CA) will potentially improve the multiquadrant applications of the robotic equipment facilitating the splenic flexure takedown. Whichever current market platform is used, the enhancement of the three-dimensional vision, degrees of freedom, and rotation in the robotic wristed arms and the high-definition resolution and vision in confined spaces help expedite robotic-assisted procedures.

The goal of this chapter is to provide detailed steps to perform an abdominoperineal resection (APR) including surgical pearls and tips acquired through our clinical experience in robotic technology.

14.2 Indications for APR

Robotic-assisted APR have the same indications as any mid or distal rectal/anal or pelvic cancer where sphincter-sparing techniques will preclude complete oncologic resection or expected quality of life with poor functional outcome would potentially cripple the patient to a fully functional recovery.

The most important contraindication to robotic APR is the physiologic inability of the patient to tolerate the stress of a major intestinal resection. Patient selection in the early learning curve may facilitate the operator to familiarize with the steps and the procedure. As the experience increases, relative contraindications such as prior abdominal or pelvic operations may no longer suppose a halt in the decision making to provide the patient with a minimally invasive technique to their rectal disease. Intestinal adhesiolysis may be performed laparoscopically upon entry or with the docked robotic arms as per surgeon and team's preference. The robotic technology is specially suited for surgery in a localized quadrant (urology, gynecology) although the introduction of the new robotic system da Vinci Xi™ (Intuitive Surgical Inc., Sunnyvale, CA) will potentially allow the exchange of the camera for working ports without undocking the robot with a new thinner profile and better ergonomic equipment.

Indications for surgery are mainly invasive adenocarcinoma to the sphincter complex and recurrence of squamous cell carcinoma; also the performance of a completion proctectomy in patients with inflammatory bowel disease when sphincter sparing and pelvic reconstruction are prohibitive is also enhanced using the robotic system. Other unusual indications would be presacral tumors with invasion to the distal rectum.

In our personal experience, unless the patient is unfit to tolerate general anesthesia, all patients with distal rectal/pelvic disease that are precluded from preservation of sphincter are routinely selected for robotic surgery. If a pelvic exenteration is required, a consideration should be made with an expert robotic-trained urologist.

14.3 Preoperative Stoma Site Marking

The placement of a permanent stoma is a significant change in personal perception as well as social withdrawal. In order for an enterostomate to fulfill an active lifestyle, it is imperative to be educated preoperatively. In 1953, Turnbull identified the importance of assessing the abdomen preoperatively in order to avoid postoperative complications from poor stoma location [1]. Current guidelines recommend for all patients a preoperative visit allowing for stoma siting and for education of the patient and, if desired, the appropriate family members [2].

Evaluation of the preoperative patient's abdomen is done in multiple positions for optimal stoma site selection: lying, standing, and sitting (Figs. 14.1, 14.2, 14.3, 14.4, 14.5, and 14.6).

These maneuvers help reduce postoperative complications such as pouch leakage, peristomal skin irritation, pain, odor, and patient/family frustration and they are currently supported with

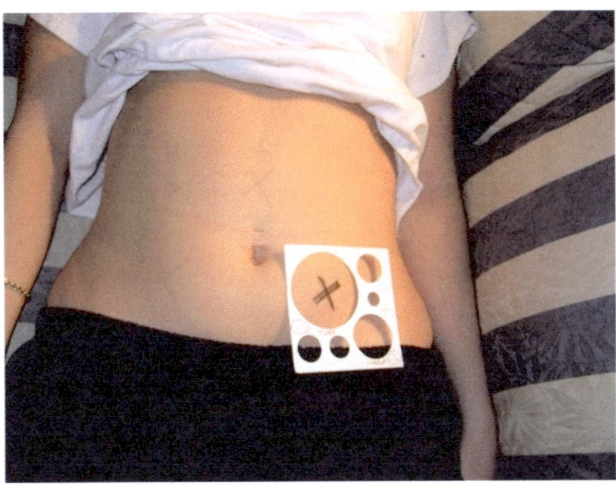

Fig. 14.1 Standard placement supine. Courtesy of Jane Carmel, MSN, RN, CWOCN

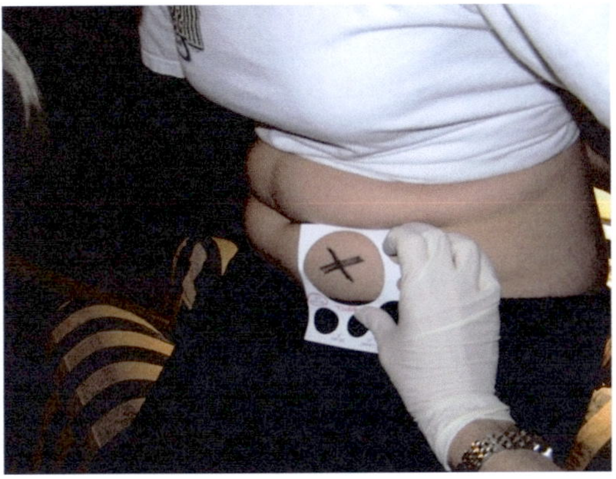

Fig. 14.2 Placement bending over. Courtesy of Jane Carmel, MSN, RN, CWOCN

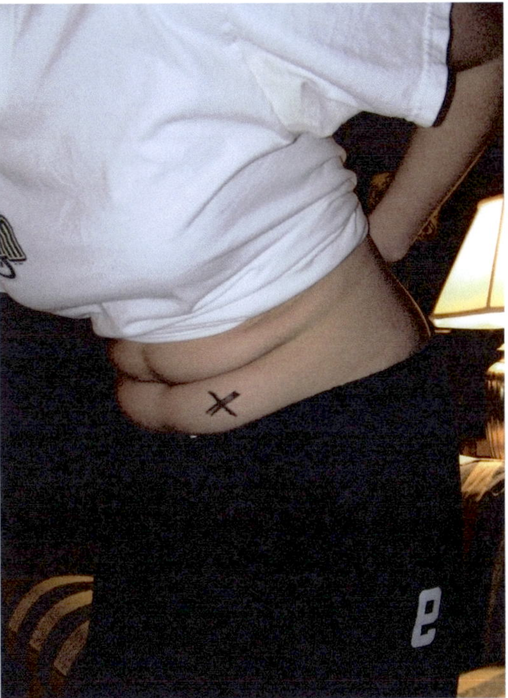

Fig. 14.3 Placement on standing position. Courtesy of Jane Carmel, MSN, RN, CWOCN

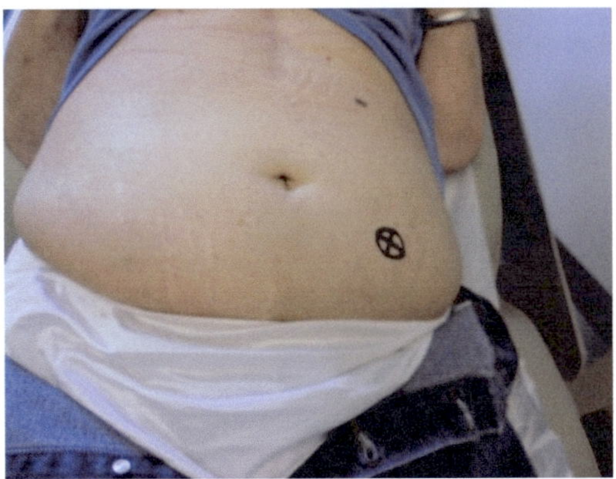

Fig. 14.4 Obese abdomen placement supine

current literature. It can enhance patient independence and return to optimal functioning [3–7].

It is important in the marking process to place the stoma within the rectus muscle and in the patient's visual field, outside of any creases, scars, wrinkles, and bony prominences and considering [8]. The guide developed by ASCRS and WOCN is noted in Table 14.1.

The usual site for an APR would be the left lower quadrant, but there are specific patient considerations (i.e., in wheelchair-bound or obese patients the optimal stoma site should be in the left upper quadrant; in patients whose profession requires them to wear specific tool belt or harness, they should bring that belt with them to be marked).

Indelible marking is the recommended method and most common since it does not leave permanent marking (tattooing) or break skin barrier (scratching) [8]. When marking for an anticipated robotic APR, since there is no midline incision, one of the trocar sites may serve as a potential stoma site; therefore, it is imperative that the

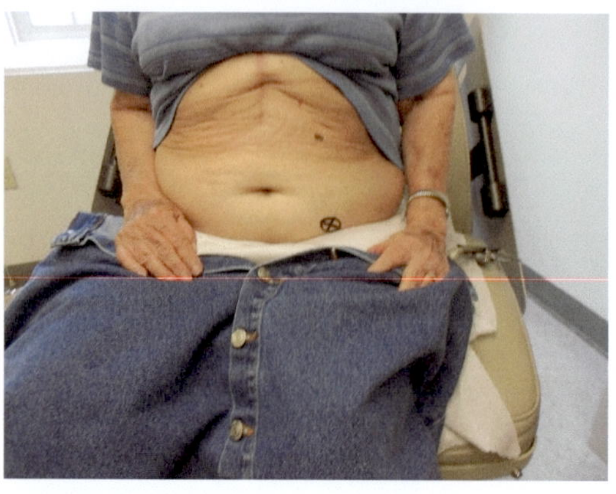

Fig. 14.5 Obese abdomen placement on sitting position

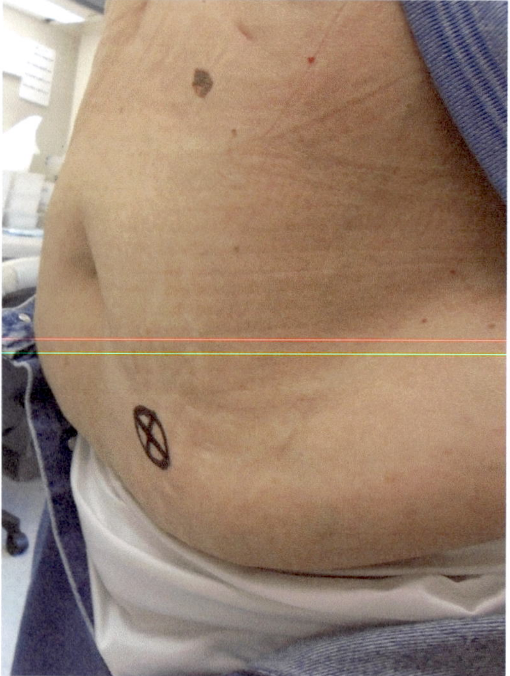

Fig. 14.6 Obese abdomen on standing position

Table 14.1 Stoma marking key points

Key points to consider
• Positioning issues: contractures, posture, mobility, e.g., wheelchair confinement, use of walker, etc.
• Physical considerations: large/protruding/pendulous abdomen, abdominal folds, wrinkles, scars/suture lines, other stomas, rectus muscle, waistline, iliac crest, braces, pendulous breasts, vision, dexterity, presence of hernia
• Patient considerations: diagnosis, history of radiation, age, occupation
• Other: surgeon preferences, patient preferences, type of ostomy or diversion, anticipated stool consistency
• Multiple stoma sites: mark fecal and urinary stomas on different horizontal planes/lines

14.4 Procedure for Robotic APR

14.4.1 Room Setup

- Appropriate preplanning and arrangements in the room will facilitate the flow of the operation, operating room space, and resource usage (Table 14.2).
  - Routine placement of the patient-side cart on the patient's left side will decrease the docking time considering side docking in the left hip (Fig. 14.7).
  - The patient bed may be angled toward the right side about 10–15°.
- The bedside assistant is on the patient's right side as the port is usually located over the right upper quadrant of the abdomen. Routinely, the instruments are passed from the surgical technician or placed in the pocket of the surgical draping.

14.4.2 Patient Positioning

- Routine combined approach is performed in these cases where the main operating surgeon will perform the abdominal part and a second surgeon will proceed through the perineal portion of the procedure when the intra-abdominal

surgeon and the WOC nurse have a direct communication. It is recommended to "bud" all stomas. This allows the effluent to readily flow into the pouching system increasing the wearing time even in situations with diarrhea stool secondary to radiation enteritis, medication side effects, clostridium difficile colitis, or other pathology.

Table 14.2 Procedure of stoma marking

Gather items needed for the procedure:
1. Marking pen, surgical marker, transparent film dressing, flat skin barrier (according to surgeon's preference and facility policy)
2. Explain stoma marking procedure to patient, and encourage patient participation and input
3. Carefully examine patient's abdominal surface. Begin with patient fully clothed in sitting position with feet on the floor. Observe the presence of belts, braces, and any other ostomy appliances
4. Examine patient's exposed abdomen in various positions (standing, lying, sitting, and bending forward) to observe for creases, valleys, scars, folds, skin turgor and contour
5. Draw an imaginary line where the surgical incision is going to be. Choose a point approximately 2 in. from the surgical incision where 2–3 in. of flat adhesive barrier can be placed
6. With the patient lying on back, identify the rectus muscle. This can be done by having the patient do a modified sit-up (raise the head up off the bed). Placement within the rectus muscle can help to prevent peristomal hernia formation and/or prolapse
7. Choose an area that is visible to the patient and if possible below the belt line to conceal the pouch
8. If the abdomen is large, choose the apex of the mound or if the patient is extremely obese, place in the upper abdominal quadrants
9. It may be desirable to mark sites on the right and left sides of the abdomen to prepare for a change in the surgical outcome (you may want to number your first choice as 1)
10. Clean the desired site with alcohol and allow to dry. Then proceed with marking the selected site with a surgical marker/pen. You may cover with transparent film dressing if desired to preserve the mark
11. Once marked, have the patient assume sitting, bending, and lying position to assess and confirm the best choice. It is important to have the patient confirm they can see the site

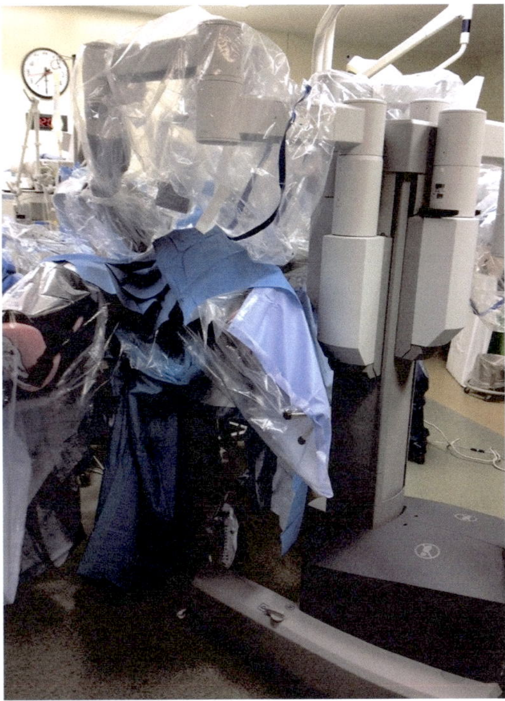

Fig. 14.7 Robotic left-hip docking

sliding noted in over 300 robotic colorectal surgeries performed at our institution; however, there are incidents reported in the literature that the patient has fully slid off the operating table [9].

- In morbidly obese patients we place elastic tape wrapped around the chest and across the shoulders.
- The anesthesia team routinely performs a "tilt" test prior to the draping of the patient to ensure proper ventilation and evaluate cardiovascular effects of the Trendelenburg positioning.

dissection has been completed. For that reason, all our patients will be placed in a modified lithotomy position. The patient is secured to the table using the Allen® Hug-U-Vac® steep trend positioner (Allen Medical Systems, Inc. Acton, MA). The advantages with this system include a patient weight capacity up to 500 lb (227 kg), enabling secure positioning in robotic surgery, the design allows easy access to the forearm and the IV lines, and the bag system securely straps to the table with no

14.5 Port Placement

- As part of our standardization protocol for the robotic team, the port placement is the same in every deep pelvic operation, rarely adding any ports, most of the time for additional laparoscopic lysis of adhesions in patients with prior major abdominal surgeries. In virgin abdomens, a supraumbilical port is placed using the standard 12 mm port under direct vision through the port using the 8 mm straight robotic camera. Once appropriate pneumoperitoneum is established, it is easier to place the remaining ports. Alternatively, a right or left upper quadrant port may be placed prior to the midline to evaluate for possible adhesions (Fig. 14.8).

- Evaluation of the abdominal cavity for possible metastatic disease is performed prior to the port placement.
- The port #1 could be 8 mm or the 13 mm robotic stapler port. It is placed at least 10 cm lateral to the umbilical port to avoid collisions, the most common place is in the right lower quadrant at the intersection of the right midclavicular line (MCL) and a line between the superior iliac crest (SIC) and the umbilicus. Port #2 (8 mm robotic port) is placed over the mirror image in the left MCL. However, for the most part, we use the outside outline of the stoma site marking by our enterostomal therapist, which will be used at the end of the operation to perform the permanent colostomy.

Port #3 is also an 8 mm port and will be placed over an area at or lateral to the left anterior axillary line and a horizontal line from the umbilicus.

- An assistant port is routinely placed in the right upper quadrant, normally a 12 mm. The clinical reasoning is twofold: if robotic stapling is not available to use one of the current market endoscopic staplers to transect the proximal specimen or in case of robotic instrument failure, we have for emergent situations a 10 mm diathermy sealing device for control of the vessels. If a robotic stapler port is placed in port #1, then a 5 mm port is used for the first assistant.
- Routine use of 10 mm camera 0° angle is done for all pelvic cases.
- Instruments used:
  - Port #1: cautery hook or scissors
  - Port #2: Cadiere grasper or fenestrated bipolar grasper
  - Port #3: intestinal graptor

14.5.1 Docking the Patient-Side Cart

The robot is docked though an imaginary line from the left SIC to the right shoulder after the patient has been placed in surgery-ready position and tilted. We routinely place the patient on 20–30° of Trendelenburg and 15° to the right. It is important to lower the table to the minimum height to facilitate the robotic arm docking. In efficient robotic teams, this maneuver can be accomplished in less than 2 min.

14.5.1.1 Exposure of the Pedicle and Pelvic Inlet (Video 14.1)

- The graptor retractor is used to cranially tent the rectosigmoid junction, and the assistant may use a laparoscopic bowel grasper to expose the groove underneath the vessels for further triangulation (Fig. 14.9). This maneuver when well performed will facilitate the entire pelvic and structure identification.
  - Use the Cadiere grasper to triangulate the tissues underneath the pedicle for blunt and sharp dissection. Using the hook with or

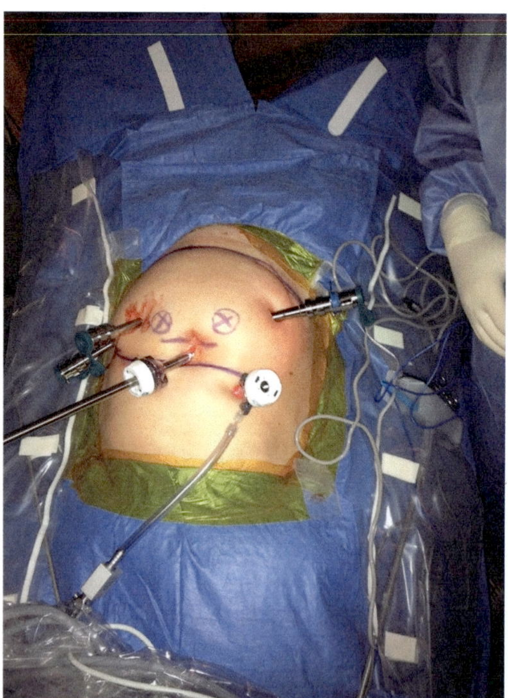

Fig. 14.8 Port placement and positioning

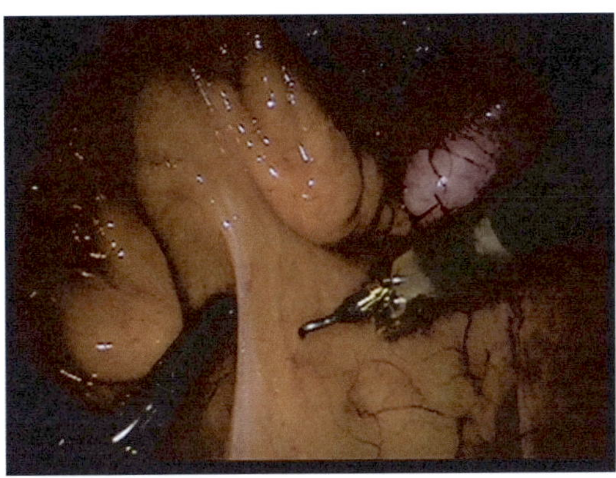

Fig. 14.9 Exposure IMA with triangulation

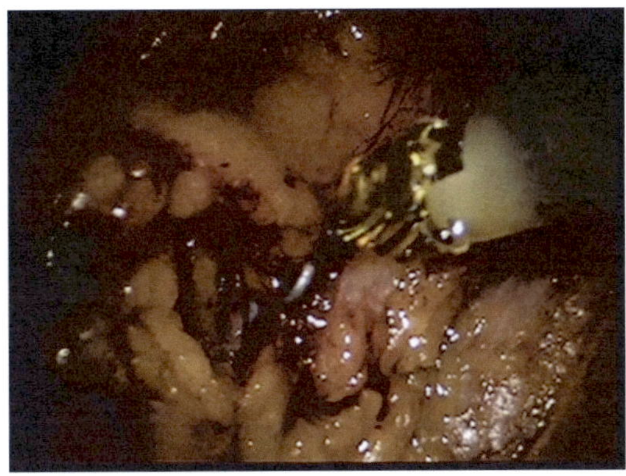

Fig. 14.11 Second window for ureter exposure lateral to IMA fully exposed

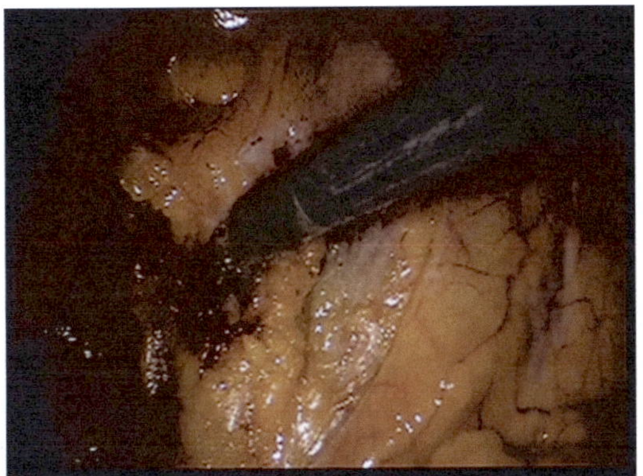

Fig. 14.10 Second window for ureter exposure lateral to IMA

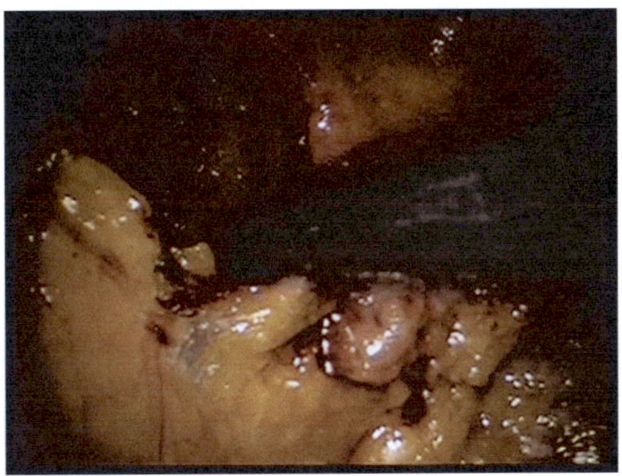

Fig. 14.12 Paracolic mobilization medial to lateral

without cautery blunt and sharp dissection is performed.

- Identification of the hypogastric nerves and separation from the IMA pedicle.
- Continuation of the medial to lateral approach with identification of the ureter at the junction with the left iliac. A common mistake is to try to find it deeper in the left retroperitoneal area caudal to the internal and external iliac bifurcation. A second window sometimes is performed lateral to the pedicle, this window many times will expose the ureter right underneath it (Figs. 14.10 and 14.11).
- Once the ureter has been identified, proximal dissection of the retroperitoneal space is done with care to avoid injury to the ureter and gonadal pedicle. For the most part

this part is truly areolar (Fig. 14.12) and blunt dissection may be performed in many cases to nearly reach the splenic flexure without the need of rotating the robotic system.

- Takedown of the pedicle (Fig. 14.13) with diathermy device can be done using:
  Arm #1 with the sealing device.
  Assistant Port using laparoscopic diathermy device from the right upper quadrant.
  After this maneuver, the paracolic gutter is further mobilized above the Gerota's fascia (Fig. 14.14).
- Exposure of the pelvis is done with the arm #3 retractor. This step is essential for full exposure of the pelvis for the posterior dissection. Our preference is to pass the

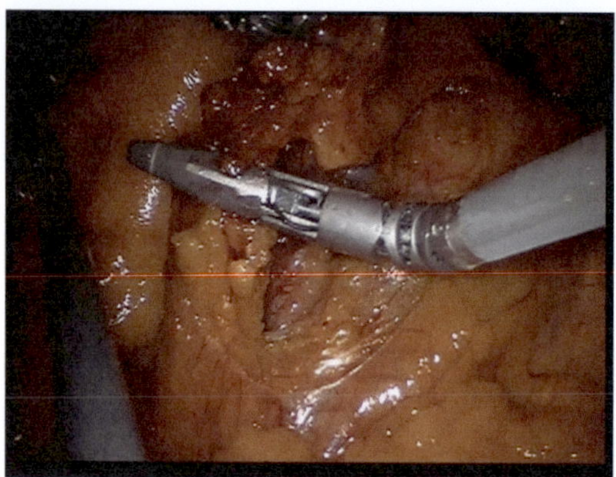

Fig. 14.13 Takedown of inferior mesenteric artery

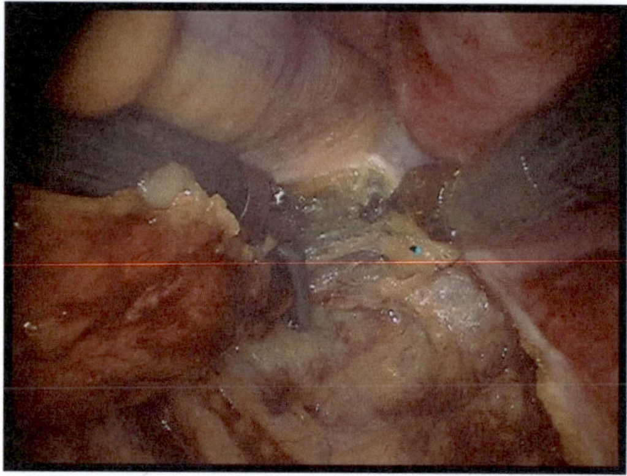

Fig. 14.15 Right pelvic inlet and distal lateral stalk mobilization

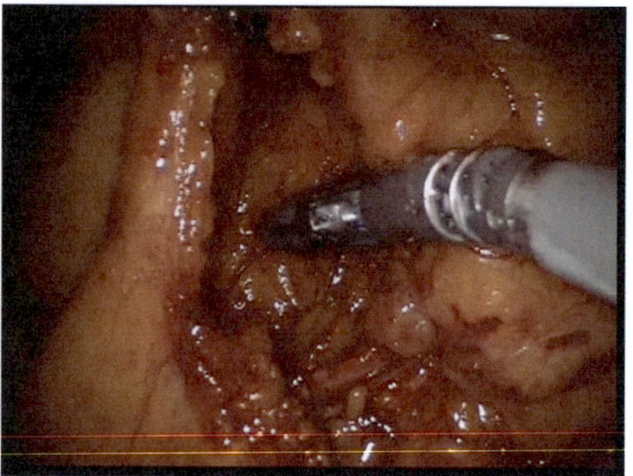

Fig. 14.14 Paracolic mobilization medial to lateral after IMA is taken

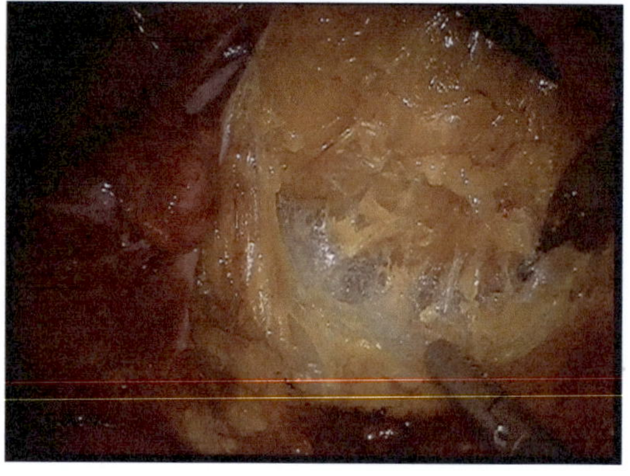

Fig. 14.16 Posterior dissection TME pelvic inlet

retractor from the lateral side through the window of the already taken vascular pedicle. Using the blades of the retractor and the arm, cranial retraction of the rectosigmoid junction is done with excellent visualization of the areolar tissue of the pelvic inlet in the mesorectal plane. It is important to identify the hypogastric nerves and preserve them posterior to our dissection plane (Fig. 14.15).

14.5.1.2 Posterior Lateral and Anterior Dissection in Minor Pelvis Plane

- This area is entered using the hook or scissors on cautery posteriorly through the areolar plane until the levator plate is entered (Fig. 14.16). We prefer to use the straight camera although

for deep curved pelvis, the last remnants of the anococcygeal ligament may be easier and visualized with the 30° angled camera. This step is operator dependent, and for the most part, the surgeon tends to use the type of camera angulation used during their laparoscopic experience. Also for deeper planes, it may be necessary at times to advance the arm #3 using the blades for anterior retraction and exposure of the posterior mesorectal plane.

- Once that is completed, the dissection is extended laterally on the right side of the pelvic inlet. Some surgeons prefer to use the sealing device and they may find the so-called lateral stalks and avoid bleeding. Others prefer the diathermy device in higher coagulation settings.

- Attention is turned to the left lateral rectal aspect, which is exposed with the aid of arm

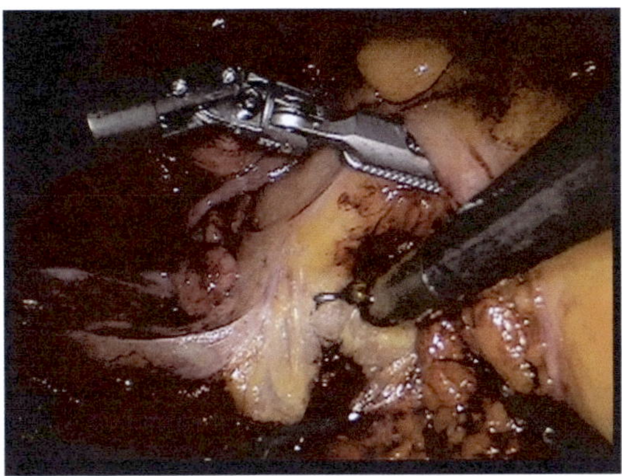

Fig. 14.17 Left pelvic inlet entrance triangulation graptor retractor

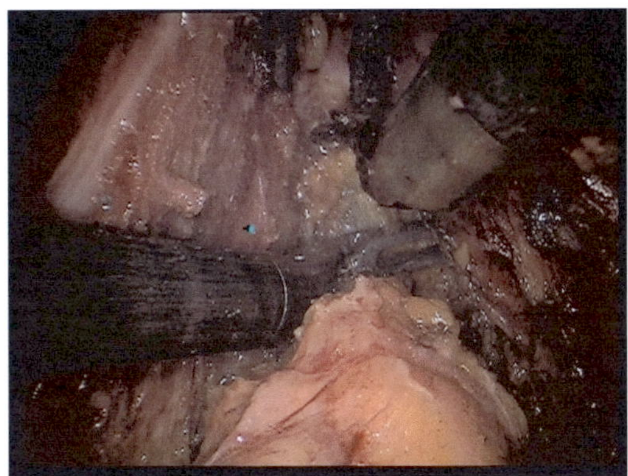

Fig. 14.19 Posterior vaginectomy on APR

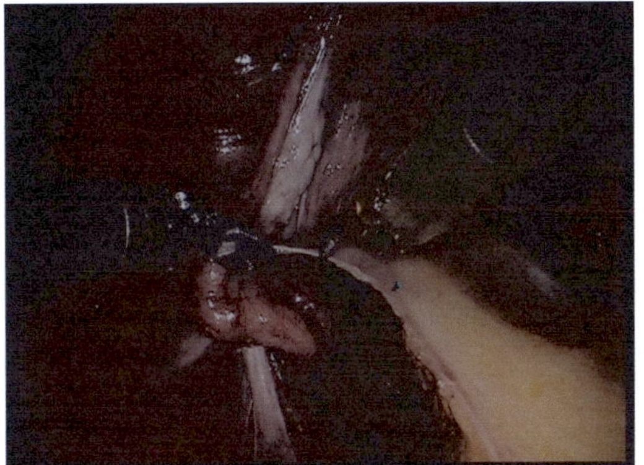

Fig. 14.18 Rectovaginal septum exposure and triangulation

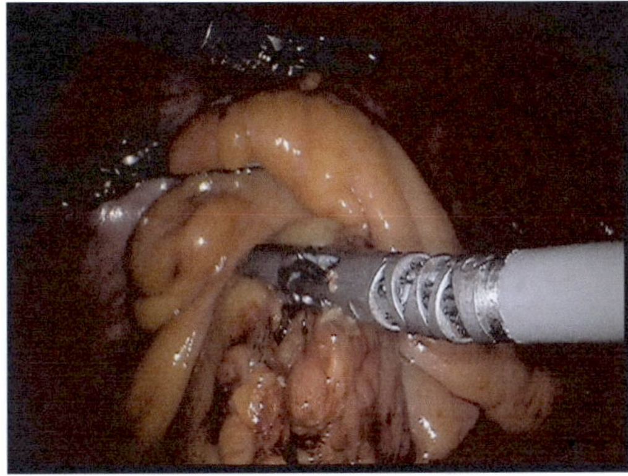

Fig. 14.20 Mesenteric takedown for proximal transection sigmoid

#3 pushing the midrectum to the left of the pelvis. Cautery is used to the level of the anal canal (Fig. 14.17).

- After the posterior and lateral areas are mobilized, the anterior part of the peritoneum is incised, and using the separated blades of the third arm, exposure of the Denonvilliers' fascia in the male or the rectovaginal septum is done (Fig. 14.18). Cautery is used to separate this areolar plane. Posterior vaginectomy can be performed in case of anterior invasion of the tumor (Fig. 14.19), guidance of the dissection with an assistant in the pelvis using digital examination.
- The dissection in many instances can be continued until the skin of the perineum is open through the abdomen. To avoid losing pneumoperitoneum, an abdominal pad can be used.

- Transection of the sigmoid colon can be done intracorporeally after the pedicle has been taken down (Fig. 14.20). Prior to that maneuver, we routinely perform fluorescent evaluation of the colon with 10 mg of indocyanine green after the pedicle has been taken to the colon chosen for transection (Fig. 14.21). If vascular flow is noted over the area, transection is then performed (Fig. 14.22).

14.5.1.3 Extracorporeal Portion of the Procedure

- In order to expedite the procedure, we routinely use a two-surgeon team. The robotic platform is decoupled from the patient, and perineal extraction and permanent colostomy are done at the same time.

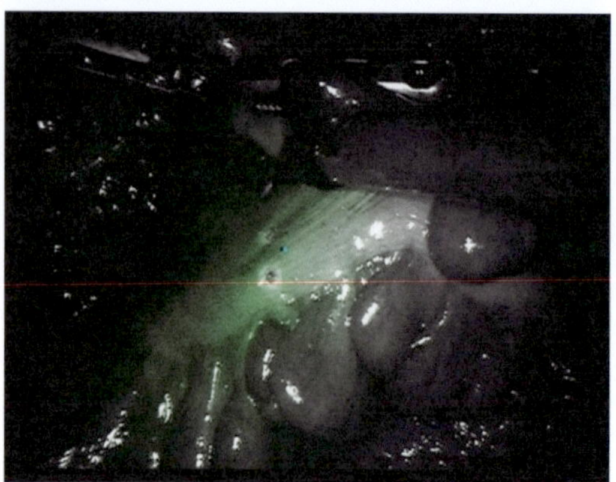

Fig. 14.21 Proximal immunofluorescence marking

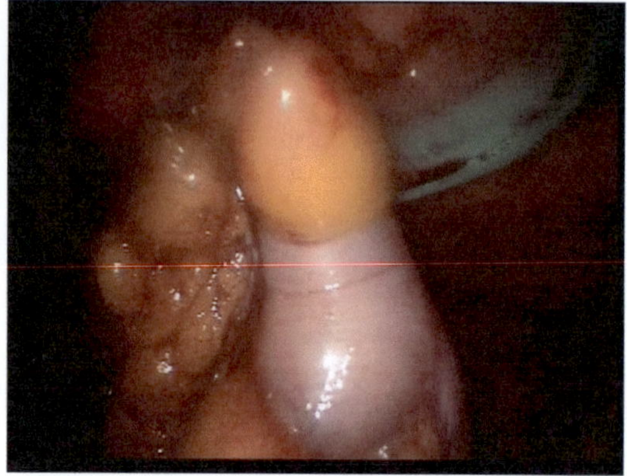

Fig. 14.23 Extraction proximal colon using wound protector retractor

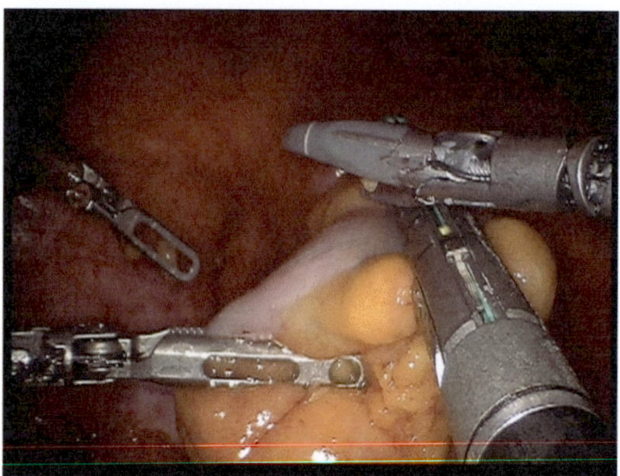

Fig. 14.22 Transection proximal colon

- The skin marked for the permanent stoma is incised and dissection is done using the Army-Navy retractors until the anterior rectus fascia is found. The fascia is opened vertically and using the clamp the muscle is split and retracted with the long blade of the retractors exposing the posterior rectus sheath. We routinely preserve the pneumoperitoneum and use the camera to guide the assistant to grab the distal end of the colon to mature. After the distal stapled colon is extracted through the stoma (Fig. 14.23), deflation of the abdomen has already occurred and the stoma is matured removing the stapled line and absorbable sutures.
- The perineal portion is done using the Beckman retractors after the skin is incised at the hair-bearing areas and the cautery until the area is connected to the pelvic dissection, first posteriorly and then laterally and anteriorly. In our experience, we have been able to dissect as low as the skin transabdominally so minimal dissection is required for extracorporealization of the rectum.
- The planes are closed in layers using absorbable sutures. If the defect is large, consideration should be given for a consultation to a plastic surgery team for rectus abdominis flap. Smaller defects may be primarily closed and we prefer to use subcuticular sutures of 4/0 PDS and dermabond for the skin sealing.
- The specimen is always sent and evaluated by the pathologist intraoperatively for clear macroscopic margins and the presence of the tumor in the specimen.

14.5.2 Patient Characteristics and Selection

The use of robotic technology has been shown to have lower rate of conversion in obese and ultralow cancers when compared to other techniques [10, 11].

Our current experience in all types of colorectal resections indicates the feasibility of the use of robotic technology, especially in obese patients as they may benefit more of the minimally invasive approach and the lower conversion to open.

Moreover, our current data indicate the same oncologic in 103 consecutive colectomies in rectal cancer when comparing BMI > 30 or less with statistically same nodal sampling, radial, and distal margins.

The patient's height implies a deeper pelvis to dissect. We routinely place the ports lower allowing the instruments to reach deeper. In the event that reach is needed once the platform has been docked, all ports may be pushed in using the port clutch system. Routinely, we do not need to take the splenic flexure on our APR, and also splenic flexure takedown is explained elsewhere in the textbook.

14.5.3 Robotic Accessories

The latest da Vinci® Surgical System Xi model (Intuitive Surgical Inc., Sunnyvale, CA) has been recently introduced in April 2014. The arms are interchangeable as well as the camera. We do not have this system to our avail but other experienced robotic surgeons seem to find this system more similar to laparoscopic technique. Also, the ability to perform multiquadrant surgery and rotate the upper part of the boom of the arm may make this new advanced model more suitable to colorectal surgery.

We routinely use the EndoWrist® One™ Vessel Sealer (Intuitive Surgical Inc., Sunnyvale, CA) for all of the vascular pedicle takedown procedures. This device allows the safely takedown of vessels up to 7 mm in diameter, as well as grasping and blunt dissection.

At the time of transecting the colon, this maneuver can be performed using current laparoscopic staplers or the EndoWrist® One Stapler 45 available at our institution. Our preference at the pelvis is to use the double row of 1.5 mm closed height of the staple.

Much debate currently exists about the use of Firefly™ (Intuitive Surgical Inc., Sunnyvale, CA) to delineate the vascular flow of the colon. Our data was published although the study was not designed to evaluate difference in leak rate; a transection margin more proximal than the marked in white light consistently showed in nearly 50 % of the rectal resections. Our department has adopted its use in all left-sided and rectal resections [12–16].

14.5.4 Other Tips and Tricks for Success

The commitment of the institution and the surgical team is a must for a successful development of a robotic program. In the beginning of the program, it is important to rehearse every step with the team as they become familiar with the instrumentation. Also, routine avoidance of opening all available instruments is mandatory in this cost-containment environment. The use of all instruments, the design of the surgery carts, and the cost analysis of the devices in comparison to current laparoscopic equivalents may help in the decision to use stapler, sealing, and suction devices.

14.5.5 In an Emergency…

A regular laparotomy tray is routinely available in the room for emergency situations. Also, laparoscopic sealing devices are in the room and are available in case the current robotic technology does not control the bleeding. It is important to have a dedicated assistant; in our institution our purely dedicated physician assistants or certified first assistant provide consistency, and each of them has experience in at least over 400 procedures done, and they are able to anticipate all the surgeon's needs and the next steps in each procedure.

14.6 The Evidence for Robotic APR

Minimally invasive rectal cancer surgery is complex with a long learning curve secondary to the bony pelvis constraints and the size of the tumor. Robotic surgery itself also has a learning curve that in recent publications has been described in 15 and 35 cases. The speed is dependent on the team's ability of docking time, surgeon's console time, and overall operating room time [12–15]. The institution's total number of procedures is also dependent on outcomes as Delaney et al. showed [16]: higher-volume surgeons and hospitals have a significant lower length of hospital stay, cost, and complications. Hence, the dedication of the institution to the technology and support of the surgeon are important.

Total mesorectal excision as described by Heald is the standard surgical technique that has shown significant decreased local recurrence [17–19]. The performance of this technique distally as the mesorectum thins out may increase the risk of rectal perforation to 22.8 %, which significantly increases the risk of local recurrence [20–22]. Several authors have recommended the performance of an extralevator dissection, and Marecik et al. described a robotic technique in five patients with intact mesorectal envelope and negative circumferential margins [23]. In high-risk patients, where there is concern of radial margin invasion or patients with malignant fistulas to vagina, we have successfully used this technique obtaining clear radial margins as well.

The most current study reporting short-term oncologic outcomes has been recently reported by Kim et al. in 200 cases [24]. Their mean distance to the anal verge was 6 cm. Twenty-seven percent received preoperative chemoradiation as per protocol. In their series, sphincter sparing was used in 186 patients (93 %) with only 6.5 % APR performed. In experienced hands, the total robotic time averaged 140 min (range 59–367) with a console time average of 135 min. The authors described an extremely low circumferential margin rate of 2.5 % and positive distal margins in 1.5 % with no conversions. The mean number of lymph nodes retrieved was 17 (range 3–83). The oncologic surveillance's mean was 29.8 months, with an overall recurrence rate of 13.7 % (18 patients) metastatic and seven local recurrences (4.5 %). The overall survival rate at 5 years was 92.0 % with a disease-free survival and the local pelvic control rates at 5 years of 81.7 % and 95.0 %, respectively.

Upon reviewing earlier laparoscopic and robotic data, the original report of the COLOR I trial had 10 % of positive circumferential margin [25]. Meta-analysis has shown similar circumferential margin rate between the robotic or laparoscopic techniques that ranges 0–7.5 % [11, 26–29]. It is clear that the current data is early and institutional/surgeon dependent although there is a trend to improved local control. Further studies are under way to further evaluate oncologic and functional outcomes.

After having selected the type of resection to be done or the supralevator, the question is how to perform the closure of the APR. Musters et al. reviewed in a meta-analysis routine APR versus extralevator. Complication rates are 15.3 % and 14.8 %, respectively, when no radiation is used preoperatively; however if used, the complication rate doubles. The use of biologic material to close significantly decreases the complications to 7.3 % [30].

14.7 Summary

This chapter describes a systematic approach to performing an APR, stressing the importance of the ergonomics in port placement and docking technique. The performance of extralevator technique robotically provides a "bird's-eye view to the levators" and potentially improves the local recurrence and decreases a circumferential margin. Current literature is still very institutional dependent and heavily linked to the surgeon's experience and learning curve.

14.8 Key Points

- The steps of the operation and technique of APR are similar to laparoscopic or robotic technique with a separate equipment needed for the perineal portion of the procedure.
- Ergonomic placement of the ports and the docking of the robot are crucial for efficiency and avoidance of intraoperative arm collisions. Planning for proper distal reach of the dissection must be taken into consideration.
- Appropriate training, simulation, and rehearsal of the case with the bedside assistant and the robotic team will expedite the procedure.

- A contingency plan for emergent conversion must be always in place including laparoscopic instrumentation in the room and a minor laparotomy tray.

References

1. Turnbull G, Erwin-Toth P. Ostomy care: foundation for teaching and practice. Ostomy Wound Manage. 1999;45(Suppl):23S–30S.
2. American Society of Colon & Rectal Surgeons and Wound Ostomy & Continence Nurses Society. ASCRS and WOCN Joint Position Statement on the Value of Preoperative Stoma. Wound, Ostomy and Continence Nurse Society. http://c.ymcdn.com/sites/www.wocn.org/resource/resmgr/docs/0807stomamarkingps.pdf?hSearchTerms=%22stoma+and+siting%22
3. Bass E, Del Pino A, Tan A, Pearl R, Orsay C, Abcarian H. Does preoperative stomal marking and education by the enterostomal therapist affect outcome ? Dis Colon Rectum. 1997;40(4):440–2.
4. Gulbiniene J, Markalis R, Tamelis A, Salazinaskas Z. The impact of preoperative stoma siting and stoma care education on patient's quality of life. Medicina (Kaunas). 2004;41(1):1045–53.
5. Park J, Del Pino A, Orsay C, et al. Stoma complications. Dis Colon Rectum. 1999;42(12):1575–80.
6. Pittman J, Baka T, Ellett M, Sloan R, Rawl SM. Psychometric evaluation of the ostomy complication severity index. J Wound Ostomy Continence Nurs. 2014;41(2):147–57.
7. Pittman J, Rawl SM, Schmidt CM, et al. Demographic and clinical factors related to ostomy complications and quality of life in veterans with an ostomy. J Wound Ostomy Continence Nurs. 2008;35(5):493–503.
8. Carmel JE, Goldberg M. Preoperative and postoperative management. In: Colwell J, Goldberg MT, Carmel J, editors. Fecal and urinary diversions: management principles. St. Louis, MO: Mosby; 2004. p. 207–39.
9. Huettner F, Pacheco PE, Doubet JL, Ryan MJ, Dynda DI, Crawford DL. One hundred and two consecutive robotic-assisted minimally invasive colectomies—an outcome and technical update. J Gastrointest Surg. 2011;15(7):1195–204.
10. deSouza AL, Prasad LM, Marecik SJ, Blumetti J, Park JJ, Zimmern A, et al. Total mesorectal excision for rectal cancer: the potential advantage of robotic assistance. Dis Colon Rectum. 2010;53(12):1611–7.
11. Scarpinata R, Aly EH. Does robotic rectal cancer surgery offer improved early postoperative outcomes? Dis Colon Rectum. 2013;56(2):253–62.
12. Kim HJ, Choi GS, Park JS, Park SY. Multidimensional analysis of the learning curve for robotic total mesorectal excision for rectal cancer: lessons from a single surgeon's experience. Dis Colon Rectum. 2014;57:1066–74.
13. Bokhari MB, Patel CB, Ramos-Valadez DI, Ragupathi M, Haas EM. Learning curve for robotic-assisted laparoscopic colorectal surgery. Surg Endosc. 2011;25(3):855–60.
14. Sng KK, Hara M, Shin JW, Yoo BE, Yang KS, Kim SH. The multiphasic learning curve for robot-assisted rectal surgery. Surg Endosc. 2013;27(9):3297–307.
15. Jimenez-Rodriguez RM, Diaz-Pavon JM, de la Portilla de Juan F, Prendes-Sillero E, Dussort HC, Padillo J. Learning curve for robotic-assisted laparoscopic rectal cancer surgery. Int J Colorectal Dis. 2013;28(6):815–21.
16. Keller DS, Hashemi L, Lu M, Delaney CP. Short-term outcomes for robotic colorectal surgery by provider volume. J Am Coll Surg. 2013;217(6):1063–9.e1.
17. Heald RJ, Moran BJ, Ryall RD, Sexton R, MacFarlane JK. Rectal cancer: the Basingstoke experience of total mesorectal excision, 1978–1997. Arch Surg. 1998;133:894–9.
18. Kapiteijn E, Marijnen CA, Nagtegaal ID, et al. Preoperative radiotherapy combined with total mesorectal excision for resectable rectal cancer. N Engl J Med. 2001;345:638–46.
19. Martling AL, Holm T, Rutqvist LE, et al. Effect of a surgical training programme on outcome of rectal cancer in the county of Stockholm. Stockholm Colorectal Cancer Study Group, Basingstoke Bowel Cancer Research Project. Lancet. 2000;356:93–6.
20. Nagtegaal ID, van de Velde CJH, Marijnen CA, et al. Low rectal cancer: a call for a change of approach in abdominoperineal resection. J Clin Oncol. 2005;23:9257–64.
21. West NP, Finan PJ, Anderin C, Lindholm J, Holm T, Quirke P. Evidence of the oncologic superiority of cylindrical abdominoperineal excision for low rectal cancer. J Clin Oncol. 2008;26:3517–22.
22. Eriksen MT, Wibe A, Syse A, Haffner J, Wiig JN, Norwegian Rectal Cancer Group, Norwegian GI Cancer Group. Inadvertent perforation during rectal cancer resection in Norway. Br J Surg. 2004;91:210–6.
23. Marecik SJ, Zawadzki M, de Souza AL, Park JJ, Abcarian H, Prasad LM. Robotic cylindrical abdominoperineal resection with transabdominal levator transection. Dis Colon Rectum. 2011;54:1320–5.
24. Hara M, Sng K, Yoo BE, Shin JW, Lee DW, Kim SH. Robotic-assisted surgery for rectal adenocarcinoma: short-term and midterm outcomes from 200 consecutive cases at a single institution. Dis Colon Rectum. 2014;57:570–7.
25. van der Pas MH, Haglind E, Cuesta MA, Fürst A, Lacy AM, Hop WC, Bonjer HJ, Colorectal Cancer Laparoscopic or Open Resection II (COLO R II) Study Group. Laparoscopic versus open surgery for rectal cancer (COLOR II): short-term outcomes of a randomised, phase 3 trial. Lancet Oncol. 2013;14:210–8.
26. Kang J, Yoon KJ, Min BS, et al. The impact of robotic surgery for mid and low rectal cancer: a case-matched

analysis of a 3-arm comparison—open, laparoscopic, and robotic surgery. Ann Surg. 2013;257:95–101.

27. Bianchi PP, Ceriani C, Locatelli A, et al. Robotic versus laparoscopic total mesorectal excision for rectal cancer: a comparative analysis of oncological safety and short-term outcomes. Surg Endosc. 2010;24:2888–94.

28. Memon S, Heriot AG, Murphy DG, Bressel M, Lynch AC. Robotic versus laparoscopic proctectomy for rectal cancer: a meta-analysis. Ann Surg Oncol. 2012;19:2095–101.

29. Guillou PJ, Quirke P, Thorpe H, Walker J, Jayne DG, Smith AM, Heath RM, Brown JM, MRC CLASICC trial group. Short-term endpoints of conventional versus laparoscopic-assisted surgery in patients with colorectal cancer (MRC CLASI CC trial): multicentre, randomised controlled trial. Lancet. 2005;365:1718–26.

30. Musters GD, Buskens CJ, Bemelman WA, Tanis PJ. Perineal wound healing after abdominoperineal resection for rectal cancer: a systematic review and meta-analysis. Dis Colon Rectum. 2014;57:1129–39.

Robotic Rectopexy

15

James W. Fleshman, Sarah Boostrom, and Gentry Caton

Abstract

Robotic rectopexy is an advancing surgical technique for the treatment of rectal prolapse. The learning curve is shorter for robotic rectopexy compared to laparoscopic rectopexy. The technical advantages provided by the robot improve visualization in the pelvis and also contribute to lower conversion rates. Operative time approaches that of the laparoscopic approach with increased experience and use of the D'Hoore's procedure. Blood loss is not significantly different. Length of hospital stay from 2 to 6 days and recurrence of 0–15 % for robotic rectopexy are equivocal to the laparoscopic technique.

Keywords

Rectal prolapse • Robotic rectopexy • Rectal procidentia • D'Hoore's procedure • Well's procedure • Laparoscopic rectopexy • Pelvic floor

15.1 Introduction

Rectal prolapse (rectal procidentia) occurs when the wall of the rectum descends out of its normal anatomic place and circumferentially or partially protrudes through the anus until it can be grossly visualized. It is associated with pelvic floor dysfunction and may present with several different symptoms.

Depending on degree of prolapse, the patient may experience fecal incontinence, constipation, mucus discharge, tenesmus, rectal bleeding, and obstructive defecation. These symptoms are rarely life threatening; however, they may contribute to extensive debility and social anxiety for the patient [1].

Rectal prolapse can occur in both men and women; however, it is predominately an affliction of elderly women. As such, surgical correction must be individually tailored to fit the patients overall medical condition, any other pelvic dysfunction which may require a multidisciplinary approach, history of constipation, as well as the patient's fecal continence. Additionally, other related diagnoses such as prolapsing hemorrhoids must be distinguished from rectal

J.W. Fleshman, M.D., F.A.C.S., F.A.S.C.R.S. (✉)
S. Boostrom, M.D., F.A.C.S. • G. Caton, M.D.
Department of Surgery, Baylor University
Medical Center, Dallas, TX, USA
e-mail: James.Fleshman@BaylorHealth.edu

© Springer International Publishing Switzerland 2015
H. Ross et al. (eds.), *Robotic Approaches to Colorectal Surgery*,
DOI 10.1007/978-3-319-09120-4_15

181

prolapse through physical exam, history, and proper diagnostic testing [2].

15.2 Workup

Various diagnostic tests may be utilized in the workup of a patient with rectal prolapse. However, diagnostic testing should be tailored to the patient's individual physical exam findings, symptoms, and risk factors. Physical exam is of greatest value for distinguishing prolapsed hemorrhoids (with radial folds of mucosa) from full rectal prolapse (circumferential mucosal folds). This can be easily accomplished by having the patient perform a Valsalva maneuver on a toilet in the clinic and observation of the protruding tissue. The length of the prolapsed tissue is important to distinguish distal mucosal prolapse (2–3 cm), from full rectal prolapse (5–15 cm). Further differentiation may also be evident as prolapsing hemorrhoidal tissue is usually located at the 3, 7, and 11 o'clock positions [2]. Colonoscopy should be always performed in order to rule out a lead point for the intussusception, such as a polyp or carcinoma. Videodefecography is useful when prolapse cannot be replicated or internal rectal intussusception is suspected. Colonic transit studies may be necessary in a patient with complaints of constipation because those with colonic inertia may benefit from partial colectomy [1]. Anorectal manometry may be helpful in patients with a history of fecal incontinence to determine baseline external sphincter function and predict whether anterior–posterior levatorplasty combined with prolapse repair would be beneficial.

15.3 Treatment

The treatment for symptomatic rectal prolapse is surgical and is the only option for cure; however, conservative treatment in those patients deemed unfit for any surgical option may be utilized. Conservative management includes dietary adjustments, with increased fiber as well as bulking agents and stool softeners to reduce straining during evacuation. Biofeedback to retrain the pelvic floor, which exhibits non-relaxation of the puborectalis muscle, may also help patients to defecate without

straining [3]. The presence of pelvic floor outlet obstruction may doom even the most radical operative treatment of rectal prolapse to failure.

15.3.1 Surgical Treatment

There have been over 100 different surgical techniques utilized for the treatment of rectal prolapse [4]. Operations for rectal prolapse can be divided into two main categories, transabdominal procedures and perineal procedures. The decision of which surgery to perform must be individualized to the patient. In general, the perineal rectosigmoidectomy (Altemeier), the mucosal sleeve resection (Delorme), or the anal encirclement (Thiersch) are best utilized in high-risk patients that are not good candidates for a transabdominal procedure [2]. The largest attempted prospective randomized study on rectopexy technique, PROSPER, was plagued with low patient accrual and was unable to demonstrate significant differences in transabdominal vs. perineal techniques [5]. Other nonrandomized studies show that there is a higher rate of recurrence in prolapse (0–44 %) compared with transabdominal techniques (0–12 %) [6]. The transabdominal approaches include those that repair the pelvic floor, those that suspend the colon or rectum to the pelvic structures, and those that involve resection of the sigmoid colon. Additionally, aspects of these operations can be combined to tailor them for the individual patient or clinical scenario. The introduction of laparoscopic approaches has changed the thought process in the selection of patients for abdominal procedures. The minimally invasive approach may remove some of the factors, which would otherwise support a perineal or transanal approach, such as a large incision that impairs breathing or the risk-inducing adhesions, which may impair fertility. In fact, many surgeons feel there is only a very small subset of patients who are so severely debilitated and at exceedingly high medical risk for an operation that perineal approaches are no longer a major alternative for rectal prolapse.

The most common of surgical approaches, as well as the one producing the lowest recurrence rate, for rectal prolapse is rectopexy with or without sigmoid resection. A 2005 multicentric study reported recurrence rates to be 1 %, 6.6 %, and 28.9 % at 1, 5, and 10 years, respectively [7]. Frykman's first description of this technique was in 1955; it involved mobilization and elevation of the rectum cephalad with fixation of the rectum to the presacral fascia, obliteration of the cul-de-sac, and sigmoid colectomy with primary anastomosis. Despite years of advancement in surgical technology, this procedure continues to be the gold standard surgical procedure for rectal prolapse [8]. Variations of this technique include non-resection of the sigmoid colon, utilization of mesh for fixation of the rectum, and limitations of the dissection to either the anterior plane, posterior plane, or both. Roblick et al. published their experience ($n=53$) of laparoscopic rectopexy with sigmoid resection for patients with preoperative constipation. They had 89 % improvement in or elimination of constipation at their 5-year follow-up [9].

Laparoscopic technique for surgical treatment of rectal prolapsed was first published in 1992 by Berman et al. and has been employed for various approaches including rectopexy, resection, and mesh repair [10]. The laparoscopic rectopexy for rectal prolapse offers short-term advantages compared to traditional open approaches: less pain, faster return to normal daily function, shorter hospitalization, and smaller scars [11, 12].

Robotic-assisted surgery is a developing technique. In 2001, Weber et al. performed the first robotic-assisted laparoscopic colectomy for benign disease [13]. Since then, robotic approaches have been employed in multiple other procedures, including abdominoperineal resection, low anterior resection, and rectopexy [14].

There are several advantages to robotic-assisted colorectal surgery. Bokhari et al. published a retrospective paper using the cumulative sum method to determine the learning curve of robotic colorectal surgery. They surmised that the learning phase was achieved after 15–25 cases [14]. This can be compared to the learning curve numbers of laparoscopic colorectal procedures which necessitate a learning curve of 55 and 62 cases for right and left laparoscopic colectomy, respectively [15]. Similarly, a recent 2012 multicenter database analyzing conventional laparoscopic surgery published a learning curve of 88–152 cases [16].

Robotic-assisted rectopexy has been shown to meet safety standards of laparoscopic rectopexy and is considered a feasible procedure for rectal prolapse [17, 18]. Makela-Kaikkonen et al. compared robotic-assisted and laparoscopic ventral rectopexy in a matched-pair study in 2013. They found no difference in operating time, blood loss, complication rate (5 %), and length of hospital stay or in patient's subjective benefit rate [19].

The complexity of rectopexy requires careful dissection in a narrow field of view, intracorporeal suturing, and identification of at-risk pelvic anatomy. Many of the visual and retraction challenges in the human pelvis can be alleviated with use of robotic technology. The technical advantages of robotic surgery include 3D visualization, reduction of human tremor, and improved dexterity with 7° of articulation of surgical instruments [17]. It also allows the surgeon to retract with an assistant third arm that he/she controls. These advantages may positively influence the relatively high 30 % conversion rates reported in laparoscopic rectal procedures [20].

As outcomes continue to be examined in robotic vs. laparoscopic surgery, the increased cost of robotic-assisted rectopexy is a factor that will need to be addressed in order for this technique to remain a viable approach. Heemskerk et al. published their first 14 cases in 2010, in which they reported a $745.09 increase in cost for robotic rectopexy compared to traditional laparoscopic technique [21].

15.3.2 Technique

Patients receive an enema the morning of surgery. A single dose of appropriate prophylactic antibiotic is given. A urinary catheter is placed after induction of anesthesia and is subsequently removed prior to reversal at the end of the case.

15.3.3 Docking and Port Placement

The patient is positioned in modified lithotomy position. The support column, with robotic arms suspended at 45-degree angles from each other on either side of the vertical camera arm, is placed between the legs of the patient. Five ports are placed using standard laparoscopic technique. First, a 12-mm port is placed just above the umbilicus in the midline for the camera robot arm #1. An 8-mm port is placed in the right lower quadrant 8 cm below the umbilical port at the lateral edge of the rectus for the right robotic arm #2 and an 8-mm port is placed opposite in the left lower quadrant for the left robotic arm #3. Two 5-mm laparoscopic assistant ports are placed in the right anterioaxillary line under the ribs and above the anterior superior iliac spine. The #4 robotic arm is placed through an 8-mm port in the anterior axillary line on the left at the level of the umbilicus. An additional 5-mm laparoscopic suprapubic port can be placed for retraction. With the ports in place, the patient is positioned into steep Trendelenburg and the robotic arms connected. The location and size of the ports may vary with surgical preference, additional procedures being performed, and the use of different surgical tools, such as a stapler.

15.3.3.1 Alternative Docking and Port Placement

The robot can also be placed on the patient's left side. A paraumbilical 12-mm port is placed to the right of the umbilicus for the camera in robotic arm #1. The #2 robotic arm is placed in the right iliac fossa, the #3 robotic arm is placed to the left of the umbilicus, and the #4 robotic arm is placed in the left iliac fossa, all 8-mm ports. An additional 12-mm laparoscopic assistant port is placed in the right midclavicular line and a 5-mm port is placed in the suprapubic region [19].

15.3.3.2 Surgical Technique

D'Hoore's ventral rectopexy can be performed anterior to Denonvilliers' fascia in males or in the rectovaginal space in females. The rectosigmoid is retracted to the left and a peritoneal incision is made on the right of the sacral promontory and extended in a J-form along the rectum. No lateral dissection should be performed in order to decrease damage to the nerve complex of the rectum. Damage to lateral nerves has been shown to cause increased constipation as well as

neurogenic impairment of the urinary bladder and genital organs [20–23]. The rectovaginal or rectoprostatic septum is then incised to the pelvic floor, approximately 2–3 cm above the dentate line [9, 17, 24–26]. The distance from the dentate line can be approximated by digital rectal exam. A 3-cm by 17-cm hockey stick-shaped nonabsorbable mesh is fixed at the straight end of the mesh to the sacral promontory by an endofascial stapler device or nonabsorbable suture. The curved portion of the mesh is then sutured to the ventral aspect of distal rectum. The posterior vaginal fornix is elevated and sutured to the anterior aspect of the mesh, closing the rectovaginal septum. The peritoneum is closed over the mesh [21].

Modified Wells' posterior rectopexy can also be performed robotically. The posterior peritoneum is opened on the right side at the level of the sacral promontory. A retrorectal dissection is performed behind the mesorectal fascia with monopolar scissors or harmonic scalpel to release the rectum from the curve of the sacrum to the level of the coccyx. The rectum is stretched from the pelvis and then fixed to the promontory by a #0 Ethibond stitch, which approximates the posterior mesorectum to the presacral fascia. Running Vicryl suture is used to close the peritoneum [16]. A suction drain is often placed to obliterate any space behind the rectum. Heemskerk et al. abandoned the Well's procedure in favor of the D'Hoore's, quoting the latter being less complex and time consuming [21].

Either posterior or anterior rectopexy can be combined with sigmoid colon resection in patients with a history of constipation. Length of proximal colon resection has not been thoroughly reported; however, Roblick et al. recommended against splenic mobilization as an intact splenic flexure suspends the colon and may contribute to improved constipation [9]. Additional procedures to suspend additional unsupported pelvic organs can also be repaired/suspended in consultation with urogynecology colleagues.

The principles of preservation of the lateral rectal ligaments and the hypogastric nerves have been linked to preventing postoperative constipation (Scaglia, Mollen, Speakman). Several of the studies reviewed in Table 15.1 reported using a combined anterior (ventral) and posterior

Table 15.1 Studies reporting rectopexy for rectal prolapse

Year	Author	n	Time with Dz	SX	Age/BMI	Mesh	Rxn	LOO	LOS	M/M	F/U	Recurrence
2004	Munz et al. [18]	6	2–12 month	Rob Post	65 years	No	None	127 min	6 days	0/0	6 month	0 %
2007	Heemskerk et al. [21]	14		Rob Ant	52 years	Yes	None	152 min	3.9 days			
2009	De Hoog et al. [29]	20		Rob A/P	56 years	Yes	None	154 min	2.6 days		1.9 year	20 %
2011	Wong et al. [17]	23		Rob Ant	61 years/27	Yes	None	221 min	5 days		6 month	0 %
2012	Faucheron et al. [25]	175	29 month	Lap Ant	58 years	Yes	None	112 min (45–370)	2.2 days	0/5.1 %	72 month	3 % at 5 years
2013	Buchs et al. [24]	5		Rob A/P	74 years/19	Some	None	170 min (120–270)	3.6 days	0/25 %	2 month	0 % at 6 month
2013	Mantoo et al. [26]	44		Rob Ant	61 years/26	Yes	None	191 min	4 days	0/2 %	6 month	7 % at 6 month
2013	Louis-Sylvestre et al. [27]	90		Rob Ant	60.9 years/24.5	Yes	None/P	246 min (180–415) Sacrocolpopexy	3.4 days	0/8 %	15 month	0 %
2013	Makela-Kaikkonen et al. [19]	20		Rob Ant	60 years/25	Yes	None	159 min	3.1 days	0/5 %	3 month	5 %
2013	Perrenot et al. [28]	77		Rob Ant	60 years/23	Yes	9	223 min	6.5 days	0/10 %	53 month	12.5 %

technique or posterior alone [18, 24, 27–29], while others adopted an anterior approach only in an effort to decrease nerve damage [17, 19, 27, 29].

Kneist et al. described intraoperative pelvic nerve monitoring in 2013 for laparoscopic rectopexy that may be developed in the future to prevent nerve damage during resection with rectopexy and posterior dissection. Further investigations to verify their ten patient prospective case series will be necessary before broader application is warranted [23].

15.4 Outcomes

Overall morbidity from robotic rectopexy in the published literature is 5–25 % with very low mortality [19, 24–28]. Morbidity may be attributed to rectal injuries, urinary infection, urinary retention, bowel obstruction, incisional hernia, hemorrhage, or wound infection.

15.5 Length of Operation

Length of operation is a factor, which is often scrutinized when evaluating new surgical techniques. For robotic surgery this time is often divided into total operative time and the time at the robotic console. Like all other approaches, the robot has a learning curve. This may be shorter for surgeons already familiar with laparoscopic approaches. Faucheron et al. reported on their laparoscopic ventral technique in 175 cases with a mean operative time of 112 min, which was a significant decrease from a median of 240 min for their first ten patients [25]. De Hoog et al. published comparative results for open ($n=47$) vs. lap ($n=15$) vs. robotic ($n=20$) rectopexy in 2009. Their operative times were 77, 119, and 154 min, respectively [29]. In a comparison of robotic vs. laparoscopic ventral rectopexy, Makela-Kaikkonen et al. reported a mean operative time of 159 min, mean preparation time of 26 min, mean console time of 115 min, and total time in OR 231 min for robotic cases. The matched-pair laparoscopic cases had a mean operative time of 153 and 234 min of total time in the OR [19].

The operative technique seems to effect the operation duration as well. Heemskerk et al. reported longer operative time with robotics vs. laparoscopic approach at 152 min vs. 113 min. However, they noted shorter times after they changed from Well's posterior technique to D'Hoore's ventral technique from 162 to 122 min in favor of D'Hoore's [21]. Wong et al. published their early robotic experience with 40 laparoscopic ventral rectopexies vs. 23 robotic ventral rectopexies. Their robotic operative time was 221 min (setup time was 17 min) compared to 162 min in the laparoscopic cases. The robotic cases had a larger BMI (27 vs. 24) and also required double-mesh implantation more often than the laparoscopic cases, which they cite as an explanation for the longer operative time [17]. Mantoo et al. compared 44 patients treated with robotic ventral rectopexy and 74 patients treated by laparoscopic approach. Operative times were 191 and 163 min, respectively. Simultaneous levatorpexies were performed in many of these cases [26]. Perrenot et al. reported on a group of 77 consecutive patients treated with robotic ventral rectopexy. Average operating time was 223 min. The last 15 of their cases had an operative time of 175 min and the learning curve was estimated to be 18 cases where the times shortened [28].

Operative time for robotic rectopexy can approach that of laparoscopic rectopexy as the surgeon and surgical time become more familiar with the overall process. Reported time should be designated as setup, console, and overall operative time to allow the surgical team to identify aspects that can decrease overall OR time.

15.5.1 Blood Loss/Conversion

Blood loss is similar for laparoscopic and robotic rectopexy. Mean blood loss during laparoscopic rectopexy has been reported as 37–45 mL and during robotic rectopexy varies from 5 to 25 mL and in many cases was too small to quantify [17, 19, 24, 26]. Generally, the blood loss has been reported to be lower with the robotic technique, but the clinical significance is likely negligible.

Conversion rates for robotic surgery have generally been quoted as lower than laparoscopy. Conversion rates as low as 6.5 % were reported (5/77) in 2013 [28]. Mantoo reported 3 out of 74 (4 %) laparoscopic procedures converted to open rectopexy due to adhesions, inability to tolerate pneumoperitoneum, and a missing needle, and 1/44 (2.2 %) robotic cases converted due to poor visualization ($p=0.085$) [26]. Wong et al. reported 4/40 (10 %) conversions during laparoscopic cases and 1/23 (4 %) in the robotic patients [17]. Heemskerk et al. reported a 1/19 (5 %) conversion rate in robotic cases and none in their 14 laparoscopic cases [21]. Faucheron reported a 1.6 % conversion rate for laparoscopic rectopexy [25]. None of these studies were randomized.

15.5.2 Length of Stay/Cost

Length of hospital stay after rectopexy contributes to a significant portion of hospital cost. Typical criteria for dismissal following rectopexy include passing flatus or having a first bowel movement, ambulating, pain control with pills, and tolerating oral intake.

Faucheron et al. reported 175 laparoscopic ventral rectopexies with a median hospital stay of 2.2 days (range, 1–12) [25]. De Hoog et al. compared open, laparoscopic, and robotic length of stay and reported 5.7 (2–30) days, 3.5 (1–14) days, and 2.6 (1–6) days, respectively, with $p<0.001$ [29]. Buchs et al. reported a mean hospital stay for robotic cases of 3.6 days (range, 2–7) [24]. Wong reported similar length of stay of 5 days for laparoscopic and robotic rectopexy [17]. Mantoo et al. also reported a shorter stay for robotic cases compared to laparoscopic 5 vs. 4 days although not statistically significant [26]. Munz and Perrenot report similar length of stay of 6 and 6.5 days for their robotic rectopexy cases [18, 28].

In a comparative study, Makela-Kaikkonen et al. published a mean length of stay at 3.1 and 3.3 days for robotic and laparoscopic rectopexy, respectively [19]. Similarly, Heemskerk et al. reported a length of hospital stay of 3.5 and 4.3 days for robotic and laparoscopic rectopexy, respectively. They further analyzed the cost of the procedures and found that the total cost to the hospital was $745.09 (16 %) more for robotic surgery. However, the decreased length of stay of the robotic cases did not offset the higher cost of the operating room costs in terms of the robot and personnel salary. This difference may decrease with improvement in the robotic learning curve as well as economics of the equipment [21].

The length of stay difference between laparoscopic and robotic rectopexy is minimal with some studies favoring laparoscopic and others robotic. As experience increases, the differences in stay are likely to equilibrate.

15.5.3 Recurrence/Resolution of Symptoms

In order for robotic rectopexy to be a viable option for rectal prolapse, recurrence rates must be comparable to laparoscopic surgery. Additionally, the resolution of the patients' preoperative complaints ought to also be followed.

Samaranayake et al. reported recurrence of 3.4 % (range 0–15 %) from pooled data in a systematic review for open or laparoscopic ventral rectopexy [30]. In a series of 175 consecutive laparoscopic cases, Faucheron et al. reported 3 % recurrence at 24 months, with no patients lost to follow-up [25].

Conversely, De Hoog et al. reported a case–control study of open vs. laparoscopic vs. robotic rectopexy in 2009 [29]. In that study they had 90 % follow-up and 2 %, 27 %, and 20 % recurrence, respectively. They found that recurrences were statistically more likely to occur in males and women of childbearing age. Their higher rate of recurrence in laparoscopic and robotic cases may be related to the use of the EMS stapler to fix mesh to the promontory. In their functional analysis, they reported equivalent decrease for all techniques in both Wexner score and IDL score (impact on daily life). Makela-Kaikkonen et al. reported short-term follow-up of 40 patients, half undergoing robotic and half undergoing laparoscopic rectopexy, in a matched paired study, recurrence of 5 % in each group at 3 months. In those same patients 80 % felt that their preoperative symptoms had resolved [19].

In a comparative nonrandomized study of 33 patients undergoing robotic or laparoscopic rectopexy, no difference was seen in postoperative incontinence based on Parks–Browning classification. Interestingly, they also reported no difference in postoperative constipation between Wells' and D'Hoore's procedure [21].

Wong et al. published a prospective comparison of short-term outcomes for laparoscopic vs. robotic rectopexy. They reported no recurrence of prolapse at 6 months in 40 laparoscopic and 23 robotic cases. Furthermore, the two groups had similar new onset postoperative urinary incontinence, which had resolved in follow-up [17]. Mantoo et al. reported on their results with 6-month follow-up and 6.8 % recurrence in the robotic group and 4 % recurrence in the laparoscopic group, without significant difference. The obstructed defecation syndrome score (ODS) improved in both groups with a statistically significant difference in the robotic group vs. the laparoscopic group. They gave no explanation for this finding. Additionally, they found that of their patients that were sexually active, most had improvement in dyspareunia regardless of technique. None of the patients had new onset sexual dysfunction [26].

Perrenot et al. published long-term follow-up of robotic rectopexy with 77 cases and mean follow-up of 52.5 months. They reported 9/77 (12.8 %) recurrences, none of which occurred when a sigmoidectomy was also performed. Fecal incontinence in their group improved from a Wexner score of 10.5 to 5 out of 20, with no worsening of fecal incontinence in any patient [28].

In most studies, robotic rectopexy compares well with laparoscopic rectopexy in recurrence and resolution of symptoms. These outcomes are likely influenced by method of fixation and length of follow-up.

15.6 Conclusion

Robotic rectopexy has been shown to be a safe and equivalent treatment for rectal prolapse compared to laparoscopic and superior to open procedures. As with any disease process, the choice of treatment should be tailored to the needs of the individual patient, based on concomitant urogynecological organ prolapse, continence, previous surgeries, and comorbidities. Lateral dissection is to be avoided; however, emerging technology may improve visualization and detection of pelvic nerves. As a surgical team's experience grows, the operative time will continue to approach that of laparoscopic operations. Costs will need to be further evaluated as technology improves, competition in the robotics market increases, and overall cost of hospital admissions is scrutinized.

References

1. Madhulika G, et al. Prolaspe, intussusception and SRUS (Internet). http://www.fascrs.org/physicians/education/core_subjects/2008/prolapse_intussusception_srus/. Accessed April 2014.
2. Beck D, Roberts P, Saclarides T, Senagore A, Stamos M, Wexner S. The ASCRS textbook of colon and rectal surgery. 2nd ed. New York: Springer; 2011.
3. Tou S, Brown S, Malik A, Nelson R. Surgery for complete rectal prolapse in adults. Cochrane Database Syst Rev. 2008;8(4):CD001758.
4. Schiedeck T, Schwander O, Scheele J, Farke S, Bruch H. Rectal prolapse: which surgical option is appropriate? Langenbecks Arch Surg. 2005;390:8–14.
5. Senapati A, Gray R, Middleton L, Harding J, Hills R, et al. PROSPER: a randomized comparison of surgical treatments for rectal prolapse. Colorectal Dis. 2013;15:858–70.
6. Madiba T, Baig M, Wexner S. Surgical management of rectal prolapse. Arch Surg. 2005;140: 63–73.
7. Raftopoulos Y, Senagore AJ, Di Giuro G, Bergamaschi R, Rectal Prolapse Recurrence Study Group. Recurrence rates after abdominal surgery for complete rectal prolapse: a multicenter pooled analysis of 643 individual patient data. Dis Colon Rectum. 2005;48(6):1200–6.
8. Frykman HM. Abdominal proctopexy and primary sigmoid resection for rectal procidentia. Am J Surg. 1955;90(5):780–9.
9. Roblick U, Bader F, Jungbluth T, Laubert T, Bruch H. How to do it—laparoscopic resection rectopexy. Langenbecks Arch Surg. 2011;396:851–5.
10. Berman I. Sutureless laparoscopic rectopexy for procidentia. Technique and implications. Dis Colon Rectum. 1992;35:689–93.
11. Solonmon M, Young C, Eyers A, Roberts R. Randomized clinical trial of laparoscopic versus abdominal rectopexy for rectal prolapse. Br J Surg. 2002;89(1):35–9.

12. Sajid MS, Siddqui MR, Baig MK. Open versus laparoscopic repair of full thickness rectal prolapse: a re-meta-analysis. Colorectal Dis. 2010;12(6):515–25.

13. Weber PA, Merola S, Wasielewski A, Ballantyne G. Telerobotic-assisted laparoscopic right and sigmoid colectomies for benign disease. Dis Colon Rectum. 2002;45(12):1689–94.

14. Bokhari M, Patel C, Ramos-Valadez D, Ragupathi M, Haas E. Learning curve for robotic-assisted laparoscopic colorectal surgery. Surg Endosc. 2011;25(3):855–60.

15. Tekkis P, Senagore A, Delaney C, Fazio V. Evaluation of the learning curve in laparoscopic colorectal surgery: comparison of right-sided and left sided resections. Ann Surg. 2005;242(1):83–91.

16. Miskovic D, Ni M, Wyles S, Tekkis P, Hanna G. Learning curve and case selection in laparoscopic colorectal surgery: systematic review and international multicenter analysis of 4,852 cases. Dis Colon Rectum. 2012;55(12):1300–10.

17. Wong MT, Meurette G, Rigaud J, Regenet N, Lehur P. Robotic versus laparoscopic rectopexy for complex rectocele: a prospective comparison of short-term outcomes. Dis Colon Rectum. 2011;54(3):342–6.

18. Munz Y, Moorthy K, Kudchadkar R, Hernandez J, Martin S, Darzi A, et al. Robotic assisted rectopexy. Am J Surg. 2004;187(1):88–92.

19. Makela-Kaikkonen J, Rautio T, Klintrup K, Takala H, Vierimaa M, Ohtonen P, et al. Robotic-assisted and laparoscopic ventral rectopexy in the treatment of rectal prolapse: a matched-pairs study of operative details and complications. Tech Coloproctol. 2013;18(2):151–5.

20. Guillou P, Quirke P, Thorpe H, Walker J, Jayne D, Smith A, et al. Short-term end points of conventional versus laparoscopic-assisted surgery in patients with colorectal cancer (MRC CLASSIC trial): multicenter randomized controlled trial. Lancet. 2005;365:1718–26.

21. Heemskerk J, de Hoog D, van Gemert W, Baeten G, Greve J, Bouvy N. Robot-assisted vs. conventional laparoscopic rectopexy for rectal prolapse: a comparative study on costs and time. Dis Colon Rectum. 2007;50(11):1825–30.

22. Speakman C, Madden M, Nicholls R, Kamm M. Lateral ligament division during rectopexy causes constipation but prevents recurrence: results of a prospective randomized study. Br J Surg. 1991;78(12):1431–3.

23. Kneist W, Kauff D, Naumann G, Lang H. Resection rectopexy—laparoscopic neuromapping reveals neurogenic pathways to the lower segment of the rectum: preliminary results. Langenbecks Arch Surg. 2013;398:565–70.

24. Buchs N, Pugin F, Ris F, Volonte F, Morel P, Roche B. Early experience with robotic rectopexy. Int J Med Robot Comput Assist Surg. 2013;9(4):61–5.

25. Faucheron JL, Voirin D, Riboud R, Waroquet P, Noel J. Laparoscopic anterior rectopexy to the promontory for full-thickness rectal prolapse in 175 consecutive patients: short and long-term follow-up. Dis Colon Rectum. 2012;55(6):660–5.

26. Mantoo S, Podevin J, Regenet N, Rigaud J, Lehur P, Meurette G. Is robotic-assisted ventral mesh rectopexy superior to laparoscopic ventral mesh rectopexy in the management of obstructed defecation? Colorectal Dis. 2013;15(8):469–75.

27. Louis-Sylvestre C, Herry M. Robotic-assisted laparoscopic sacrocolpopexy for Stage III pelvic organ prolapse. Int Urogynecol J. 2013;24(5):731–3.

28. Perrenot C, Germain A, Scherrer M, Ayav A, Brunaud L, Bresler L. Long-term outcomes of robot-assisted laparoscopic rectopexy for rectal prolapse. Dis Colon Rectum. 2013;56(7):909–14.

29. De Hoog D, Heemskerk J, Nieman F, van Gemert W, Baeten G, Bouvy N. Recurrence and functional results after open versus conventional laparoscopic versus robot-assisted laparoscopic rectopexy for rectal prolapse: a case-control study. Int J Colorectal Dis. 2009;24(10):1201–6.

30. Samaranayake C, Luo C, Plank A, Merrie A, Plank L, Bissett I. Systematic review on ventral rectopexy for rectal prolapse. Colorectal Dis. 2010;12(6):504–14.

Robotic Transanal Surgery (RTS)

16

Matthew Albert, Sam Atallah, and Roel Hompes

Abstract

Robotic transanal surgery (RTS) is a relatively new application of the robot in the endoluminal treatment of rectal diseases especially rectal neoplasms. RTS was facilitated by the development of flexible transanal ports for TAMIS (transanal minimally invasive surgery) that permit docking of the robotic system to allow more complex endoluminal dissection and suturing. Although the technique is in its infancy, newer robotic platforms in the next several years should further enhance the feasibility of endoluminal surgeries potentially even more proximal in the colon.

Keywords

Robotic transanal surgery • Transanal endoscopic surgery (TEM) • Transanal minimally invasive surgery (TAMIS)

Electronic supplementary material: The online version of this chapter (doi: 10.1007/978-3-319-09120-4_16) contains supplementary material, which is available to authorized users. Videos can also be accessed at http://link.springer.com/book/10.1007/978-3-319-09120-4_16.

M. Albert, M.D., F.A.C.S., F.A.S.C.R.S. (✉)
S. Atallah, M.D., F.A.C.S., F.A.S.C.R.S. (✉)
Department of Colorectal Surgery, Florida Hospital, 661 E. Altamonte Drive, Suite 220, Altamonte Springs, FL 32701, USA
e-mail: Matthew.albert.md@flhosp.org; sam.atallah.md@flhosp.org

R. Hompes, M.D.
Department of Colorectal Surgery, Oxford University Hospitals, Oxford, UK

16.1 Introduction

The feasibility of robotic transanal surgery has been five decades in the making beginning in the 1960s when Sir Alan Parks first described the surgical technique of per anal excision for the removal of rectal neoplasms [1]. A decade later Gerhard Buess developed and performed transanal endoscopic microsurgery (TEM) [2]. Despite its limitations, TEM has clearly demonstrated to be superior than traditional transanal surgery with improved reach, visualization, and the ability to perform nonfragmented precise tumor resections [3–8].

In 2009, transanal minimally invasive surgery (TAMIS) was developed utilizing concepts from the past decades' enthusiasm for NOTES coupled with the desire for improvements in multiport surgery leading to the development of single-incision laparoscopic platforms [9]. Using soft flexible access channels combined with traditional laparoscopic insufflators, the benefits and novelties of high visualization endoluminal surgery using traditional laparoscopic instruments within a stable distended rectum became immediately apparent [10–14]. Moreover, these new affordable transanal access platforms expedited the realization of transanal access to perform retrograde total mesorectal excision (taTME), initially conceptualized in 2006 using the prior rigid rectoscopes [15]. Currently, transanal TME has consumed rectal cancer surgeons around the world, pushing the boundaries of sphincter preservation, along with techniques to improve the minimally invasive approach to dissection of the lower third of the rectum while minimizing circumferential resection margin (crm) positivity [16–18].

Simultaneously, robotic enthusiasts noting the benefits of rectal dissection in the confined space of the pelvis became intrigued with the possibilities of transferring these advantages to endoluminal surgery within the rectum. Robotic-assisted transanal endoscopic surgery and robotic transanal total mesorectal excision have both been accomplished; however, many of the potential gains are offset by the difficult robotic docking and instrument collision. Newer robots with significant functional improvements will overcome these obstacles and most likely play a significant role in the evolution of endoluminal rectal cancer surgery in the next decade.

16.2 Indications

The use of local excision for the treatment of rectal neoplasms has expanded over the last decade. The National Comprehensive Cancer Network (NCCN) guidelines and the American Society of Colon and Rectal Surgeons (ASCRS) recent practice parameters for the treatment of rectal cancer both state that local excision is an acceptable treatment modality for early favorable cancers without high-risk features [19]. The most defining feature of an early rectal cancer suitable for local excision is the absence of lymph node disease; however, currently radiologic assessment is still challenging and often inconclusive. Depth of tumor invasion is a potent predictor of lymph node metastasis as T1 cancers with invasion restricted to the submucosa are less likely to metastasize [20–22]. Additionally small cancers, less than 3 cm in diameter, are less likely to have nodal disease, and the absence of poor differentiation, tumor budding, and vascular or lymphatic invasion is also associated with reduced incidence of nodal disease (Table 16.1). This guidance has been bolstered by a recent analysis of Surveillance, Epidemiology, and End Results (SEER) data demonstrating that the local excision of T1 rectal cancer does not affect cancer-specific survival when compared to radical surgery [23]. The indications for local excision may also be broadened

Table 16.1 Histopathologic features of low- and high-risk early rectal cancer

	Low-risk ERC	High-risk ERC
Absolute factors		
Morphology	– Polypoid	– Ulcerated
	– Sessile	– Flat raised
Tumor grade	G1–G2	G3–G4/signet ring
Depth of invasion	Haggitt 1–3	Haggitt 4
	T1sm1	T1sm2–3
Lympho-vascular invasion	No	Yes
Resection margin	R0	Rx or R1
Relative factors		
Tumor budding	–	+
Mucinous histology	–	+
Position in distal 1/3 rectum	–	+
Tumor size	<3–4 cm	>3–4 cm
Cribriform-type structural atypia	–	+

ERC early rectal cancer

to include cT0 lesions in patients with locally advanced rectal cancer after neoadjuvant therapy for the purpose of confirming mural pathologic response (cPR/ypT0) [24–26].

All patients who are surgical candidates for per anal excision, TEM, or TAMIS are similarly suitable for robotic transanal excision. Neoplasms in the upper, mid, and lower rectum can all be removed utilizing a robotic transanal approach; however, this approach is optimal for tumors in the range of 6–10 cm from the anal verge. Although very low-lying lesions, whose distal margin sits below the edge of the access channel, may be amenable to robotic excision, one would have to strongly consider the benefits or advantages of this.

Perhaps the most valuable indication for robotic transanal surgery would be in the treatment of complex benign disorders such as rectourethral fistula or rectal anastomotic revisions that would benefit from the magnified three-dimensional image and tremor-free intuitive instrument movement to perform accurate hemostatic dissection with improved suturing capabilities (Video 16.1). However, while robotic transanal surgery (RTS) is in its development, it is more appropriate that less intricate cases are chosen at the start of a surgeons' learning curve, i.e., benign mid-rectal polyps or excision of a scar following the endoscopic removal of a malignant polyp (Video 16.2).

16.3 Robotic Approach for Resection of Rectal Neoplasms

All patients who have been selected to undergo RTS resection must have also undergone colonoscopy to assess for synchronous lesions and to obtain a biopsy of the rectal lesion.

A pragmatic approach suitable for most practices is to assess the primary tumor clinically and then radiologically with rectal ultrasound and increasingly now MRI to identify those with unexpected advanced T-stage and more importantly evidence of nodal involvement. On this basis an early rectal cancer most suitable for local excision should be <3 cm in diameter, freely mobile, ultrasound stage T1, and well or moderately differentiated on biopsy, lack lymphovascular invasion and mucinous architecture, and be free from nodal disease on MRI. A significant proportion of rectal lesions treated by local excision are only confirmed as malignant on the final postoperative pathology. This can make staging of the mesorectum later difficult as a result of regional postsurgical changes both in the wall and potentially lymph nodes. Avoidance of this situation is critical; the threshold for preoperative imaging by MRI or ultrasound even in benign-appearing lesions should be low, especially when high-grade dysplasia is present by biopsy [27]. Carcinoembryonic antigen level (CEA) and CT body imaging is also performed to assess for tumor metastasis. Patients with stage IV disease or locally advanced lesions are not candidates for robotic transanal surgery unless the objective is palliation.

Preoperative preparation is according to institutional guidelines; broadly speaking patients receive bowel preparation the day before the planned surgery to ensure minimal contamination of the operative field, in particular if peritoneal entry is anticipated. Preoperative antibiotics are administered prior to the initiation of surgery and standard deep venous thrombosis prophylaxis is undertaken.

All procedures are performed under general anesthesia; a peripheral nerve block around the anus consisting of 20-mL 0.5 % bupivacaine can be administered to aid in relaxation of the sphincters and improve postoperative analgesia.

Patient positioning is not dictated by tumor location with various setups having been reported irrespective of this. For obvious reasons the prone position avoids any conflict of the robotic arms with the patients' lower extremities. While lithotomy and the lateral approach are less cumbersome and provide better access to the airway for the anesthesiologist, there is the potential for conflict of the robotic arms, particularly in obese patients. In lithotomy position particularly, docking requires strategically moving the legs and stirrups around the robotic arms.

While the robotic setup might seem cumbersome and time-consuming, the docking time

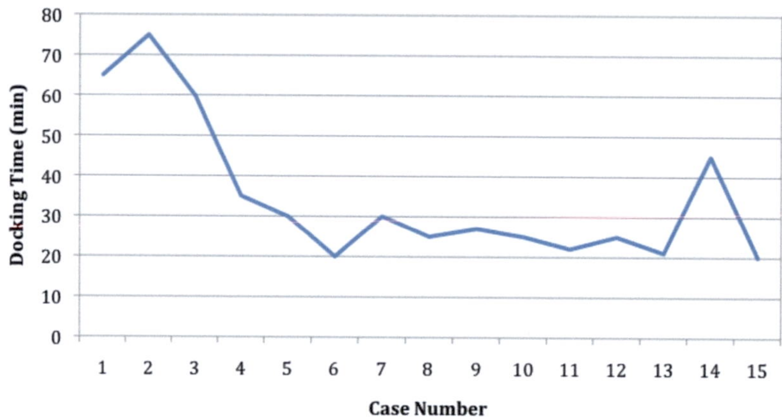

Fig. 16.1 Demonstration of the learning curve for the docking procedure. *With permission from Hompes R, Rauh SM, Ris F, Tuynman JB, Mortensen NJ. Robotic Transanal Minimally Invasive Surgery for local excisions of rectal neoplasms. Br J Surg 2012;101:578–81.* © *Blackwell Science in 2012* [28]

significantly reduces with experience [28–30]. In the cohort recently reported by Hompes et al., the mean docking time for the last five cases was less than half of the first five cases (22 min vs. 52 min, respectively), and it is the authors' opinion that the setup will not be a major impediment to the use of the robot for transanal procedures (Fig. 16.1) [31].

To date all robotic intraluminal cases have been performed through a GelPOINT path (Applied Medical Inc., Rancho Santa Margarita, CA, USA) or transanal glove port. The GelPOINT path consists of a 4-cm long access channel with a 4 cm diameter, combined with a gel cap seal and 3–4 working 12-mm ports. The transanal glove port is a novel less-expensive creation utilized for transanal access where an airtight channel is created using an Alexis retractor (Applied Medical), plastic anoscope, and sterile surgical glove with trocars fabricated through the digits. The setup of the glove port is demonstrated in Video 16.3. Interestingly, the glove port may facilitate the robotic setup, enabling flexibility by permitting docking of the cannulas away from the limited perianal workspace. Furthermore, the glove port allows for a wide axis of movement for instruments inside the rectum enabling them to be used more widely apart or easily rotated and/or crossed. It is this latter feature which is of particular interest for the robotic approach. The crossed setup for the cannulas with switched robotic arm control allows for additional intraluminal reach while still maintaining completely intuitive control. Also, inherent to this setup is the maximal separation of the robotic arms externally reducing collision between the robotic arms and/or camera. We have found that external conflict was more common in proximal lesions and with the use of the 5-mm robotic instruments, since they lack the robotic Endo-Wrist® technology, and the crossed setup proved particularly helpful to eliminate this. The benefit of the 5-mm instruments is their narrower profile, which allows for easy transition from a crossed setup to a parallel setup without any help from the bedside assistant (Video 16.4). Furthermore, the elbows of the joints can help to stent the rectal lumen in case of an unstable pneumorectum or to get access to a lesion proximal to a rectal valve of Houston.

After introduction of the transanal platform, the robot (da Vinci® Si Surgical System, Intuitive Surgery, Sunnyvale, CA, USA) is side-docked with the forks of the robotic cart parallel with and lining up with the caudal base of the table (Fig. 16.2, Video 16.3). A pneumorectum of 10–15 mmHg is established using a standard laparoscopic carbon dioxide insufflator. The robotic instruments are introduced into the rectum under direct vision (Video 16.1); the robotic cannulas can be positioned in parallel or crossed (with reversed arm control assignments) depending on

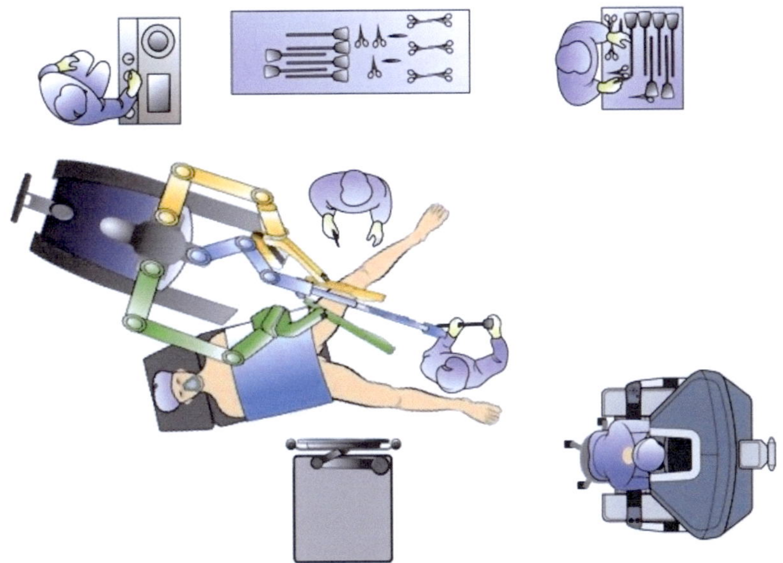

Fig. 16.2 Room setup and docking position for the robot and patient for RTS performed in the lithotomy position

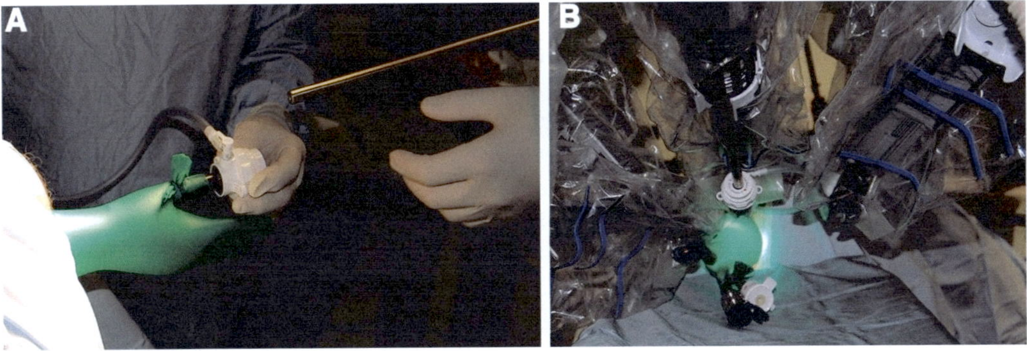

Fig. 16.3 (**a**) 12-mm camera port is inserted through the thumb of the glove ("thumbs-up position"), and after establishing a pneumorectum, the access to the rectum is assessed. (**b**) After docking of the camera, two 8-mm ports are inserted into the tips of two fingers

the height and location of the lesion within the rectum. Standard setup entails the use of an 8.5-mm robotic 30° camera in various positions; however, the 30° upward camera positions in our experience circumvent collisions of the robotic arms, in particular with the parallel setup. With the 30° upward camera positions, insertion of the camera through the thumb of the surgical glove ("thumbs-up" position of the camera) avoids excessive strain on the glove material and avoids tearing of the glove (Fig. 16.3a, b). A variety of

8-mm EndoWrist® instrumentation or 5-mm instrumentation can be used, including monopolar permanent cautery hook, Maryland bipolar forceps, DeBakey forceps, and a small or large needle driver. A bedside surgeon provides endoluminal assistance with a laparoscopic grasper, disposable suction-irrigation device, or scissors.

The technique of robotic transanal resection is identical to resection performed with other advance platforms. A robotic 5-mm hook cautery and Maryland grasper initially are placed in the two operating trocars. The console surgeon then performs a full-thickness local excision, first by demarcating the perimeter of the lesion with generally a 1-cm margin using monopolar energy. For evacuation of smoke, a bedside assistant uses a 5-mm laparoscopic suction-irrigator device passed directly through the GelPOINT cap without the need for a trocar or through the fourth finger of the glove. Simple short bursts of suction maintain image clarity without collapsing the rectal lumen. The specimen may be tented gently using a robotic Maryland grasper, while hook cautery allows for full-thickness excision. Importantly, the CO_2 insufflation provides a natural "pneumo-dissection," thereby augmenting the ease and clarity of local excision using robotic transanal surgery. To retrieve the resected specimen, the robot must be dismounted from the GelPOINT path interface. The lesion can be retrieved with a 5-mm grasper, the lid to the port simply removed allowing for specimen extraction. When the glove port is used, the specimen can be stored in the pouch of the glove and retrieved at the end of the procedure.

Closure of the full-thickness rectal wall defect, which is generally recommended, is then performed. The hook cautery and Maryland grasper are exchanged with one or two robotic needle drivers. Robotic intraluminal suturing is then carried out using a V-Loc 180 absorbable wound closure device (Covidien, Mansfield, MA). This allowed for suturing without the need for intraluminal knot tying, since the unidirectional barbs on the suture self-lock as they pass through the rectal wall. The defect can be closed with a single running V-Loc stitch, thereby completing the operation (Videos 16.1 and 16.2).

As with any new technique, it is imperative that the quality of the resection is not compromised and safety of the patient is ensured. In the authors' experience, the patients had comparable outcomes compared to the benchmarks set with transanal endoscopic surgery, and procedures were effectively and safely undertaken. While the postoperative follow-up is short, to date no local or distant recurrences were found.

Clearly there is still room for improvement of both the robotic instruments and transanal platform. Future optimization of this technique including the ideal setup (crossed vs. parallel) and type of instrumentation (8 mm vs. 5 mm) for the various lesion locations within the rectum and new developments in robotic platforms will increase its application for patients with advanced rectal lesions, offering rectal preserving therapy. Again while we describe here the use of the transanal robotic platform for local excision of rectal tumors, the stability and intraluminal versatility of this platform will lend itself perfectly to more advanced transanal procedures, transanal total mesorectal excision (taTME) perhaps being one of them.

16.4 Surgical Approach for Robotic Transanal TME

taTME is a newer technique used to facilitate dissection of the middle and lower third of the rectum. Although it is still in its infancy, with no long-term data, the approach seems to have many advantages over both open and laparoscopic rectal resection. Early data has consistently shown high negative circumferential margin (CRM) rates in addition to high-quality complete mesorectal specimens [16–18]. Robotic-assisted transanal surgery for total mesorectal excision (RATS-TME) is performed with a hybrid approach, relying on laparoscopic assistance for colon, upper rectum, and splenic flexure mobilization in addition to pedicle ligation. The abdominal approach can be performed prior to the initiation of the transanal approach; however, many choose to start the operation from below. The legs are elevated in Allen stirrups to the high-dorsal lithotomy position and the perineum is then prepped and draped appropriately. For low-lying lesions, the approach begins under direct vision and an intersphincteric resection is performed prior to robotic docking. The distal rectum is then closed with a running continuous suture of 2–0 Prolene. Alternatively, standard total mesorectal excision can be initiated with the access channel secured into the rectum from the outset and a Prolene purse string suture placed just above the anorectal ring. The gel cap is secured to the access channel and CO^2 insufflation is turned on. Generally, transanal TME can be performed with the insufflator set at 8–10 mm of pressure, as the volume is smaller to fill as compared to the robotic transanal excision as described above. For robotic-assisted transanal TME, patients are positioned in moderate Trendelenburg, and the lower extremities are then returned to the low, modified lithotomy position to allow the robotic cart to be docked without encroachment. The robotic approach and cart docking is identical to that previously described. A 30° 8-mm HD robotic camera lens and 2 working arms— a 5-mm hook-monopolar cautery and a 5-mm Maryland grasper—are used for the dissection and these instruments are docked through the GelPOINT transanally. A bedside assistant again can utilize a laparoscopic suction-irrigator device mainly aiding smoke removal.

Working in a retrograde fashion from the distal rectum proximally, the mesorectum is dissected circumferentially maintaining the surgical tenants of total mesorectal excision. During the dissection of the distal 5 cm of rectum, the working space is limited and movement of the robotic arms fairly constrained. As the dissection progresses, however, there is usually an increase in the working space within the pelvis, and with the aid of pneumo-dissection, robotic taTME is significantly easier particularly in the mid-rectum. The upper rectum is more challenging to dissect using RATS-TME, as working angles necessary to complete the dissection are difficult to obtain, especially posterior.

As with the approach from above, the posterior and then lateral planes along the pelvis are established first, saving the anterior dissection for last. If the anterior dissection is carried out first, the rectum will be drawn posteriorly by gravity, making the posterior dissection extremely difficult.

Specimen extraction and anastomosis can all be performed transanally or for bulkier specimens through a Pfannenstiel incision or potential ostomy site if one is planned for temporary fecal diversion.

16.5 The Evidence for Robotic Transanal Surgery: Local Excision and taTME

The use of the robot endoluminally through a transanal approach only became feasible in 2009 with the development of TAMIS and the first approved flexible platforms designed specifically for transanal access (GelPOINT path, Applied Medical). Clinical data therefore remains limited. Further hindering the numbers lies in the inherent difficulty and limitations of the current robotic setup, which may offset the perceived benefits of increased endoluminal dexterity.

Atallah was the first to pursue robotic transanal surgery in 2010, first in a dry-lab setup and shortly thereafter in cadavers using variable approaches to docking ultimately settling on a parallel-docking approach with the patient in lithotomy position [29, 30]. Hompes and Mortensen in 2012 described an effective, cheap, and potentially improved technique through the adaptation of a transanal "glove port" for robotic access and subsequently published the largest series of robotic transanal surgery with 16 cases in May 2014 [31]. Various other case reports from the USA and Europe similarly have shown feasibility in a small number of patients (Table 16.2) [29, 30, 32–41]. No short- or long-term data exists regarding patient outcomes, recurrence rates, quality of resection, or survival. However, one would hope that outcomes equivalent to other advanced transanal platforms could be demonstrated, as this belies the principles of its intended purpose: to improve the ease, visualization, and quality of resection through the use of robotic micro instrumentation. Ultimately superior outcomes will be required to justify the increased cost of this technique, amounting to 1000 € (US$1700) per case in Hompes' paper.

Robotic taTME is even more in its infancy with three references in the literature but with increasing discussion and enthusiasm, perhaps in anticipation of new robotic platforms [35–37, 40–42].

Table 16.2 Current published series of robotic transanal surgery

Author	Date	Country	PLAT	PROC	Model	n	BEN	MAL	DAV	SIZE	MRG	MES	LN	DOCK	OT	LOS	FU	Remarks
Atallah [29]	Sept 2011	USA	TAMIS-GP	TAMIS	Cadaver	2	N/A	N/A	N/A	N/A	N/A	N/A	N/A	Right shoulder	35	N/A	N/A	First case of RTS
Atallah [30]	May 2012	USA	TAMIS-GP	TAMIS	Human	1	0	1	7	3	Free	N/A	N/A	Right shoulder	105	1	1.5	First human case of RTS
Hompes [35]	May 2012	UK	Glove	TAMIS	Cadaver	2	N/A	N/A	N/A	N/A	N/A	N/A	N/A	Parallel right	–	N/A	N/A	First report of using a glove for interface
Bardakcioglu [32]	Dec 2012	USA	TAMIS-GP	TAMIS	Human	1	1	0	8	1.5	Free	N/A	N/A	Parallel left	–	0	–	Second human case of RTS
Atallah [36]	June 2013	USA	TAMIS-GP	RATS-TME	Human	1	0	1	4	3.4	Free	Near complete	0/35	Parallel right	87	3	1.5	First report of using RTS for transanal TME
Vallribera [37]	Aug 2013	Spain	Glove	TAMIS	Human	1	1	0	6	2.5	Free	N/A	N/A	Lateral	180	1	–	First small series on RTS using glove
Buchs [34]	Aug 2013	Switzerland	Glove	TAMIS	Human	3	0	3	10.2	3.2	Free	N/A	N/A	Lateral	110	3	2	Description of lateral approach to RTS
Gomez-Ruiz [38]	Feb 2014	Spain	TAMIS-GP	RATS-TME	Cadaver	4	N/A	N/A	N/A	N/A	N/A	Complete	–	Left	82 (robotic)	N/A		First experiment for RATS-TME One case ligation of IMA and IMV transanally
Hompes [28]	Apr 2014	UK	Glove	TAMIS	Human	16	6	10	8	5.3	13 free/3 positive	N/A	N/A	Side	108	1.3	–	Largest series of robotic TAMIS
Atallah [39]	Apr 2014	USA	TAMIS-GP	TAMIS	Human	1	0	1	4	–	Free	N/A	N/A	Side	93	1	1.5	Video vignette
Gomez-Ruiz [40]	May 2014	Spain	TAMIS-GP	RATS-TME	Human	1	0	1	5	6.7	Free	Complete	29	Left side	420	6	–	Article in Spanish
Verheijen [41]	May 2014	Netherlands	TAMIS-GP	RATS-TME	Human	1	0	1	8	3	Free	Complete	–	Left hip	205	3	1.5	
Atallah [42]	June 2014	USA	TAMIS-GP	RATS-TME	Human	3	0	3	2.5	2.5	Free	1 complete 2 near complete	30	Right parallel	376	4.3	3	Largest series of three RATS-TME
Total (m)						37												

PLAT platform used for transanal approach, *GP* GelPOINT path transanal access platform, *n* number of lesions resected, *BEN* number of benign cases included on the study, *MAL* number of malignant cases included on the study, *DAV* distance of lesions from anal verge, *SIZE* largest diameter of surgical specimen (cm), *MRG* number of patients with positive margins, *MES* intactness of mesorectum, *LN* average number of lymph nodes harvested, *DOCK* robot docking position, *OT* operative time (min), *PO* intraoperative and postoperative complications, *CNV* number of conversion from robotic to other transanal approaches, *PO* intra- and postoperative complications, *LOS* length of stay (days), *FU* follow-up measured (months), *(m)* mean

Despite the few reports on robotic transanal surgery to date, the procedure is feasible, is safe, and can be used as a tool to perform endoluminal excision as with TEM and TAMIS. The availability of the next-generation robot, da Vinci Xi and da Vinci SP (Intuitive Surgical), will immediately improve upon the setup limitations incurred with prior systems potentially increasing its use.

16.6 Conclusions

RTS illustrates a novel approach to the resection of well-selected and appropriately staged rectal neoplasia. En bloc resection of the rectum, with the technique of robotic-assisted taTME, represents a newer direction for RTS. A potential key advantage of RTS over TAMIS or TEM is the ability of the console surgeon to perform intricate surgery more easily within the narrow, cylindrical lumen. The EndoWrist movement allows for greater intraluminal dexterity. This, together with magnified 3D optics, enhances the surgeon's ability to perform transanal local excision with improved precision in addition to more complex tasks such as intraluminal suturing. RTS is a new approach to transanal access. Its ability to accomplish intricate tasks with ease makes this technique attractive for more complex cases (transanal repair of fistula), where traditional platforms remain challenging.

Robotic transanal surgery is a technique still in its infancy, and its application for rectal surgery has not yet been fully defined. New single-port robotic platforms and improved instrumentation will greatly facilitate docking and ease of use in the next year, while the rationale and techniques for rectum-preserving strategies in rectal cancer become better defined. Safety, effectiveness, and financial aspects of robotic transanal surgery have to be further evaluated and confirmed before widespread application.

16.7 Key Points

- The local excision of rectal neoplasms utilizing advanced transanal platforms beginning with TEM in 1983, and TAMIS in 2009, has consistently shown improved outcomes with lower recurrence rates than traditional per anal technique.
- Differences in local recurrence outcomes are largely due to enhanced access to the lesion, restored visualization, stable pneumorectum, and improved instrumentation permitting an improved resection as compared to traditional transanal excision (TAE).
- The utilization of a surgical robot to improve upon current surgical techniques could potentially expound upon the discrepancy in local recurrence rates and outcomes.
- Surgical technique, and specifically robotic setup, is somewhat more challenging and less standardized than the previous chapters given the youthfulness of the procedure.
- Robotic transanal surgery is enabled through use of the current da Vinci SI robotic platform (Intuitive Surgical, Sunnyvale, CA), concurrently with a flexible transanal access port (GelPOINT path, Applied Medical, Rancho Santa Margarita, CA) or glove port.
- Transanal total mesorectal excision (taTME) was first conceptualized on rigid platforms in cadavers in 2006 and since evolved into clinical practice for the treatment of benign and malignant neoplasms of the rectum with equivalent outcomes in short-term follow-up.
- Robotic transanal TME has been performed in humans yet remains experimental and difficult with the current robotic platforms.
- Robotic transanal excision and robotic transanal TME are cutting-edge applications exploiting the robot in the evolving treatment of rectal cancer; however, these surgical procedures expose all of the limitations of current robotic platforms: mainly the issues with robotic docking and working within a more confined space without arm crossing and robotic arm collision.
- Newer robotic platforms (da Vinci Xi, Intuitive Surgical), available commercially in late 2014, employ years of technological design advancements to overcome the current limitations of robotic transanal surgery and will potentially transform endoluminal colon surgery in the next decade.

References

1. Parks AG, Rob C, Smith R, Morgan CN. Benign tumours of the rectum. In: Rob C, Smith R, Morgan CN, editors. Clinical surgery, vol. 10. England, London: Butterworths; 1966. p. 541.

2. Buess G, Hutterer F, Theiss J, Böbel M, Isselhard W, Pichlmaier H. [A system for a transanal endoscopic rectum operation]. Chirurg. 1984;55:677–80.

3. Saclarides TJ, Smith L, Ko ST, et al. Transanal endoscopic microsurgery. Dis Colon Rectum. 1992;35: 1183–91.

4. Palma P, Horisberger K, Joos A, et al. Local excision of early rectal cancer: is transanal endoscopic microsurgery an alternative to radical surgery? Rev Esp Enferm Dig. 2009;101:172–8.

5. Winde G, Nottberg H, Keller R, et al. Surgical cure for early rectal carcinomas (T1) transanal endoscopic microsurgery vs. anterior resection. Dis Colon Rectum. 1996;39:969–76.

6. Heintz A, Mörschel M, Junginger T. Comparison of results after transanal endoscopic microsurgery and radical resection for T1 carcinoma of the rectum. Surg Endosc. 1998;12:1145–8.

7. Moore JS, Cataldo PA, Osler T, et al. Transanal endoscopic microsurgery is more effective than traditional transanal excision for resection of rectal masses. Dis Colon Rectum. 2008;51:1026–30; discussion 30–1.

8. Middleton PF, Sutherland LM, Maddern GJ. Transanal endoscopic microsurgery: a systematic review. Dis Colon Rectum. 2005;48:270–84.

9. Atallah S, Albert M, Larach S. Transanal minimally invasive surgery: a giant leap forward. Surg Endosc. 2010;24:2200–5. Epub 21 Feb 2010.

10. Martin-Perez B, Andrade-Ribeiro GD, Hunter L, Atallah S. A systematic review of transanal minimally invasive surgery (TAMIS) from 2010 to 2013. Tech Coloproctol.2014;18:775–88.doi:10.1007/s10151-014-1148-6. Epub 2014 May 7.

11. Albert M, Atallah S, deBeche-Adams T, Izfar S, Larach S. Transanal minimally invasive surgery (TAMIS) for local excision of benign neoplasms and early-stage rectal cancer: efficacy and outcomes in the first 50 patients. Dis Colon Rectum. 2013;56:301–7.

12. Lim SB, Seo SI, Lee JL, Kwak JY, Jang TY. Feasibility of transanal minimally invasive surgery for mid-rectal lesions. Surg Endosc. 2012;26:3127–32. doi:10.1007/s00464-012-2303-7. Epub 2012 Apr 28.

13. McLemore EC, Weston LA, Coker AM, et al. Transanal minimally invasive surgery for benign and malignant rectal neoplasia. Am J Surg. 2014;208:372–81. doi:10.1016/j.amjsurg.2014.01.006. Epub 2014 Apr 1.

14. Schiphorst AH, Langenhoff BS, Maring J, Pronk A, Zimmerman DD. Transanal minimally invasive surgery: initial experience and short-term functional results. Dis Colon Rectum. 2014;57:927–32.

15. Whiteford MH, Denk PM, Swanström LL. Feasibility of radical sigmoid colectomy performed as natural orifice translumenal endoscopic surgery (NOTES) using transanal endoscopic microsurgery. Surg Endosc. 2007;2:1870–4.

16. Atallah S, Albert M, Debeche-Adams T, Nassif G, Polavarapu H, Larach S. Transanal minimally invasive surgery for total mesorectal excision (TAMIS-TME): a stepwise description of the surgical technique with video demonstration. Tech Coloproctol. 2013;17:321–5. doi:10.1007/s10151-012-0971-x. Epub 2013 Feb 2.

17. de Lacy AM, Rattner DW, Adelsdorfer C, et al. Transanal natural orifice transluminal endoscopic surgery (NOTES) rectal resection: "down-to-up" total mesorectal excision (TME)—short-term outcomes in the first 20 cases. Surg Endosc. 2013;27:3165–72.

18. Velthuis S, Nieuwenhuis DH, Emiel T, et al. Transanal versus traditional laparoscopic total mesorectal excision for rectal carcinoma. Surg Endosc. 2014;28(12): 3494–9.

19. Monson JR, Weiser MR, Buie WD, et al. Practice parameters for the management of rectal cancer (revised). Dis Colon Rectum. 2013;56:535–50.

20. Nascimbeni R, Burgart LJ, Nivatvongs S, Larson DR. Risk of lymph node metastasis in T1 carcinoma of the colon and rectum. Dis Colon Rectum. 2002;45(2):200–6.

21. Tytherleigh MG, Warren BF, Mortensen N. Management of early rectal cancer. Br J Surg. 2008; 95:409–23.

22. Kikuchi R, Takano M, Takagi K, et al. Management of early invasive colorectal cancer. Dis Colon Rectum. 1995;38:1286–95.

23. Bhangu A, Brown G, Nicholls RJ, et al. Survival outcome of local excision versus radical resection of colon or rectal carcinoma: a Surveillance, Epidemiology, and End Results (SEER) population-based study. Ann Surg. 2013;258:563–9; discussion 569–71.

24. Garcia-Aguilar J, Shi Q, Thomas Jr CR, et al. A phase II trial of neoadjuvant chemoradiation and local excision for T2N0 rectal cancer: preliminary results of the ACOSOG Z6041 trial. Ann Surg Oncol. 2012; 19:384–91.

25. Kundel Y, Brenner R, Purim O, et al. Is local excision after complete pathological response to neoadjuvant chemoradiation for rectal cancer an acceptable treatment option? Dis Colon Rectum. 2010;53:1624–31.

26. Kim CJ, Yeatman TJ, Coppola D, et al. Local excision of T2 and T3 rectal cancers after downstaging chemoradiation. Ann Surg. 2001;234(3):352–8; discussion 358–9.

27. Serra-Aracil X, Caro-Tarrago A, Mora-López L, Casalots A, Rebasa P, Navarro-Soto S. Transanal endoscopic surgery with total wall excision is required with rectal adenomas due to the high frequency of adenocarcinoma. Dis Colon Rectum. 2014;57(7): 823–9.

28. Hompes R, Rauh SM, Ris F, Tuynman JB, Mortensen NJ. Robotic transanal minimally invasive surgery for local excisions of rectal neoplasms. Br J Surg. 2012;101:578–81. doi:10.1002/bjs.9454.

29. Atallah SB, Albert MR, deBeche-Adams TH, Larach SW. Robotic TransAnal minimally invasive surgery in a cadaveric model. Tech Coloproctol. 2011;15:461–4.
30. Atallah S, Parra-Davila E, deBeche-Adams T, Albert M, Larach S. Excision of a rectal neoplasm using robotic transanal surgery (RTS): a description of the technique. Tech Coloproctol. 2012;16:389–92.
31. Hompes R, Ris F, Cunningham C, Mortensen NJ, Cahill RA. Transanal glove port is a safe and cost-effective alternative for transanal endoscopic microsurgery. Br J Surg. 2012;99:1429–35.
32. Bardakcioglu O. Robotic transanal access surgery. Surg Endosc. 2012;27:1407–9.
33. Valls FV, Bassany EE, Jimenez-Gomez LM, Chavarria JR, Carrasco MA. Robotic transanal endoscopic microsurgery in benign rectal tumour. J Robotic Surg. 2014;8:277–80. doi:10.1007/s11701-013-0429-9.
34. Buchs NC, Pugin F, Volonte F, Hagen ME, Morel P, Ris F. Robotic transanal endoscopic microsurgery: technical details for the lateral approach. Dis Colon Rectum. 2013;56:1194–8.
35. Hompes R, Rauh SM, Hagen ME, Mortensen NJ. Preclinical cadaveric study of transanal endoscopic da Vinci surgery. Br J Surg. 2012;99:1144–8.
36. Atallah S, Nassif G, Polavarapu H, et al. Robotic-assisted transanal surgery for total mesorectal excision (RATS-TME): a description of a novel surgical approach with video demonstration. Tech Coloproctol. 2013;17:441–7.
37. Vallribera Valls F, Espín Bassany E, Jiménez-Gómez LM, Ribera Chavarría J, Carrasco MA. Robotic transanal endoscopic microsurgery in benign rectal tumour. J Robotic Surg. 2014;8:277–80. doi:10.1007/s11701-013-0429-9.
38. Gomez Ruiz M, Martin Parra I, Calleja Iglesias A, et al. Preclinical cadaveric study of transanal robotic proctectomy with total mesorectal excision combined with laparoscopic assistance. Int J Med Robot 2014. doi:10.1002/rcs.1581
39. Atallah S, Quinteros F, Martin-Perez B, Larach S. Robotic transanal surgery for local excision of rectal neoplasms. J Robot Surg. 2014;8(2):193–4. doi:10.1007/s11701-014-0463-2.
40. Gomez Ruiz M, Palazuelos CM, Martin Parra JJ, et al. New technique of transanal proctectomy with completely robotic total mesorectal excision for rectal cancer. Cir Esp. 2014;92:356–61.
41. Verheijen PM, Consten EC, Broeders IA. Robotic transanal total mesorectal excision for rectal cancer: experience with a first case. Int J Med Robot. 2014;10(4):423–6. doi:10.1002/rcs.1594. Epub 2014 May 8.
42. Atallah S, Martin-Perez B, Pinan J, Quinteros F, Schoonyoung H, Albert M, Larach S. Robotic transanal total mesorectal excision: a pilot study. Tech Coloproctol.2014;18(11):1047–53.doi:10.1007/s10151-014-1181-5. Epub 2014 Jun 24.

Single-Docking Totally Robotic Low-Anterior Resection or Pull-Through Intersphincteric Resection

17

Hsin-Hung Yeh, Nak Song Sung, and Seon Hahn Kim

Abstract

Laparoscopic total mesorectal excision (TME) for rectal cancer is still technically demanding procedure with high conversion rates because of the narrow and confined pelvic space. Its pitfall of laparoscopy to rectal surgery can be overcome with application of the da Vinci robotic platform which has several advantages including three-dimensional magnified vision, stable camera platform, tremor elimination, stable traction, and articulating EndoWrist. Recent several studies for robotic rectal surgery have demonstrated a lower conversion rate and comparable short-term operative and oncologic outcomes comparing with laparoscopy. It is no doubt that well-organized randomized trials are still needed; however, it is certain that the robotic system is very effective for rectal cancer surgery.

Keywords

TME • Rectal cancer • da Vinci • Laparoscopic • Robotic

Electronic supplementary material: The online version of this chapter (doi: 10.1007/978-3-319-09120-4_17) contains supplementary material, which is available to authorized users. Videos can also be accessed at http://link.springer.com/book/10.1007/978-3-319-09120-4_17.

H.-H. Yeh, B.Med., F.R.A.C.S. • S.H. Kim, M.D., Ph.D. (✉)
Department of Colorectal Surgery, Korea University Anam Hospital, Seoul, Korea
e-mail: deanyeh@ausdoctors.net; drkimsh@korea.ac.kr

N.S. Sung, M.D.
Department of Surgery, Division of Colorectal Surgery, Korea University Anam Hospital, Seoul, South Korea
e-mail: tjdskrthd@daum.net

17.1 Introduction

Total mesorectal excision (TME) is an essential technique to gain proper oncologic outcomes for treatment of rectal cancer [1], A recent meta-analysis demonstrated a comparable oncologic adequacy of laparoscopic surgery for rectal cancer compared to open surgery, but it still showed a wide range of conversion rate (0–32.4 %) [2]. It implies underlying technical difficulty of laparoscopic surgery in the treatment of rectal cancer because of confined and complex pelvic space. Robotic system offers several advantages including the 3D eye magnified vision, enhanced dexterity, and stable operating platform so that it enables the surgeon to dissect the "holy plane" during TME more precisely. Several robotic approaches for rectal cancer such as hybrid, double docking, and single docking are currently utilized [3–5]. Since we introduced the da Vinci robotic system at our institution in 2007, we have developed a single-docking totally robotic technique that does not require movement of the patient cart during the entire dissection of low-anterior resection (LAR) or intersphincteric resection (Videos 17.1 and 17.2) (ISR) [3]. We have standardized and simplified our robotic technique to make it a safe and feasible operation for rectal cancer through our consecutive experiences of more than 300 operations. In this chapter, we describe our stepwise surgical technique and tips of totally robotic LAR or ISR currently used at our institution.

17.2 Procedure Overview

17.2.1 Equipment

- Camera—0° camera is used (30° down or up camera when needed).
- Three robotic arms.
  - Arm 1: hot shears (monopolar curved scissors)
  - Arm 2: Maryland bipolar forceps
  - Arm 3: Cadiere forceps
    The reason why Cadiere forceps is preferred over other graspers is due to its size. Its smaller size makes it easier to maneuver in a tight pelvis. It also has lower grasping pressure compared to other graspers, such as the ProGrasp forceps. It decreases the risk of inadvertent tissue injury.
- Hem-o-lok clips (Weck Closure System, Research Triangle Park, NC, USA)
- Laparoscopic stapling device via assistant
- Optional instruments
  - Harmonic curved shears
  - Robotic stapling device
  - Robotic vessel-sealing device

17.2.2 Patient Positioning and Room Setup for Totally Robotic LAR or ISR

The patient is placed in a modified lithotomy position using stirrups. The legs are lowered so the thigh is at the same level as the torso. The Trendelenburg position with the patient tilted left side up allows the omentum and the small bowel loops to fall away from operative field due to gravity. Often, 15–20° head down and 15–20° right-side down are required. The right side of the greater omentum should also be positioned over the liver (Fig. 17.1a).

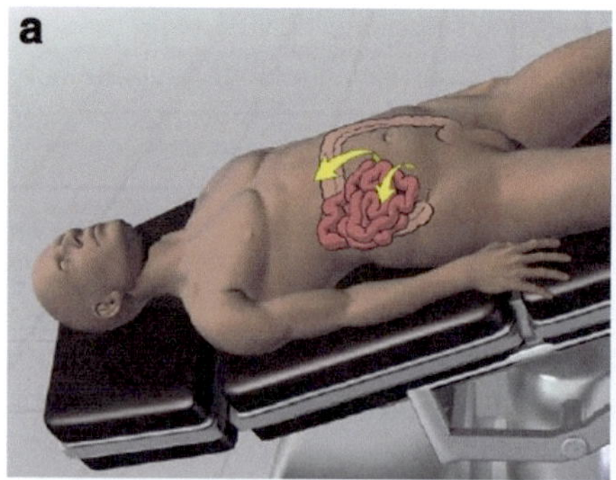
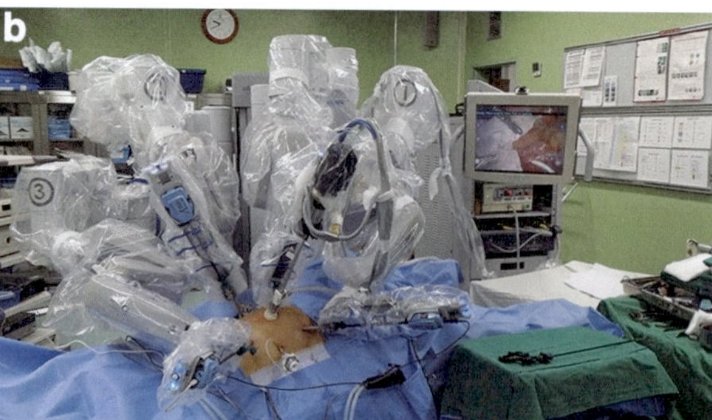

Fig. 17.1 (**a**) Patient positioning for single-docking totally robotic LAR or ISR. (**b**) The robotic setup for single-docking totally robotic LAR or ISR

As the patient will remain in this position for a significant amount of time, care should be taken to ensure the patient would not slide on the operating table during the case. In our institution, we use a surgical beanbag mattress to keep the patient in place.

The patient cart is positioned and docked obliquely at left side of the patient. Also note the robotic arms are well fanned out to minimize external collision (Fig. 17.1b).

During the operation, both the assistant and the scrub nurse should stand on the patient's right side. This allows them access to the robotic instruments. The video cart is placed toward the right foot of the patient to allow visualization of the video screen.

17.2.3 Trocar Placement

Pneumoperitoneum can be established via either Veress needle, direct optical entry, or direct cutdown. Our preferred method is direct cutdown.

Our standard robotic setup includes five instrument ports in addition to the camera port (Figs. 17.2 and 17.3). RLQ port is usually placed at McBurney's point. It is important to avoid bony structures such as the iliac crest to allow maximum range of motion for the robotic arm. Another consideration is also given if covering ileostomy is required as this port site will be used for ileostomy.

RUQ port is placed 2 cm from the costal margin and just medial to the midclavicular line. Left-side ports are placed along left midclavicular line. The LUQ port is placed at a lower level to the RUQ port to avoid clashing during colonic dissection.

The assistant port is placed in right-flank position between the RUQ and camera port.

Trocar placement is of importance to prevent problems during the operation. Distance between camera/instrument and target anatomy and the distance between the instrument ports are also important. The camera port should be at least 15 cm from target anatomy. The distance between the instrument ports on the same side of the patient should be at least 8 cm apart. The angle between the two right-side instrument ports should be as wide as possible (Fig. 17.4). Correct trocar placement will prevent clashing of the instrument arms during surgery.

17.2.4 Initial Laparoscopy

- Full initial diagnostic laparoscopy is performed looking for evidence of peritoneal or metastatic disease.
- Divide any adhesions that may limit mobilization and exposure.
- The aim is to expose the left colon, base of the mesentery, and inferior mesenteric artery (IMA) and vein (IMV).

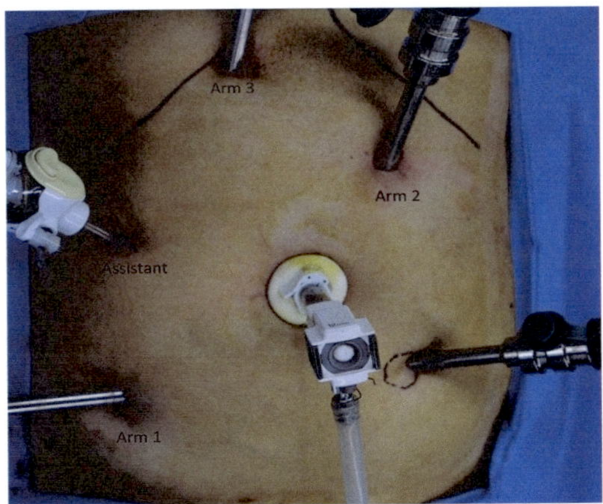

Fig. 17.2 Port placement for abdominal phase

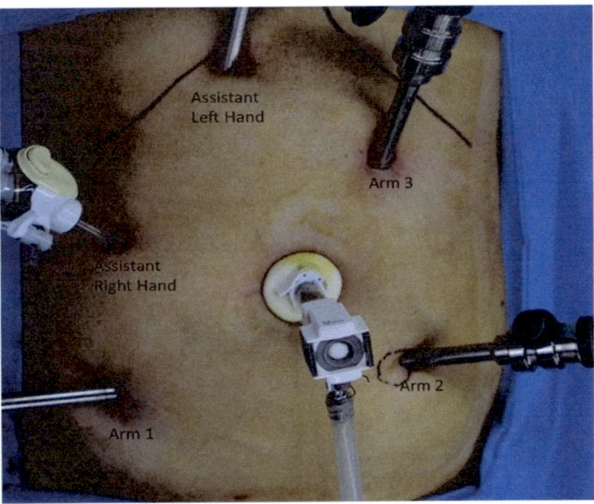

Fig. 17.3 Port placement for pelvic phase

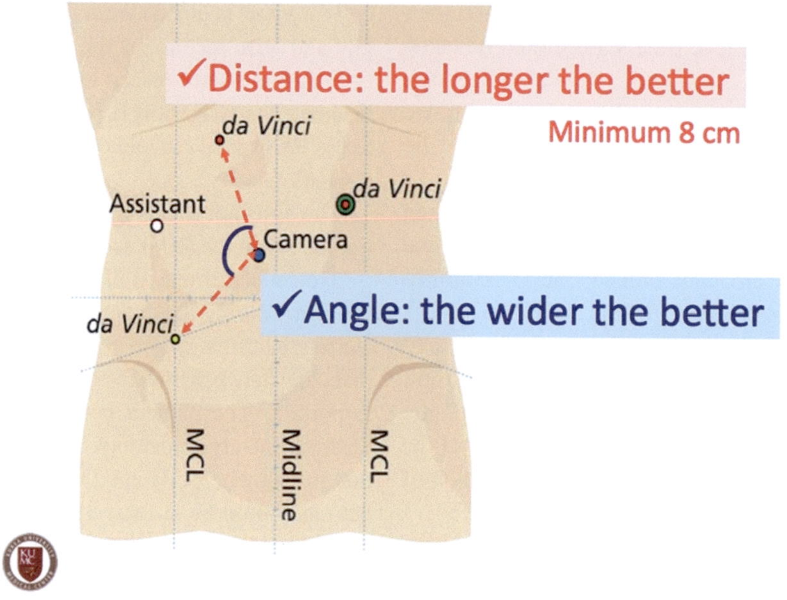

Fig. 17.4 Diagram showing the angle between the robotic ports in RUQ and RLQ should be as wide and long as possible

- The omentum is retracted above the stomach and the liver along with the transverse colon. The weight of the omentum, along with Trendelenburg position, helps keep the transverse colon way from operative field.
- Retract small bowel loops medially and toward RUQ.
- Assess the left colon and sigmoid. Sometimes the mobilization of the splenic flexure may not be necessary if there is redundant sigmoid colon.
- One or two pieces of small gauze may be placed intraperitoneally to help retract the small bowel.
- In female patients, the uterus is best retracted away using sutures.

17.2.5 Docking: Single vs. Double

Various robotic techniques have been described in literature, including hybrid, double docking, and single docking. The authors have developed the single-docking technique over many years involving significant patient numbers and believe this method provide excellent exposure. This is the method we shall describe in detail.

17.2.5.1 Hybrid Approach

The splenic flexure and left colon is mobilized laparoscopically. The patient cart is then docked either at an angle on the patient's left side or between the legs for pelvic dissection.

17.2.5.2 Double Docking

Two separate dockings include the initial docking for mobilization of splenic flexure and the second docking for sigmoid and pelvic dissection. An alternate technique recently described is to undock the patient cart, but rather than move the patient cart, the patient bed is moved instead into the new position.

17.2.5.3 Single Docking

The patient cart is obliquely placed on the patient's left. The central column of the patient cart should line up along an imaginary line between the camera port and the left anterior superior iliac spine.

Moving the robotic arms into different ports allows both dissection of the left colon/splenic

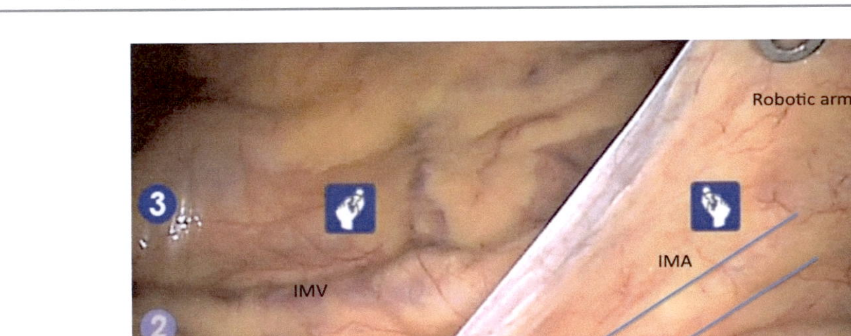

Fig. 17.5 Exposure of the IMA. Arm 2 retracts the sigmoid mesentery toward anterior abdominal wall, leaving both arms 1 and 3 for dissection

flexure and pelvic dissection. Docking on the patient's left also allows access to the patient's perineum, enabling the surgeon to check his/her dissection by digital examination without undocking the patient cart.

17.3 Abdominal Dissection

17.3.1 Port Placement (Fig. 17.2)

- Instrument arm 1: monopolar curved scissors through the RLQ port.
- Instrument arm 2: Maryland bipolar forceps through the LUQ port.
- Instrument arm 3: Cadiere forceps through the RUQ port.
- The assistant utilizes a grasper and a sucker through the assistant port on the right flank.

17.3.2 Medial-to-Lateral Approach

This is the standard practice of this department.

The sigmoid colon mesentery is lifted up using arm 2 to reveal the base of the mesentery and IMA (Fig. 17.5). The assistant uses a non-toothed grasper to retract the small bowel away from operative field. Mesentery above sacral promontory is incised and dissected using arms 1 and 3. The IMA is identified and skeletonized. The aorta is used as a landmark for dissection of the IMA. Keep the aorta horizontal while visualizing the IMA. A D3 dissection is performed by dissecting a cuff of the mesentery at least 1 cm around the origin of the IMA and included in the specimen, while the periaortic sympathetic nerve plexus is preserved (Fig. 17.6). Once skeletonized, the IMA is ligated at its origin with Hem-o-lok clips. This can be performed either by the assistant or via the robotic arm. Using the robotic arm does require exchanging the instrument arm but does have the advantage of better rotation and angulations provided by the robotic wrist. It is best if the IMA is not ligated flush against the aorta. A short cuff is recommended in case of bleeding.

We have also developed a technique for patients with cardiovascular diseases whereby the IMA is ligated at a low level while preserving the left colic vessels but oncological resection is not compromised by including the same mesenteric tissue in the final specimen. This is done by carefully skeletonizing the IMA, dissecting

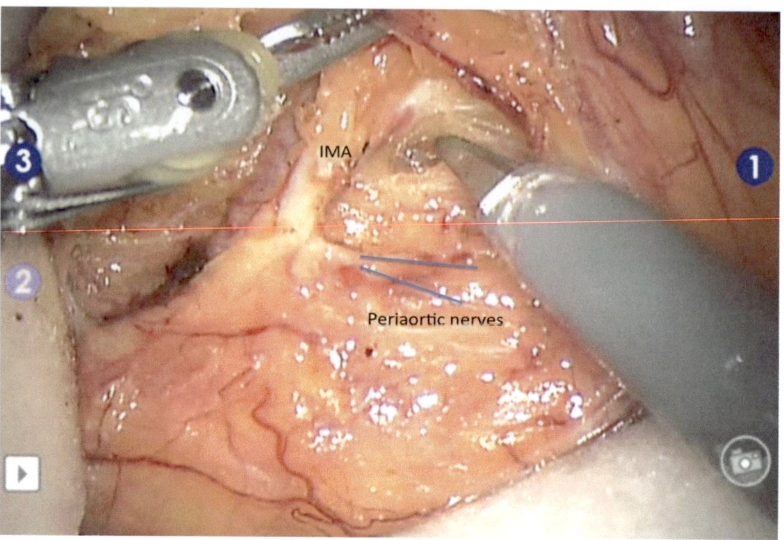

Fig. 17.6 The IMA is skeletonized and the periaortic sympathetic nerves are preserved

mesenteric tissue from the IMA, until the left colic artery is identified. Mesenteric tissue is dissected off the left colic pedicle to allow the IMA to be ligated above the left colic branch.

It is of importance to identify the nerves and preserve them. The 3-dimensional view is very helpful in identifying the nerves. By skeletonizing the IMA, the nerves are better identified and preserved. The assistant may assist with retraction with a sucker or grasper.

The IMA is then lifted toward the anterior abdominal wall and the descending colon and sigmoid mesentery is dissected from the retroperitoneum. Dissection is performed by using a sharp dissection. The plane between the mesentery and the Gerota's fascia can be identified using both traction and countertraction of both arms 2 and 3. Sometimes the plane can be better identified by gentle pushing using the instrument arms. It is important to constantly reposition arm 2 to help with retraction. Arm 2 should be retracting the mesentery upward toward anterior the abdominal wall. This allows arm 3 to be used for countertraction. Any bleeding can be controlled using bipolar in the left robotic arm (arm 3) or the monopolar scissors in the right arm (arm 1).

Dissection of the colonic mesentery off the retroperitoneum is continued proximally toward the splenic flexure. The IMV is identified on the lateral side of the duodenum and dissected.

Before ligation of the IMV, the arc of Riolan (otherwise known as the meandering artery) should be sorted. The arc of Riolan, when present, may be significant in affecting the blood supply provided by the marginal artery. If required, the IMV should be ligated to ensure the arc of Riolan remains intact (Fig. 17.7). Ligation of the IMV does not affect oncological outcome but provides mobilization of the left colon to reach the pelvis during anastomosis.

The boundaries of medial dissection are the inferior border of the pancreas proximally and the aorta medially. Laterally, dissection is carried out as far laterally as possible until the visualization of the psoas muscle. The left ureter should be visualized crossing the left iliac vessels and preserved.

If the splenic flexure is mobilized, proximal dissection is extended above the pancreas and lesser sac entered inferiorly during medial dissection. This is done by incising the peritoneum overlying the transverse colon mesentery at the level of the pancreas. Dissection of the mesentery off the superior aspect of the pancreas will lead you into the lesser sac. Once lesser sac is entered, the transverse colon mesentery can be dissected off its attachment to the anterior aspect of the

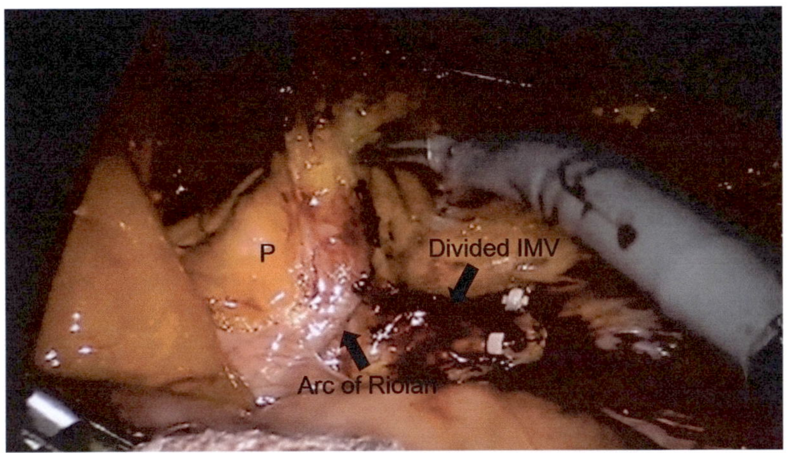

Fig. 17.7 Preservation of arc of Riolan. *P* pancreas

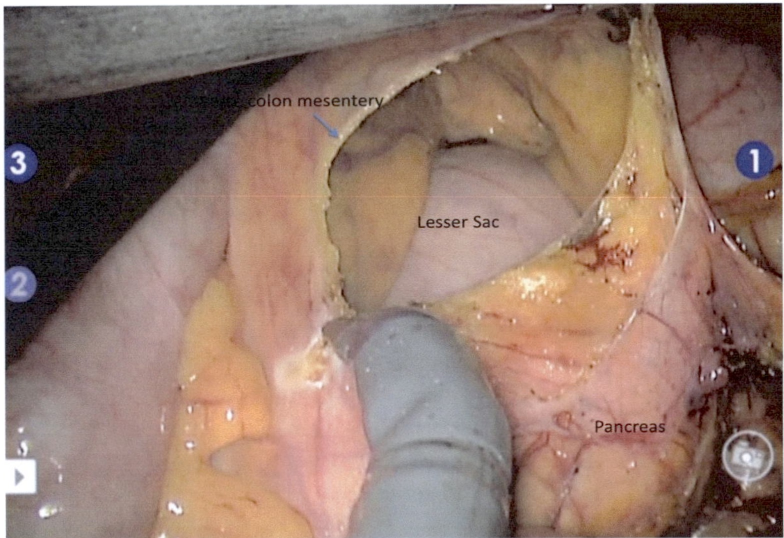

Fig. 17.8 Medial dissection above the pancreas to enter the lesser sac and dissection of the transverse colon mesentery off the pancreas. The *black-colored* instrument is the assistant's grasper

pancreas (Fig. 17.8). The assistant places the grasper into the lesser sac and lifts the transverse colon mesentery upward. This dissection is carried laterally toward the splenic flexure. This is identified by the omentum that attaches to the tail of the pancreas.

Once medial dissection is complete, lateral dissection can be performed. The sigmoid colon is separated from its peritoneal attachments commencing at the sigmoid notch by dissecting along the line of Toldt. The colon is retracted medially and inferiorly (i.e., toward the RLQ) by the assistant and left for the surgeon's left robotic arm to be used for countertraction (Fig. 17.9). If the medial dissection is adequate, lateral dissection should quickly join the dissection as previously done medially.

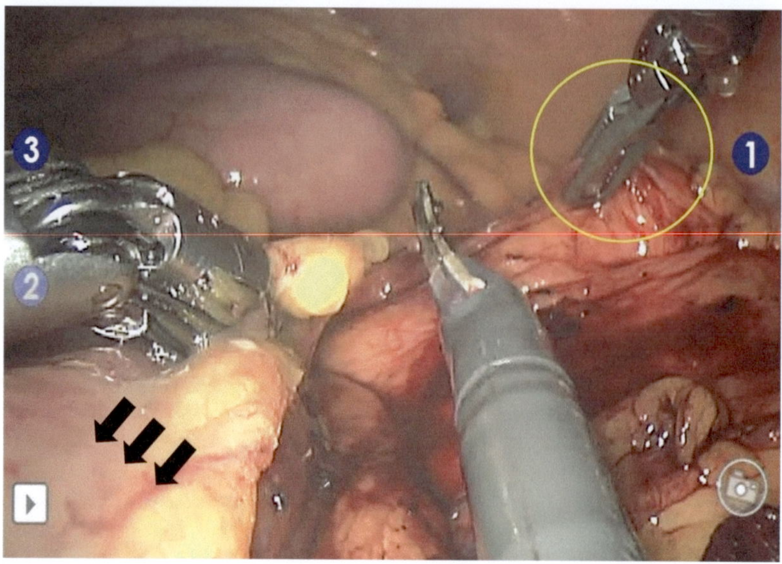

Fig. 17.9 The descending colon is retracted medially and inferiorly by the assistant (*arrows*) and surgeon's left robotic arm is used for countertraction (*yellow ellipse*) during lateral dissection

17.3.3 "Hand-On-Hand" Technique

During repositioning of instruments, communication between the surgeon and assistant is important. We use a "hand-on-hand" technique. The surgeon retracts the colon/mesentery into the desired position, and then the assistant comes in with his/her instrument to replace of the surgeon's robotic arms. It is important that only one person moves at a time to avoid losing the established retraction, i.e., surgeon moves, then assistant moves. This also reduces unnecessary movement and the risk of inadvertent injury.

17.3.4 Splenic Flexure Mobilization

The splenic flexure is mobilized by first continuing the lateral dissection of the left colon toward the spleen. It is important to constantly reposition the assistant so adequate traction on the left colon is maintained during dissection. One will then encounter the attachment of the greater omentum onto the proximal left colon. By using robotic arm 2 to lift the greater omentum toward the anterior abdominal wall, the greater omentum is dissected off the splenic flexure using robotic arms 1 and 3. Once the omentum is dissected off the colon, the lateral attachments of the splenic flexure may be divided to fully mobilize the splenic flexure. The greater omentum is then further dissected off the transverse colon toward the midline. This is best performed by lifting the omentum using robotic arm 2 and countertraction provided by the assistant.

Most of the dissection of the greater omentum off the transverse colon requires only two robotic arms. There may be excessive clashing especially toward the middle of the transverse colon. If there is excessive clashing between robotic arms 2 and 3, arm 2 may be removed. Dissection using only arms 1 and 3 usually is adequate.

17.4 Pelvic Dissection

17.4.1 Port Placement (Fig. 17.3)

- Instrument arm 1: monopolar curved scissors through the RLQ port.
- Instrument arm 2: Maryland bipolar forceps through the LLQ port.
- Instrument arm 3: Cadiere forceps through the LUQ port.

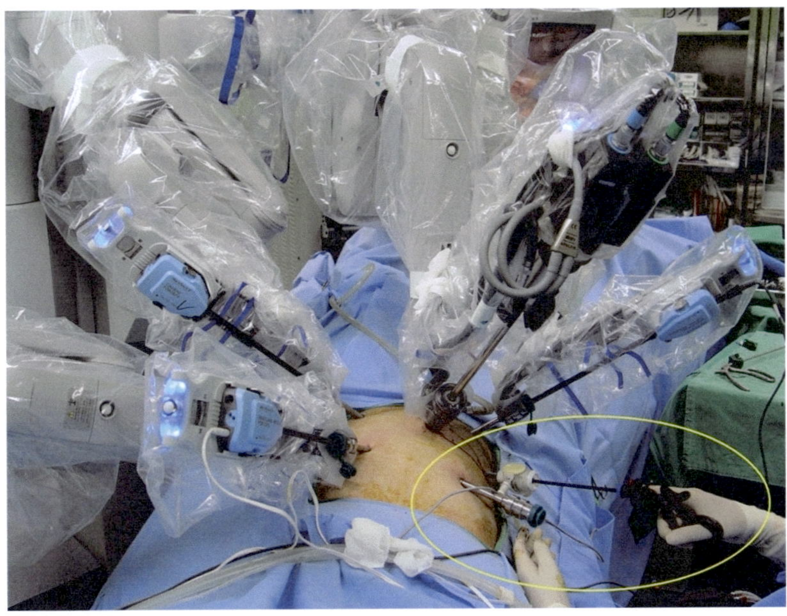

Fig. 17.10 An overview from the patient's head side after repositioning the robotic arms for the pelvic dissection. Note the two trocars available for the assistant on the right side of the patient (*yellow ellipse*). Also note the robotic arms are well fanned out to minimize external collision

- The assistant utilizes a grasper and a sucker through the RUQ and the assistant port on the right flank.

Once colonic dissection is complete, one turns its attention to the pelvis.

Robotic arms are swapped to its new position by repositioning the arms without completely undocking the patient cart (Figs. 17.3 and 17.10).

The rectum is lifted out of the pelvis by upward retracting the sigmoid colon by the assistant toward the spleen. This can be done with a grasper or by using nylon tape to wrap around the rectosigmoid junction (Fig. 17.11). This frees the surgeon to use both arms 2 and 3 for retraction, with one retracting and the other providing countertraction. The assistant has access to two instrument ports to provide retraction of the colon, retraction of the small bowel if necessary, and suction of any fluid or smoke from the diathermy. Usually, the assistant would have a grasper in the left hand and a sucker in the right hand. The assistant uses his/her left hand to retract the colon, while the right hand is used to retract the small bowel or provide countertraction.

The TME plane is identified, and with adequate traction, there should be a relatively bloodless plane. Dissection posteriorly first along the sacrum is followed by lateral dissection with division of the lateral peritoneal folds. Anterior dissection is left last as it is usually most difficult.

Arm 2 is used to retract the rectum upward toward the anterior abdominal wall. The left-hand arm (arm 3) can be used to provide further retraction or countertraction. Note that retraction can be done by either opening the instrument or using the wrist of the instrument to push the tissue away. A layer of alveolar tissue can be seen to demonstrate the avascular plane of TME when adequate retraction is achieved. It is important to keep the dissection close to the mesorectal fascia.

The hypogastric nerves are identified during posterior dissection and preserved.

The key is adequate retraction and sticking close to the TME plane on the rectal side.

During lateral dissection, robotic arm 2 is usually used to provide lateral traction on the pelvic sidewall, while the assistant uses the sucker to retract the rectum medially (Fig. 17.12).

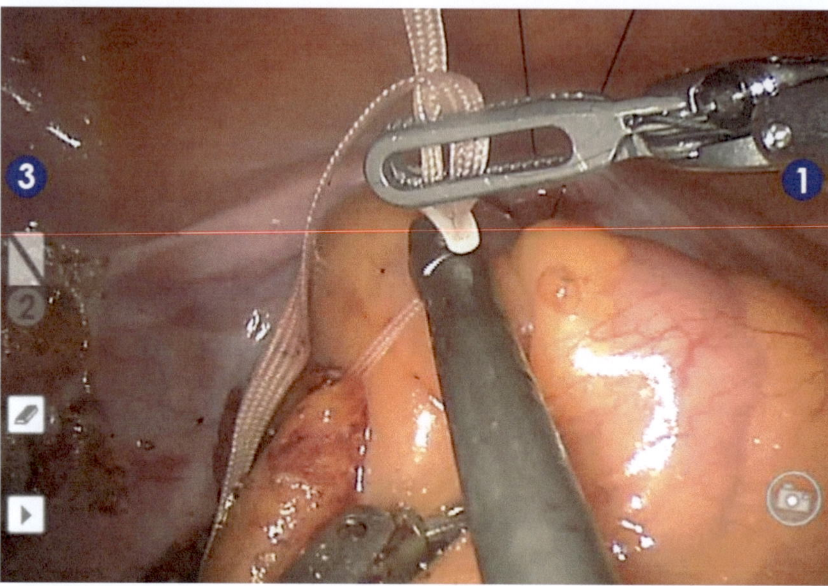

Fig. 17.11 A nylon tape around the rectosigmoid colon to assist with retraction of the rectum out of the pelvis using the RUQ port. Also note the stitch in the anterior peritoneal reflection to assist with exposure in the narrow male pelvis

Fig. 17.12 Lateral pelvic dissection demonstrating positions of each robotic arms

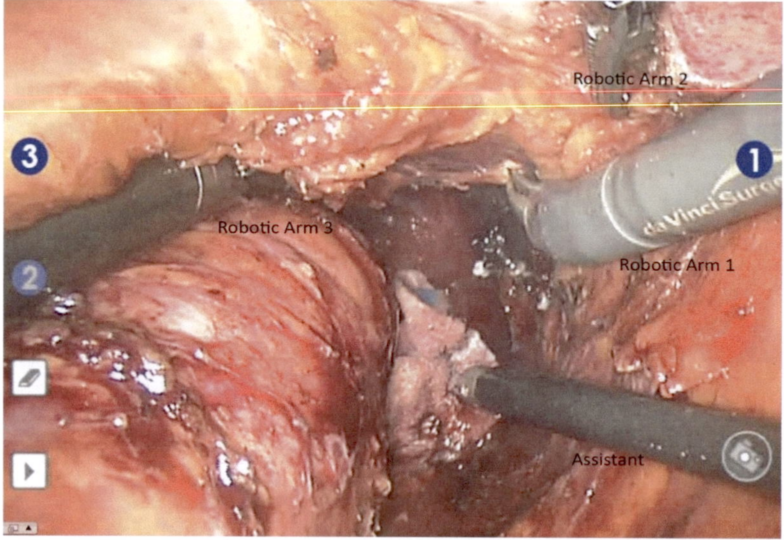

Adequate traction is vital to provide good exposure as this is the key to identifying the correct TME plane laterally.

To assist with exposure anteriorly, peritoneum overlying the bladder near the peritoneal reflection can be hitched up toward the anterior abdominal wall using a straight needle. Robotic arm 2 can assist with further retraction of the peritoneum overlying the bladder, while arm 3 pushes down on the rectum to provide countertraction.

Seminal vesicles are identified and dissection continued along the Denonvilliers' fascia. Unless

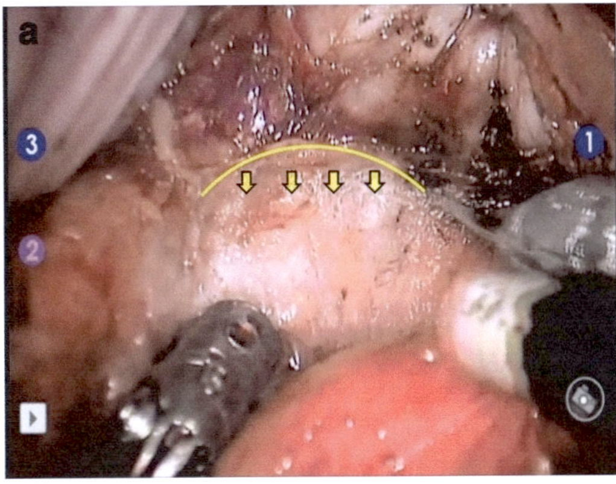

Fig. 17.13 (**a**) The dissection plane is behind the Denonvilliers' fascia (*yellow line*) to preserve the neurovascular bundle that lies immediately anterior to the fascia. (**b**) The dissection plane is anterior to the Denonvilliers' fascia (*yellow line*) to achieve a negative circumferential margin, when tumor involves the anterior rectum

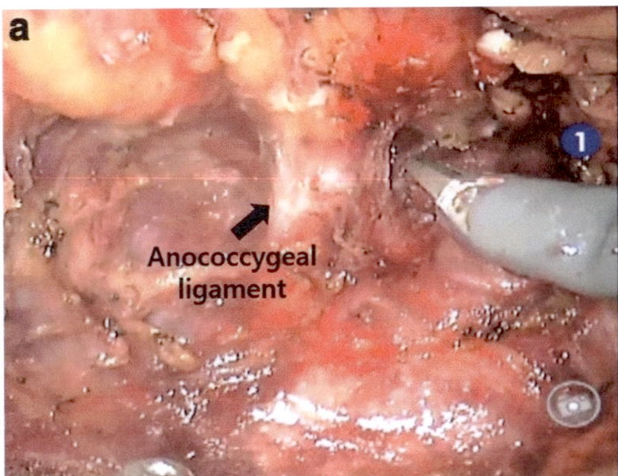

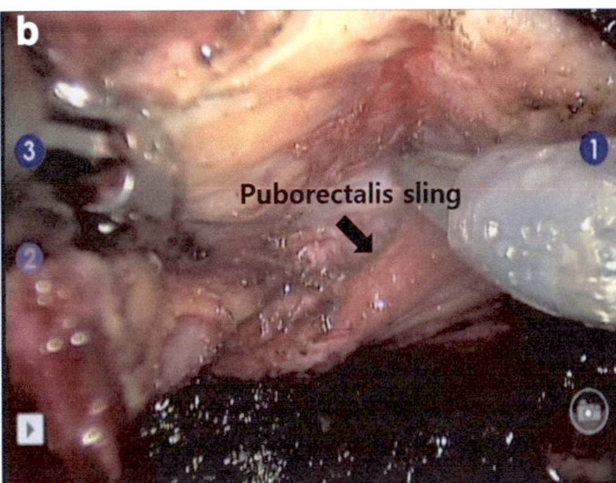

Fig. 17.14 Two principles of trocar placement. (**a**) Anococcygeal ligament should be divided for intersphincteric resection. (**b**) Puborectalis sling is identified and dissected off

the fascia needs to be resected en bloc for oncological reasons (i.e., anterior rectal cancer), dissection should leave the Denonvilliers' fascia behind to preserve the neurovascular bundle that lies immediately anterior to the fascia (Fig. 17.13a).

It is also important to note that there is usually a vessel that crosses the fascia anteriorly from the prostate toward the mesorectum. This is often the source of bleeding if not adequately controlled. When tumor involves the anterior rectum, the dissection plane should be anterior to the Denonvilliers' fascia to achieve a negative circumferential margin (Fig. 17.13b).

Instruments in arms 2 and 3 can be swapped at any time to provide better retraction. As the da Vinci eliminates any physiological tremor, dissection with the left hand can be utilized. Hot shear can be swapped to arm 3 for dissection, especially on the left side.

Dissection is continued until the identification of the pelvic floor. This can be easily identified as the muscle fibers of the pelvic floor will contract when touched with diathermy. The extent of the dissection can be confirmed on digital examination.

For intersphincteric dissection, two anatomical landmarks—the anococcygeal ligament posteriorly (Fig. 17.14a) and the puborectalis slings bilaterally—are identified (Fig. 17.14b). The anococcygeal ligament has to be divided to enter the intersphincteric plane. Dissection is continued as low as possible and then completed from below.

During pelvic dissection, it can be very easy to develop "tunnel vision" in the narrow pelvis. It is easy to become disorientated as the camera can rotate, especially early in the learning curve. It is advisable to frequently bring the camera back for an overview of the pelvis and reorientate. Another tip is to look for the camera icon in the surgeon console, located in the middle of the top part of the screen. It shows the level and orientation of the camera.

17.5 Rectum Transection for Low-Anterior Resection

Once pelvic dissection is completed, the patient cart is at this stage undocked and moved away from the patient. The rectum is resected by a conventional laparoscopic manner. The da Vinci has recently added a stapling device to its robotic arm but it is unavailable in our institute at the time of writing this chapter. The RLQ port is swapped to a 12 mm port and a laparoscopic stapler is used for resection of the distal rectum. In difficult narrow pelvis, the patient cart can be partially undocked. The camera is left in situ to provide stable view of the distal rectum. Arm 2 is left in situ to provide anterior retraction of the pelvis. Arms 1 and 3 are undocked. The RLQ port is again swapped to a 12 mm port and resection performed as above (Fig. 17.15a, b).

17.5.1 Extraction of Specimen

Wound extraction may be performed either through the left iliac fossa or the umbilical incision. Usually, the left lower quadrant port site is preferred due to lower rate of incisional hernia in the published literature. Wound protector (such as Alexis) is used and the specimen is externalized. Decision is made regarding the length of resection. Usually this is determined by the location of the IMA with the resection performed in line with the IMA. The mesenteric vessels are ligated. The marginal artery is identified and cut to check for adequate blood flow before ligation. Proximal colonic resection is then performed using a hard bowel clamp and a knife in a usual fashion.

17.5.2 Anastomosis

Standard double-stapling technique is used. A purse string is placed using nonabsorbable sutures to the proximal colon. The anvil of the circular stapling device is placed in the proximal colon and secured with the purse string. The colon is placed back into the peritoneal cavity and pneumoperitoneum is reestablished. This can be done by placing a glove over the Alexis wound protector or by twisting the wound protector and then closed with soft bowel clamp. If the umbilical wound was used for specimen extraction, the tip of a finer of the glove is cut

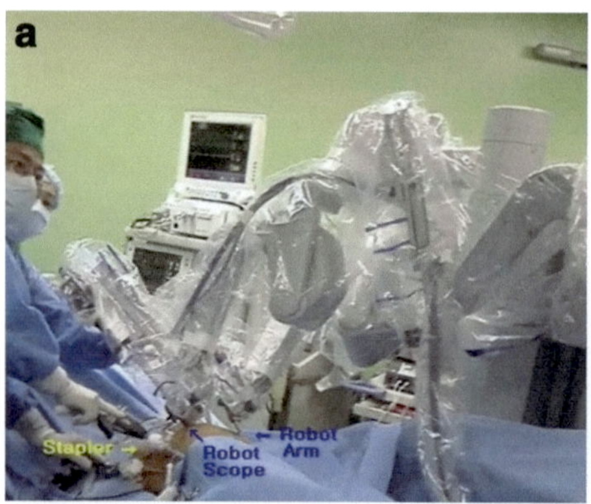

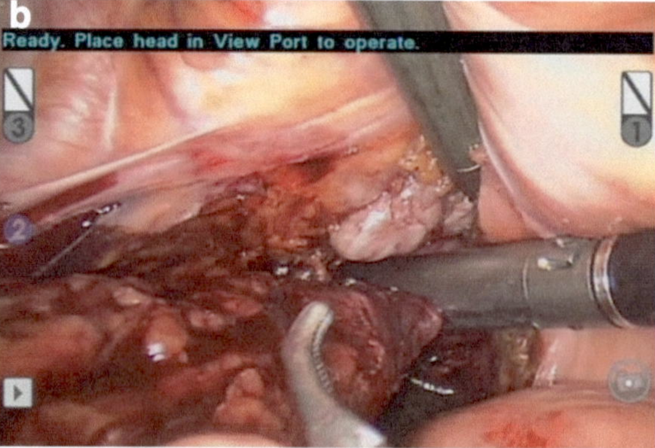

Fig. 17.15 (**a**) Outside view during the rectal transection. (**b**) Inside view during the rectal transection

and camera port placed into the finger. This is usually secured with a suture to ensure it is airtight.

The bowel is retracted from the pelvis so good view of the staple line is obtained. The stapler is introduced into the rectum via the anus by the assistant under direct vision and direction of the surgeon. Once in a good position, the stapler is opened to enable the spike of the stapler to come through the rectal stump. The anvil is placed over the spike and a click should be audible. One should also feel the anvil click into place. The spike is then retracted into the stapler closed until the green zone is reach on the indicator. Before firing, it is important to check the orientation of the colon and to ensure the mesentery is not twisted. This is done easily by making sure the tinea of the colon is facing up. It is our practice to hold that position for at least 15 s before the safety is removed and the stapler fired. The stapler is then opened slightly before being removed from the patient. Often the stapler needs to be rotated slightly clockwise and anticlockwise to disengage the bowel from the stapler before withdrawal. The donuts are then checked for completeness. A leak test is then performed. This is done by filling the pelvis with saline, compressing the proximal colon with a grasper, while the assistant blows air into the rectum with an empty syringe. Leakage of air detected by bubbles would be indicative of a positive test and suggests some compromise of the anastomosis.

17.6 Intersphincteric Resection

When performing an intersphincteric resection, a "pull-through" approach of specimen extraction and a hand-sewn coloanal anastomosis can be used. In this method, resection of the colon or rectum is not performed during robotic dissection but the left colic artery should be divided robotically to reach the specimen out through the anus. In a high lithotomy position, the anus is exposed with interrupted everting sutures (Fig. 17.16).

Once intersphincteric dissection is completed from the perineal side, the rectum and proximal colon is delivered via the anus. Proximal resection of the colon is then made after ligation of the mesenteric vessels. This is done by a linear stapling device. A side-to-end anastomosis is preferred so the staple line is secured with interrupted absorbable sutures. An enterotomy is made on the antimesenteric border of the colon 3 cm away from the distal end, and full thickness of the colon is anastomosed to the sphincter muscles and anal mucosa using 3-0 absorbable sutures.

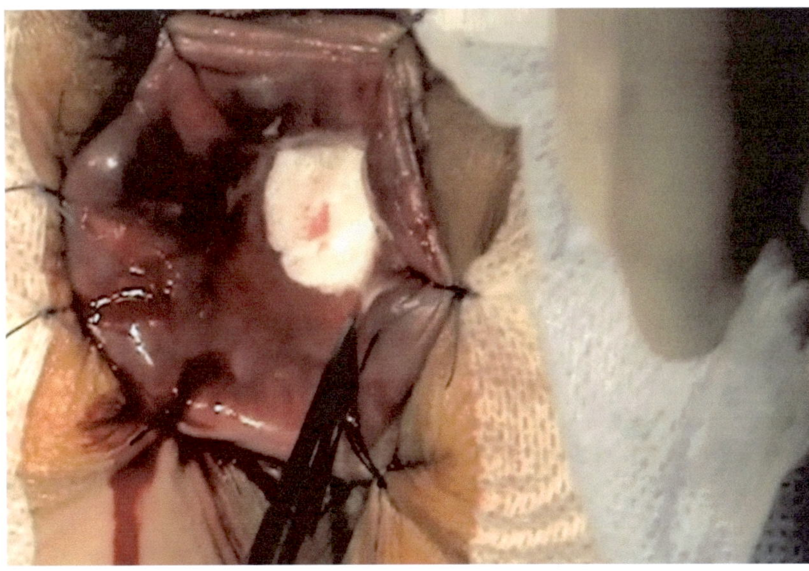

Fig. 17.16 Preparation of the anus with interrupted sutures for perineal approach

17.6.1 Covering Ileostomy

Covering ileostomy is not routinely used in anterior resection at our institution.

- Indication for covering ileostomy includes:
  - Neoadjuvant radiotherapy
  - Intersphincteric resection and hand-sewn coloanal anastomosis
  - Ultralow-anterior resection (double-stapled anastomosis within 1 cm from the dentate line)
  - Technical difficulty during the case including incomplete donuts or positive air leak test

If required, the right lower quadrant port site is used for ileostomy. Trephine is incised over the port site and dissected down to the fascia. The fascia is incised vertically and muscle blunted split transversely. The peritoneum is incised and loop of terminal ileum brought out through the trephine. Orientation of terminal ileum is confirmed on laparoscopy. Loop ileostomy is matured after the closure of all abdominal wounds and dressing applied.

17.6.2 Wound Closure

Wound is closed in a usual manner. For the specimen extraction site, we prefer layered closure using interrupted absorbable sutures. Fascia is closed over the 12 mm trocar site.

17.7 Technical Tips

- Standardize the operation; do the same operation every time.
- Good exposure leads to better visualization which equates to successful surgery.
- Maximum use of patient position prior to docking; ensure maximum head down and tilt to help move the small bowel out of operative field.
- Communication with the assistant is vital; this applies to the way retraction is performed as well as change of instruments.
- The two most common problems faced during the initial learning curve are external collision and internal exposure.
- Correct positioning of trocar is vital to minimize external collision and provide better ergonomics of the robotic arms during surgery.
- The elbows and shoulders of the robotic arms should be spread out like a fan to minimize external collision. Most of the external collision can be fixed by repositioning the elbows of the robotic arms.
- Understand the concept of remote center; adequate distance between target organ and instrument port means smaller range of motion outside the patient's body, avoiding external collision of instruments.
- Utilize the master clutch to avoid clashing of the surgeon's controls. Experienced surgeons utilize the master clutch more to ensure adequate space is maintained between the workspaces of his/her two hands.
- Undock a robotic arm if excessive clashing occurs and all other maneuvers to resolve the clashing fail.
- Poor internal exposure is mainly due to the small bowel in operative field or due to inadequate traction/countertraction.
- Don't be afraid of using sponges or gauze in the operative field to assist with retraction; it is quite a useful tool to keep the small bowel away from the operative field.
- Use the assistant effectively to improve exposure. The assistant should be either retracting the small bowel away from operative field or assist with retraction.
- Remember, robotic pelvic surgery is a "six-hand" operation: four surgeon hands (including camera arm) and two assistant hands.

17.8 Summary

In general, there are three approach methods in robotic rectal surgery including hybrid, double docking, and single docking, as we mentioned in this chapter. Since we started to apply the robotic system for rectal cancer surgery at our institution in July 2007, we have developed and tried to standardize our single-docking totally robotic surgery.

Several systemic review articles reported currently have demonstrated that the robotic surgery was a safe and feasible method in terms of clinical and short-term oncologic outcomes, even though they had some limitations with heterogeneity of collected data and mostly nonrandomized controlled trials [6–8]. We reported our 200 consecutive data about robotic surgery from patients with rectal cancer in which median distance from the anal verge was 6 cm recently. It also showed an acceptable morbidity (7.5 %), a low rate of positive circumferential resection margin (CRM) (2.5 %), and excellent survival data in stage III (5-year overall survival, 88.6 %) [9]. We still need well-constructed randomized controlled trial to prove its certain role with evidence, but in view of the results achieved so far, the robotic system may have definite advantages including better local control in mid-low rectal cancer or narrow confined pelvic space.

Another concern for robotic system application in rectal cancer surgery is whether we can get better functional outcomes such as sexual and voiding function with avoidance of autonomic nerve injury. Laparoscopic itself is not a predisposing factor to nerve injury, but Jayne et al. demonstrated that laparoscopic rectal resection did not adversely affect bladder function, but there was a trend toward worse male sexual function which may be explained by the higher rate of TME comparing to open surgery in the MRC CLASICC trial [10]. They have also found that conversion to open surgery was independent predictors of postoperative male sexual dysfunction [10]. There has not been much available data about functional outcomes in robotic rectal surgery, but several studies have reported low conversion rates of robotic surgery for rectal cancer [4, 5, 8, 11]. We can expect better functional outcomes from these results.

Although current studies have shown quite promising results with robotic rectal surgery, well-constructed studies are still required to prove its safety, efficacy, and long-term functional and oncologic benefit. In addition, we have to make effort to develop adequate training programs and solve the high-cost issues.

References

1. Heald RJ, Husband EM, Ryall RD. The mesorectum in rectal cancer surgery–the clue to pelvic recurrence? Br J Surg. 1982;69(10):613–6.
2. Arezzo A, Passera R, Salvai A, Arolfo S, Allaix ME, Schwarzer G, et al. Laparoscopy for rectal cancer is oncologically adequate: a systematic review and meta-analysis of the literature. Surg Endosc. 2014;29(2):334.
3. Choi DJ, Kim SH, Lee PJ, Kim J, Woo SU. Single-stage totally robotic dissection for rectal cancer surgery: technique and short-term outcome in 50 consecutive patients. Dis Colon Rectum. 2009;52(11):1824–30.
4. Kwak JM, Kim SH, Kim J, Son DN, Baek SJ, Cho JS. Robotic vs laparoscopic resection of rectal cancer: short-term outcomes of a case-control study. Dis Colon Rectum. 2011;54(2):151–6.
5. Patriti A, Ceccarelli G, Bartoli A, Spaziani A, Biancafarina A, Casciola L. Short- and medium-term outcome of robot-assisted and traditional laparoscopic rectal resection. JSLS. 2009;13(2):176–83.
6. Mak TW, Lee JF, Futaba K, Hon SS, Ngo DK, Ng SS. Robotic surgery for rectal cancer: a systematic review of current practice. World J Gastrointest Oncol. 2014;6(6):184–93.
7. Scarpinata R, Aly EH. Does robotic rectal cancer surgery offer improved early postoperative outcomes? Dis Colon Rectum. 2013;56(2):253–62.
8. Xiong B, Ma L, Zhang C, Cheng Y. Robotic versus laparoscopic total mesorectal excision for rectal cancer: a meta-analysis. J Surg Res. 2014;188(2):404–14.
9. Hara M, Sng K, Yoo BE, Shin JW, Lee DW, Kim SH. Robotic-assisted surgery for rectal adenocarcinoma: short-term and midterm outcomes from 200 consecutive cases at a single institution. Dis Colon Rectum. 2014;57(5):570–7.
10. Jayne DG, Brown JM, Thorpe H, Walker J, Quirke P, Guillou PJ. Bladder and sexual function following resection for rectal cancer in a randomized clinical trial of laparoscopic versus open technique. Br J Surg. 2005;92(9):1124–32.
11. Baik SH, Kwon HY, Kim JS, Hur H, Sohn SK, Cho CH, et al. Robotic versus laparoscopic low anterior resection of rectal cancer: short-term outcome of a prospective comparative study. Ann Surg Oncol. 2009;16(6):1480–7.

Part IV

Challenges and Training

Complications Unique to Robotic Surgery

Robert K. Cleary

Abstract

The robotic platform offers the colon and rectal surgeon an opportunity to perform colorectal procedures with better vision, with instruments that articulate and are more precise, and in a comfortable sitting position. These advantages overcome some of the technical disadvantages of laparoscopy and may ultimately allow more patients the opportunity for minimally invasive surgery, especially those requiring total mesorectal excision for low- and mid-rectal cancers. There are nuances with this unique platform that colorectal surgeons and other robotic operating room personnel should be familiar with to ensure thorough preparation, allow proactive intervention, and thereby maximize patient safety and best outcomes. This chapter identifies and recommends management options for some of the nuances and unique complications related to robotic colon and rectal surgery.

Keywords

Laparoscopic • Laparoscopy • Robot • Robotic surgery • Colorectal • Colon and rectal

18.1 Introduction

The spectrum of perioperative robotic complications is generally the same as those encountered for open and laparoscopic procedures.

Like laparoscopy, robotic surgery is characterized by small abdominal wall incisions for port access, carbon dioxide (CO_2) insufflation for pneumoperitoneum, resection of a segment or all of the colon and rectum, and extraction of the specimen. Though comparisons show that robotic and laparoscopic complication rates are similar, the literature is not consistent in this regard. Halabi et al. showed in a retrospective review of the 2009–2010 National Inpatient Sample database that morbidity, anastomotic leaks, and ileus were similar when comparing robotic and

R.K. Cleary, M.D. (✉)
Department of Surgery, St Joseph Mercy Hospital
Ann Arbor, Division of Colon & Rectal Surgery,
5325 Elliott Dr, MHVI #104, Ann Arbor,
MI 48106, USA
e-mail: Robert.Cleary@stjoeshealth.org

© Springer International Publishing Switzerland 2015
H. Ross et al. (eds.), *Robotic Approaches to Colorectal Surgery*,
DOI 10.1007/978-3-319-09120-4_18

laparoscopic colorectal procedures [1]. In contrast, analysis of the 2008–2009 National Inpatient Sample database revealed lower complication rates and mortality for robotic colorectal surgery when compared to laparoscopic and open colorectal surgery [2]. Analysis of this same 2008–2009 database by other authors demonstrated that postoperative infections, fistulas, and thromboembolic complications were more common, while anastomotic leaks, ileus, and pneumonia were less common with robotic colorectal surgery when compared to laparoscopic colorectal surgery [3].

Only 45 % of elective colon surgery and 10 % of elective rectal surgery is done by the laparoscopic approach [1]. The learning curve for laparoscopic surgery has been estimated to be 50–70 cases, while the learning curve for robotic surgery has been estimated to be 20–32 cases, even for those who lack laparoscopic experience. Articulating instruments that allow more precise movements at more advantageous angles, without the need for an experienced assistant to provide a stable image and steady retraction, contribute to this shorter robotic learning curve [4–7].

Many of the available studies evaluating learning curves use operative time and conversion rates as the measured parameters. These data points may not be the best learning curve measures because with experience, surgeons may schedule more complicated cases that do not result in decreased operative times and conversions. A study comparing a novice robotic surgeon with little laparoscopic experience (<30 cases) and a novice robotic surgeon with significant laparoscopic experience (>300 cases) showed that robotic perioperative and oncologic outcomes were not different based on laparoscopic experience, suggesting that surgeons practicing open surgery may transition to the robot without first demonstrating laparoscopic proficiency [7]. Another study demonstrated that higher robotic surgeon volumes were associated with fewer complications, shorter

hospital length of stay, and lower costs [8]. A systematic review of the laparoscopic and robotic learning curves revealed that studies to date portray a multifaceted and ill-defined learning curve. The authors of this review concluded that a multidimensional assessment of surgical skills that may predict satisfactory outcomes, such as the cumulative sum analysis methodology (CUSUM), should be used in future studies to evaluate learning curves in the clinical setting [9, 10].

Current robotic systems are characterized by the master-slave platform with the surgeon sitting at a console. The disadvantage of this system is the loss of haptic feedback and the inability of the surgeon to sit at the patient operating table. The surgeon must rely on visual cues to limit the risk of visceral traction and crush injuries [4]. It is important to keep all instruments within the visual field thereby limiting the risk of injury to bowel, blood vessels, and other structures [11, 12]. These injuries may be particularly prone to occur early in the learning curve if instruments are allowed to stray outside the field of vision [5]. A stray instrument must be looked for with the camera rather than trying to bring the stray instrument into the field of view. When all instruments are within the visual field, this loss of haptic feedback is offset to a certain extent by the robotic high-definition view of pressure applied during dissection.

Visual compensation for this loss of haptic feedback during robotic surgery has been studied using visual cues and is based on research involving sensory integration. Authors have suggested that the sense of vision can affect the sense of touch and compensate for the lack of tactile information [13]. Techniques for simulating haptic sensations such as friction, stiffness, and texture on virtual objects are based on human perceptions, have been tested, and are referred to as pseudo-haptic feedback [14]. The visual cues obtained as robotic instruments touch intra-abdominal structures have been referred to as surgical synesthesia [5, 13, 14].

18.2   Trocar Injuries and Hernias

Trocar injuries can occur with laparoscopic and robotic surgery, and trocar placement is similar with both platforms. In a study comparing direct trocar, Veress needle, and open approaches, there were fewer trocar injuries to bowel and blood vessels using the open approach (open 0 %, direct trocar 2.9 %, Veress 0.6 %) [15]. Placement of the first trocar is most likely to cause organ injury as the remaining trocars are placed under laparoscopic vision. Much of the trocar injury literature is from the gynecologic and urologic laparoscopic arena [16, 17]. In a review of 40 litigated cases of laparoscopic bowel injury, it was found that the initial trocar was the most common cause of bowel injury. The Hasson open technique did not eliminate this complication. Delayed recognition of the injury was the major consideration with regard to liability [16].

Some modify trocar placement in obese individuals. Schwartz recommended initial placement of the Veress needle in the left upper quadrant in morbidly obese patients to decrease the risk for trocar injury to viscera [18]. Others have recommended optical-tip trocars [19]. An approach to trocar placement that eliminates the risk of enterotomy and other visceral injuries has not yet evolved.

Trocars sites are at risk for herniation. The incidence varies from 0.65 to 5.4 % and reports on the clinical impact of this complication vary throughout the literature [19, 20]. The incidence of trocar-site hernias may be underestimated because many are asymptomatic hernias and may remain undetected. Reported risk factors for trocar-site hernia include chronic obstructive pulmonary disease, smoking, obesity, large trocar size, midline trocar sites, incomplete fascial closure, lengthy operations, and bladed trocars. However, none of these risk factors have been conclusively demonstrated to cause trocar-site hernias on multivariate analysis. Eighty-six percent of hernias occur at trocar sites ≥10 mm, while only 2.7 % occur at sites ≤8 mm. Patients presenting with symptomatic trocar-site hernias may have incarcerated or strangulated small bowel and operative repair may require small bowel resection with the attendant risks [19].

In a review of 624 obese patients who underwent laparoscopic bariatric surgery without closure of any trocar-site fascia, 1.6 % developed trocar-site hernias at a mean of 15 months. None had intestinal obstruction or other complications related to the hernias [20]. A retrospective review of 647 laparoscopic colorectal procedures over 3 years revealed that 1.23 % of patients developed trocar-site hernias, all of which were symptomatic and all of which required operative repair. These authors recommended primary closure of trocar-site defects ≥10 mm [19]. A Medline search of 11,699 laparoscopic procedures that included 477 colorectal operations demonstrated that 1.47 % developed trocar-site hernias at a mean follow-up of 71.5 months. These authors also recommended primary closure of fascial defects ≥10 mm [21].

Others have reported higher rates of trocar-site hernias when following patients with imaging studies. In a study of 102 laparoscopic and 48 robotic Roux-en-Y gastric bypasses for morbid obesity, 39.3 % of laparoscopic and 47.9 % of robotic procedures developed trocar-site hernias, most of which were identified by ultrasonic rather than by physical examination or clinical presentation. Only two patients with hernias required operative intervention, both in the laparoscopic group [22]. In a review of 498 robotic prostatectomies, two port-site hernias were identified, both of which were located at the 12 mm supraumbilical trocar site. In this study, routine port placement included two 12 mm, three 8 mm, and one 5 mm port. Only the midline 12 mm supraumbilical trocar-site fascia was closed.

The risk for incisional hernias in midline wounds, especially at the umbilicus, is reported to be up to 10–15 %. These midline-wound hernia rates are higher than other locations such as the Pfannenstiel incision and other wounds off the midline, where the risk is less than 5 %. As a result of these data, some authors do not close 12 mm trocar-site fascial defects off the midline [23, 24]. There are conflicting reports, though, with respect to hernia size and location as reflected by case reports of hernias at 8 mm robotic trocar sites [25]. Though the literature varies with regard to conclusions about the incidence and prevention of trocar-site hernias, most surgeons close trocar-site fascial incisions greater than 8 mm at every location. And it is important to keep in mind that hernias may occur even after trocar-site fascial closure [23].

18.3 Intraoperative Enterotomy

Injuries to the intestinal tract during robotic surgery not caused by trocar placement are uncommon. Existing series are largely in the urologic and gynecologic literature [26]. The incidence of rectal injuries during prostatectomy is 0.17 % and compares favorably with open and laparoscopic prostatectomy [27]. Colon and rectal surgeons should be familiar with this complication as they may be consulted for repair. If recognized intraoperatively, simple suture closure of small bowel and colon injuries is usually safe and effective. In patients with ulcerative colitis undergoing robotic proctectomy, an unintentional proctotomy in a diseased rectum deep in the pelvis may be best visualized and suture repaired with the robot, rather than converting to a laparoscopic or an open procedure.

18.4 Converting to an Open Procedure

Conversions to open surgery occur less frequently after robotic than after laparoscopic colorectal resection [1, 28–35]. The COLOR II randomized controlled trial comparing laparoscopic and open surgery for rectal cancer was composed of surgeons with considerable laparoscopic expertise. Even so, the conversion rate for laparoscopy was 17 % in this study [36]. In a large national database analysis, the robot was associated with a 59 % reduction in conversion in the abdomen and 90 % reduction in conversion in the pelvis, when compared to laparoscopy [1]. In a study comparing robotic and laparoscopic rectal resection for cancer, Patriti

reported a 19 % conversion rate for laparoscopy compared to no conversions with the robot. This difference was remarkable in that the robot group was composed of a majority of patients with previous abdominal surgery and low rectal neoplasms requiring preoperative chemoradiation and total mesorectal excision [28].

A meta-analysis of four randomized controlled trials comparing robotic and laparoscopic colorectal surgery demonstrated that conversion for robotic colorectal procedures was 1.8 % compared to 9.5 % for laparoscopic colorectal operations [33]. In an analysis of a large regional protocol-driven externally audited database characterized by definitions for data entry, Tam et. al. found that conversion in the pelvis for robotic procedures was 7.8 % versus 21.2 % for laparoscopy (p<0.001), and 9.0 % for the robot in the abdomen compared to 16.9 % for laparoscopy (p=0.06) [34]. Conversions early in an operation, done to avoid complications, are associated with fewer complications than conversions done in response to intraoperative bleeding or enterotomies [37, 38].

There are rare occasions when conversion is required because of urgent intraoperative complications related to bleeding or enterotomies. Bleeding may occur when dissecting the inferior mesenteric artery during the course of a sigmoid resection or low-anterior resection. This is the time when the art of surgery demands poise and thoughtfulness, deciding between calm and control of bleeding with instruments, versus urgent de-docking and laparotomy. Often the bleeding vessel can be clamped with a fenestrated bipolar grasper or Maryland forceps and a locking clip or vessel sealer applied. If blood loss has not been significant and hemostasis has been obtained, then the procedure may proceed as planned. If bleeding has been temporarily controlled, but definitive hemostasis with clips or energy has not been obtained, a laparoscopic instrument through the assistant port may substitute for the robotic instrument, allowing de-docking and laparotomy in a controlled fashion with hemostasis. Alternatively, the robotic instrument may be left clamped on the vessel, while the other robotic instruments are removed and the respective robotic arms detached from the trocars. Though the robot arm providing hemostasis remains at the operating table in this case, these maneuvers typically leave enough room for laparotomy and open control of the bleeding. A hex wrench attached to the robot is used to release the instrument from the vessel at the appropriate time (D.C. Coffey, M.D., personal communication).

It is critically important that the bleeding vessel is dissected out and visualized well enough to ensure no other structures, like the ureter, are injured while gaining hemostasis. It is also important not to dissect structures not easily visualized because of bleeding, and this may be the critical factor that convinces the operating surgeon to convert to open. Though it is important not to persist to the point of significant blood loss, often blood loss appears more than it is because of the magnified image. If there is any doubt, however, de-docking the robot and laparotomy to control hemorrhage is the prudent choice. It is important to have open instruments readily available for any minimally invasive procedure to address urgent complications like bleeding.

Another important bleeding scenario is presacral hemorrhage during a robotic total mesorectal excision for rectal neoplasia. Though bleeding can sometimes be controlled with energy sources, it is best at times not to persist in this effort and instead place a small sponge and/or hemostatic agent on the bleeding vessel. A robotic instrument or suction device allows pressure to be maintained. It may be worth waiting 5–10 min once the bleeding is controlled before releasing pressure and then assessing for persistent bleeding. If the bleeding vessel, usually a torn vein, is controlled with the sponge, it is sometimes possible to continue with other parts of the procedure and reassess later. Often the bleeding will resolve spontaneously with patience. If the bleeding is not well controlled or persists despite the above maneuvers, conversion may be the prudent option.

Converting to an open procedure requires removing the robotic instruments under direct vision, detaching the robotic arms from the trocars, removing the robot from the patient bedside, providing open instruments, and proceeding with laparotomy. This can be a time-consuming process and if the conversion is for bleeding can

lead to considerable blood loss and hemodynamic compromise. Though it may not be practical for every institution to do so, procuring a circulating nurse, scrub nurse or technician, and anesthesia nursing team dedicated to robotics and familiar with preparation, malfunctions, and operative approaches may decrease the risk for morbidity during these urgent and emergent scenarios. A reflective role-playing exercise to include all relevant operating room caregivers and to simulate the emergent need to convert may help prevent morbidity in this situation [5].

18.5 Inadequate Pneumoperitoneum

Inadequate distention of the abdomen with carbon dioxide (CO_2) gas results in a poorly visualized operative field and can result in organ injury. Several possible explanations for inadequate pneumoperitoneum should be considered including an open port allowing the loss of CO_2 gas, a disconnected gas line, a port that has retracted into the subcutaneous tissue or out of the abdominal wall altogether, an empty gas tank, and rarely, inadequate muscle relaxation. The operation should be temporarily paused when visualization is obscured and inadequate pneumoperitoneum should be considered as the cause. A stepwise progression of consideration of the above etiologies should be performed with expectation that the cause for inadequate pneumoperitoneum will be identified and the operation then safely resumed [5]. In the obese patient, a second gas insufflator utilizing a robotic gas port may resolve the problem. Rarely, a procedure may need to be converted to open because of inadequate visualization of the operative field.

18.6 Inability to Deliver Small Bowel from the Pelvis

Early in the course of high- and low-anterior resections, and after thorough exploration of the abdomen, it is important to displace the small bowel to the right upper quadrant, allowing visualization of relevant anatomy and allowing the planned operative techniques to proceed. This is usually accomplished by strategic use of the Trendelenburg position and left-to-right rotation of the operating table. Natural fusion planes between the terminal ileum, terminal ileal mesentery, pelvic structures, and pelvic sidewalls, as well as adhesions from previous pelvic surgery or appendectomy, may make this maneuver difficult. Inadequate muscle relaxation may also make this challenging. If the Trendelenburg position and anesthetic muscle relaxation does not keep the small bowel in the right upper quadrant, taking time to divide offending adhesions using laparoscopic techniques will often be the remedy. Alternatively, these adhesions can be divided after docking the robot and using robotic techniques. However, the operating surgeon should be confident that the assistant will be able to deliver the small bowel out of the pelvis without the attached robotic arms impeding progress. Pausing to detach a robotic arm to assist in this maneuver is also an option.

A fatty omentum may make it difficult to retract the small bowel from the pelvis to the right upper quadrant during high- and low-anterior resections, thereby obscuring relevant anatomy. Displacing the omentum cephalad to the transverse colon is ideal but often not possible. Dividing omental attachments to the lateral sidewall and descending colon, the strategic use of the Trendelenburg position, and the strategic use of the bedside assistant with a laparoscopic instrument through the assistant trocar, may allow more effective omental displacement (D.C. Coffey, MD, personal communication).

18.7 Difficulty Delivering/ Retracting an Obese or Noncompliant Rectum

Total mesorectal excision is the critical part of the oncologic operative technique for low- and mid-rectal cancers, the quality of which affects circumferential margins and local recurrence. It is important to dissect in a plane between the fascia propria of the rectum and presacral fascia to ensure complete en bloc removal of the entire lymph node-containing mesorectum to affirm the best oncologic outcomes. This can be quite a challenge in an individual with an obese or non-compliant irradiated rectum.

Operative visualization is optimized by third-arm fixed retraction with a robotic grasper. It is also commonly necessary for the bedside assistant to provide cephalad and lateral retraction through an assistant port. This maneuver can be made more effective by routing an umbilical tape or similar structure around the rectosigmoid junction, which can be grasped by the assistant and retracted cephalad. The assistant port is typically in the right upper quadrant and is 5 or 12 mm depending on which port is used for the stapling device. For technically challenging pelvic operations, a skilled assistant using two assistant ports can help significantly and sometimes preclude the need for conversion. If the surgeon employs a technique that includes rotation of a robotic arm from the subcostal 8 mm trocar to a left lower quadrant 8 mm trocar for the pelvic dissection, this maneuver then leaves the subcostal 8 mm trocar as a second assistant port. If a second 8 mm trocar is not available for the assistant, simply adding an addition 5 mm trocar for this purpose is a reasonable option.

18.8 Trendelenburg Complications

The steep Trendelenburg position and CO_2 pneumoperitoneum for prolonged periods of time can result in alterations in cerebrovascular, respiratory, and hemodynamic parameters. Some of the associated potential complications include subcutaneous emphysema, facial and laryngeal edema, venous gas embolism, brachial plexus injuries, peripheral neuropathy, and ocular disturbances [39, 40].

18.8.1 Elevated CO_2

Carbon dioxide (CO_2) insufflation provides pneumoperitoneum, allowing visualization of the abdominal cavity structures necessary for minimally invasive abdominal surgery. The pressure exerted by CO_2 pneumoperitoneum elevates the diaphragm and can decrease functional residual volume, tidal volume, and pulmonary compliance. The steep Trendelenburg position required during sigmoid resection and low-anterior resection, along with obesity and preexisting cardiopulmonary comorbidities—especially chronic obstructive pulmonary disease—accentuates these pulmonary-function abnormalities. CO_2 is rapidly absorbed into the bloodstream across peritoneal surfaces and is ultimately exhaled by the lungs. Hypercarbia may have deleterious effects on cardiac and pulmonary function. The compensatory mechanisms that allow the patient to hyperventilate and exhale CO_2 are not present during general anesthesia and hypercarbia may therefore persist without appropriate intervention.

Hypercarbia from CO_2 insufflation may result in acidosis. The anesthesia care team should be prepared to increase the respiratory rate and/or tidal volume based on end-tidal CO_2 levels and correlate with arterial blood gases when indicated, with the understanding that end-tidal CO_2 levels may be lower than arterial CO_2 levels. Preoperative arterial blood gases and pulmonary-function tests may be necessary in those with pulmonary dysfunction for comparison with intraoperative values. Intraoperative communication between the anesthesiologist and surgeon is essential. If increasing minute ventilation does not suffice, decreasing CO_2 insufflation pressures to 10–12 mmHg may decrease pulmonary dysfunction. Pausing during the procedure to detach instruments and trocars, release the pneumoperitoneum, and place the patient in the reverse Trendelenburg position for 5–15 min may allow the end-tidal CO_2 to recover and permit the procedure to proceed. If these interventions do not ameliorate the elevated CO_2, conversion to open may be necessary [41].

18.8.2 Subcutaneous Emphysema

Subcutaneous emphysema is a complication of CO_2 insufflation and may be more common in older patients who have prolonged operations greater than 200 min and in those with end-tidal CO_2 ≥ 50 mmHg. This complication of laparoscopic and robotic surgery is usually not life threatening and typically resolves with the conclusion of CO_2 insufflation. Subcutaneous emphysema can prolong hypercarbia and so mechanical ventilation should continue until hypercarbia resolves, to decrease the work of spontaneous breathing in the recovery room. Rarely, subcutaneous emphysema may lead to pneumothorax, pneumomediastinum, and pneumopericardium [39].

18.8.3 Venous Gas Embolism

This complication should be suspected with any unexplained deterioration in hemodynamic status. There is typically an abrupt change in the end-tidal CO_2 tracing. If gas embolism is recognized as a possibility, the patient should be placed in the left lateral decubitus and head-down position. This position ameliorates air obstruction to right ventricular blood flow by placing the right ventricular outflow tract inferior to the right ventricular cavity, allowing the air to migrate superiorly out of the way of the outflow tract. There are case reports of venous gas embolism in the robotic prostatectomy literature. It is likely rare in the setting of robotic colorectal surgery, but surgeons should be aware of this complication because it is life threatening [39, 42].

18.8.4 Ischemic Optic Neuropathy

Another serious complication to consider is optic neuropathy from increased intraocular pressures and ischemia to the optic nerve. This complication can result in blindness. A systematic review of 142 patients revealed that visual loss from ischemic neuropathy has been reported after lengthy robotic operations and is typically bilateral. Three cases of visual loss after laparoscopic colorectal operations in prolonged steep Trendelenburg position have been described. All of these cases were colorectal procedures that lasted longer than 6 h [43]. The most likely etiologic factor is a combination of hypotension, increased central venous pressure, increased systemic vascular resistance, and resultant increased ocular pressure from the steep Trendelenburg position. Along with intra-abdominal carbon dioxide insufflation, this may cause decreased ocular perfusion pressure and decreased oxygen delivery to the optic nerve. Those with glaucoma may be at increased risk [40].

In addition to ischemic ocular neuropathy, these changes may lead to conjunctival edema thereby preventing effective eyelid closure and resulting in corneal exposure and traumatic abrasions, the incidence of which is thought to be 0.3–13.5 % of robotic prostate operations [39, 40]. Some authors recommend preoperative ophthalmologic assessment, intraoperative fluid restriction, and periodic breaks from the steep Trendelenburg position as preventative measures [43, 44]. The increased use of robotic procedures in the steep Trendelenburg position with carbon dioxide pneumoperitoneum may increase the incidence of ocular complications, and therefore, robotic colorectal surgeons should be aware of this possibility.

18.8.5 Peripheral Neuropathy

Patients undergoing prolonged abdominopelvic operative procedures are at risk for lower extremity neuropathy, the incidence of which ranges from 0.3 to 3.0 %. Prolonged pelvic operations in steep Trendelenburg tilt may cause lower extremity compartment syndrome and upper extremity neuropathies. These injuries may take several months to resolve or be permanent, may leave residual impairment, may require intensive physical therapy, and may significantly impair quality of life. The lithotomy position, the Pfannenstiel incision, minimally invasive surgery, prolonged operative times, and obesity may be risk factors for neuropathy. Velchura et al., in a retrospective review of a prospective database, revealed that the only independent risk factor for peripheral neuropathy in those undergoing minimally invasive surgery was obesity. This complication occurred in 3.6 % of patients undergoing robotic rectal dissection in this series, perhaps because this group had longer operative times than the laparoscopic and open groups. Most patients recover from neuropathy in the immediate postoperative period, though one patient in this series had persistent symptoms for 1 year [45].

Measures to prevent peripheral neuropathy include padding extremities, periodically changing the patient position to neutral, and avoiding steep prolonged operating table tilts.

18.9 Robot Malfunction

Because robotic systems are more complex than laparoscopic instrument counterparts, they may be more susceptible to malfunction during the course of an operation [46, 47]. These system failures may be related to the robotic instruments, robotic arms, optical system, power errors, and robotic console. Buchs et al. prospectively reviewed 526 abdominal robotic procedures and found the incidence of system failures to be 3.4 %, with a cited range in the literature of 0.4–4.5 %. Half of the failures were related to instruments, all of which were related to the harmonic scalpel tip. There was one conversion to laparoscopic due to light-source failure. The system shut down in one case and was successfully resolved by turning the system off and rebooting and without consequence to the operation. Excluding the instrument failures, the malfunction rate was 1.7 %. There was no morbidity or mortality related to system failure. The conversion rate because of system failure was 0.2 %. There were more malfunctions before the year 2011 (4.2 %) than after 2011 (2.4 %). The authors concluded that robotic malfunction rates are low and are decreasing in incidence with the evolution of advanced systems [46].

The robotic operating team should be familiar with maneuvers utilized to respond to robotic system issues. These maneuvers include pushing the stop button if the system fails to obey a command or releasing the robotic instruments from the arms. Thorough stepwise inspection and testing of the system should be performed prior to each operation, analogous to a pilot checking cockpit instruments.

When the robotic arms collide outside of the patient, the instruments may lose degrees of freedom.

This is typically resolved by having the bedside assistant remove and reinsert the instrument, thereby reseating the instrument. If this issue persists after reseating the instrument, it may be defective and should be replaced. If the operating surgeon has the impression of not being in control of the camera and instruments, it is likely because the camera control button is activated. The blinking light on the instrument indicates this. Pressing this button will inactivate the clutch and return control of the camera and instruments to the operating surgeon. The inability to control a particular instrument usually means the clutch button on that particular instrument is activated and blinking. Pressing the button to deactivate the clutch will return control of that particular instrument to the operating surgeon.

If an instrument grasping tissue needs to be removed and the console surgeon is unable to release the instrument grasp of the tissue, a hex wrench is available to manually open the jaws of the instrument. This is done by inserting the wrench into the appropriate receptacle on the instrument that accommodates the wrench, located in the relevant instrument at the patient bedside.

System issues that are not immediately or readily apparent are often resolved by restarting the system. The manufacturer provides troubleshooting flowcharts that assist with vision and connection issues.

It is likely that the incidence of system malfunction will continue to decrease with the continued advancement of robotic surgical systems and with more experienced operating room personnel devoted to preparation, setup, and proper instrument handling. Literature to date suggests that the incidence of robotic malfunction is low, that the incidence has decreased with each succeeding generation of robot technology, and that occurrences can typically be handled safely [46, 47].

18.10 Conclusion

There is a need for a minimally invasive approach that provides good outcomes with a shorter learning curve and that is more ergonomically appealing to the operating surgeon. The penetration of robotics into colon and rectal surgery is rising rapidly. The continued development of advanced optic systems, precision instruments, and ergonomic platforms has several advantages for the patient and allows the surgeon to operate in a comfortable position. As robotics are more widely adopted into the practice of colon and rectal surgery, it is important that surgeons are familiar with potential complications unique to this platform to ensure the advancement of quality and patient safety.

18.11 Key Points

- Robotic complications that are similar to laparoscopic complications include those that are a result of minimally invasive trocar placement and the establishment of pneumoperitoneum.
- The robotic system is more complex than laparoscopy and there are complications and nuances unique to this complex system.
- Familiarity with these unique robotic nuances and complications will proactively contribute to patient safety and good outcomes.

References

1. Halabi WJ, Kang CY, Jafari MD, Nguyen VQ, Carmichael JC, Mills S, Stamos MJ, Pigazzi A. Robotic-assisted colorectal surgery in the United States: a nationwide analysis of trends and outcomes. World J Surg. 2013;37:2782–90.
2. Salman M, Bell T, Martin J, Bhuva K, Grim R, Ahuja V. Use, cost, complications, and mortality of robotic versus nonrobotic general surgery procedures based on a nationwide database. Am Surg. 2013;79: 553–60.
3. Tyler JA, Fox JP, Desai MM, Perry WB, Glasgow SC. Outcomes and costs associated with robotic colectomy in the minimally invasive era. Dis Colon Rectum. 2013;56:458–66.
4. Peterson CY, Weiser MR. Robotic colorectal surgery. J Gastrointest Surg. 2014;18:398–403.
5. Ramamoorthy S, Obias V. Unique complications of robotic colorectal surgery. Surg Clin North Am. 2013;93:273–86.

6. Kim YW, Lee HM, Kim NK, Min BS, Lee KY. The learning curve for robot-assisted total mesorectal excision for rectal cancer. Surg Laparosc Endosc Percutan Tech. 2012;22:400–5.

7. Kim I, Kang J, Park YA, Kim NK, Sohn SK, Lee KY. Is prior laparoscopy experience required for adaptation to robotic rectal surgery?: feasibility of one-step transition from open to robotic surgery. Int J Colorectal Dis. 2014;29:693–9.

8. Keller DS, Hashemi L, Lu M, Delaney CP. Short-term outcomes for robotic colorectal surgery by provider volume. J Am Coll Surg. 2013;217:1063–9.e1.

9. Melich G, Hong YK, Kim J, Hur H, Baik SH, Kim NK, Liberman AS, Min BS. Simultaneous development of laparoscopy and robotics provides acceptable perioperative outcomes and shows robotics to have a faster learning curve and to be overall faster in rectal cancer surgery: analysis of novice MIS surgeon learning curves. Surg Endosc. 2015;29:558–68.

10. Barrie J, Jayne DG, Wright J, Czoski-Murray CJ, Collinson FJ, Pavitt SH. Attaining surgical competency and its implications in surgical clinical trial design: a systematic review of the learning curve in laparoscopic and robot-assisted laparoscopic colorectal cancer surgery. Ann Surg Oncol. 2014;21:829–40.

11. Cundy TP, Gattas NE, Yang GZ, Darzi A, Najmaldin AS. Experience related factors compensate for haptic loss in robot-assisted laparoscopic surgery. J Endourol. 2014;28(5):532–8.

12. Simorov A, Otte RS, Kopietz CM, Olevnikov D. Review of surgical robotics user interface: what is the best way to control robotic surgery? Surg Endosc. 2012;26(8):2117–25.

13. Tewari AK, Patel ND, Leung RA, Yadav R, Vaughan ED, El-Douaihy Y, Tu JJ, Amin MB, Akhtar M, Burns M, Kreaden U, Rubin MA, Takenaka A, Shevchuk MM. Visual cues as a surrogate for tactile feedback during robotic-assisted laparoscopic prostatectomy: posterolateral margin rates in 1340 consecutive patients. BJU Int. 2010;106:528–36.

14. Lécuyer A. Simulating haptic feedback using vision: a survey of research and applications of pseudo-haptic feedback. Presence (Camb). 2009;18:39–53.

15. Shayani-Nasab H, Amir-Zargar MA, Mousavi-Bahar SH, Kashkouli AI, Ghorban-Poor M, Farimani M, Torabian S, Tavabi AA. Complications of entry using direct trocar and/or Veress needle compared with modified open approach entry in laparoscopy: six-year experience. Urol J. 2013;10(2):861–5.

16. Vilos GA. Laparoscopic bowel injuries: forty litigated gynaecological cases in Canada. J Obstet Gynaecol Can. 2002;24(3):224–30.

17. Bishoff JT, Allaf ME, Kirkels W, Moore RG, Kavoussi LR, Schroder F. Laparoscopic bowel injury: incidence and clinical presentation. J Urol. 1999;161(3):887–90.

18. Schwartz ML, Drew RL, Andersen JN. Induction of pneumoperitoneum in morbidly obese patients. Obes Surg. 2003;13(4):601–4.

19. Moran DC, Kavanagh DO, Sahebally S, Neary PC. Incidence of early symptomatic port-site hernia: a case series from a department where laparoscopy is the preferred surgical approach. Ir J Med Sci. 2012;181:463–6.

20. Pilone V, DiMicco R, Hasani A, Celentano G, Monda A, Vitiello A, Izzo G, Iacobelli L, Forestieri P. Trocar site hernia after bariatric surgery: our experience without fascial closure. Int J Surg. 2014;12:S83–6.

21. Owens M, Barry M, Janjua AZ, Winter DC. A systematic review of laparoscopic port site hernias in gastrointestinal surgery. Surgeon. 2011;9(4):218–24.

22. Scozzari G, Zanini M, Cravero F, Passera R, Rebecchi F, Morino M. High incidence of trocar site hernia after laparoscopic or robotic Roux-en-Y gastric bypass. Surg Endosc. 2014;28:2890–8.

23. Park MG, Kang J, Kim JY, Hur H, Min BS, Lee JY, Kim NK. Trocar site hernia after the use of 12-mm bladeless trocar in robotic colorectal surgery. Surg Laparosc Endosc Percutan Tech. 2012;22:e34–6.

24. Samia H, Lawrence J, Nobel T, Stein S, Champagne BJ, Delaney CP. Extraction site location and incisional hernias after laparoscopic colorectal surgery: should we be avoiding the midline? Am J Surg. 2013;205:264–7.

25. Lim SK, Kim KH, Hong SJ, Choi YD, Rha KH. A rare case of interparietal incisional hernia from 8 mm trocar site after robot-assisted laparoscopic prostatectomy. Hernia. 2014;18:911.

26. Hung CF, Yang CK, Cheng CL, Ou YC. Bowel complication during robotic-assisted laparoscopic radical prostatectomy. Anticancer Res. 2011;31(10): 497–501.

27. Wedmid A, Mendoza P, Sharma S, Hastings RL, Monahan KP, Walicki M, Ahlering TE, Porter J, Castle EP, Ahmed F, Engel JD, Frazier HA, Eun D, Lee DI. Rectal injury during robot-assisted prostatectomy: incidence and management. J Urol. 2011; 186(5):1928–33.

28. Patriti A, Ceccarelli G, Bartoli A, et al. Short- and medium-term outcome of robot-assisted and traditional laparoscopic rectal resection. JSLS. 2009;13:176–83.

29. Baik SH, Kwon HY, Kim JS, et al. Robotic versus laparoscopic low anterior resection of rectal cancer: short-term outcome of a prospective comparative study. Ann Surg Oncol. 2009;1480–87.

30. deSouza AL, Prasad LM, Marecik SJ, et al. Total mesorectal excision for rectal cancer: the potential advantage of robotic assistance. Dis Colon Rectum. 2010;53:1611–17.

31. Bianchi PP, Ceriani C, Locatelli A, et al. Robotic versus laparoscopic total mesorectal excision for rectal cancer: a comparative analysis of oncological safety and short-term outcomes. Surg Endosc. 2010;24:2888–94.

32. D'Annibale A, Pernazza G, Monsellato I, et al. Total mesorectal excision: a comparison of oncological and functional outcomes between robotic and laparo-

scopic surgery for rectal cancer. Surg Endosc. 2013;27:1887–95.

33. Liao G, Zhao Z, Lin S, Yuan Y, Du S, Chen J, Deng H. Robotic-assisted versus laparoscopic colorectal surgery: a meta-analysis of four randomized controlled trials. World J Surg Oncol. 2014;12:122. doi:10.1186/1477-7819-12-122.

34. Tam MS, Kaoutzanis C, Franz MG, Hendren S, Mullard AJ, Krapohl G, Vandewwarker JF, Lampman RM, Cleary RK. Conversion rates are lower with robotic than with laparoscopic colorectal resection: a population-based study. Dis Colon Rectum. 2014;57:E237–8.

35. Papanikolaou IG. Robotic surgery for colorectal cancer: systematic review of the literature. Surg Laparosc Endosc Percutan Tech. 2014;24:478.

36. van der Pas MH, Haglind E, Cuesta MA, Fürst A, Lacy AM, Hop WC, Bonjer HJ. Colorectal cancer Laparoscopic or Open Resection II (COLOR II) study group. Lancet Oncol. 2013;14(3):210–8.

37. Caputo D, Caricato M, LaVaccara V, Capolupo T, Coppola R. Conversion in mini-invasive colorectal surgery: the effect of timing on short term outcome. Int J Surg. 2014;12:805–9.

38. Yang Y, Wang F, Zhang P, Shi C, Zou Y, Qin H, Ma Y. Robot-assisted versus conventional laparoscopic surgery for colorectal disease focusing on rectal cancer: a meta-analysis. Ann Surg Oncol. 2012;19:3727–36.

39. Gainsburg DM. Anesthetic concerns for robotic-assisted laparoscopic radical prostatectomy. Minerva Anestesiol. 2012;78:596–604.

40. Kan KM, Brown SE, Gainsburg DM. Ocular complications in robotic-assisted prostatectomy: a review of pathophysiology and prevention. Minerva Anestesiol. 2014 [Epub ahead of print].

41. Deveney KE. Pulmonary implications of CO_2 pneumoperitoneum in minimally invasive surgery. In: Whelan RL, Fleshman JW, Fowler DL, editors. The SAGES manual of perioperative care in minimally invasive surgery. New York: Springer; 2006. p. 360–5.

42. Coulter TD, Wiedemann HP. Gas embolism. N Engl J Med. 2000;342:2000–2.

43. Mizrahi H, Hugkulstone CE, Vyakarnam P, Parker MC. Bilateral ischaemic optic neuropathy following laparoscopic proctocolectomy: a case report. Ann R Coll Surg Engl. 2011;93:e53–4.

44. Gkegkes ID, Karydis A, Tyritzis SI, Iavazzo C. Ocular complications in robotic surgery. Int J Med Robot Comput Assist Surg. 2014. doi:10.1002/rcs.1632.

45. Velchura VR, Domajnko B, desousa A, Marecik S, Prasad LM, Park JJ, Abcarian H. Obesity increases the risk of postoperative peripheral neuropathy after minimally invasive colon and rectal surgery. Dis Colon Rectum. 2014;57:187–93.

46. Buchs NC, Pugin F, Volonté F, Morel P. reliability of robotic system during general surgical procedures in a university hospital. Am J Surg. 2014;207:84–8.

47. Agcaoglu O, Aliyev S, Taskin HE, Chalikonda S, Walsh M, Costedio MM, Kroh M, Rogula T, Chand B, Gorgun E, Siperstein A, Berber E. Malfunction and failure of robotic systems during general surgical procedures. Surg Endosc. 2012;26:3580–3.

Robotic Approaches in the Obese Patient

Ajit Pai, Slawomir J. Marecik, John J. Park, and Leela M. Prasad

Abstract

Obesity is a rapidly increasing epidemic throughout the developed world, and the obese form a significant proportion of patients presenting for colorectal surgery. The laparoscopic approach in these patients, especially those with malignancy, is difficult and has higher morbidity rates, significant propensity for conversion and poorer oncologic outcomes in some studies. The robotic platform provides attractive benefits including superior vision, stable retraction and unmatched instrument dexterity, all of which facilitate minimally invasive surgery in the obese though it continues to remain difficult. The greatest benefit of the robotic technique is seen in the performance of total mesorectal excision in the obese individual with a distal rectal cancer.

Keywords

Obesity • Colorectal surgery • Robotic surgery • Minimally invasive surgery • Colectomy • Digestive system

A. Pai, MD, FACS
S.J. Marecik, MD, FACS, FASCRS
Division of Colon and Rectal Surgery, Advocate
Lutheran General Hospital, Park Ridge, IL, USA

University of Illinois at Chicago College of Medicine,
Chicago, IL, USA

J.J. Park, MD, FACS, FASCRS (✉)
Division of Colon and Rectal Surgery, Advocate
Lutheran General Hospital, Park Ridge, IL, USA

Associate Professor of Surgery, Chicago Medical
School at Rosalind Franklin University of Medicine
and Science, Chicago, IL, USA
e-mail: jpark18@aol.com

L.M. Prasad, MD, FACS, FASCRS
Department of Surgery, Advocate Lutheran General
Hospital, Park Ridge, IL, USA

University of Illinois College of Medicine at
Chicago, Park Ridge, IL, USA

Division of Colon and Rectal Surgery, Advocate
Lutheran General Hospital, Park Ridge, IL, USA

© Springer International Publishing Switzerland 2015
H. Ross et al. (eds.), *Robotic Approaches to Colorectal Surgery*,
DOI 10.1007/978-3-319-09120-4_19

19.1 Introduction

Obesity is the most common chronic preventable disease in the western world and is a rapidly growing epidemic in the United States. *Obesity is a risk factor for diverticular disease and cancer and thus is a major concern for surgeons dealing with colorectal diseases, being grossly overrepresented and in fact representing the 'normal' patient presenting to these physicians.*

Laparoscopic surgery for colorectal diseases including cancer, diverticular disease and inflammatory bowel disease is now well established as safe, feasible and, in cancers, with oncologic outcomes comparable to open surgery [1, 2]. Improved perioperative outcomes including earlier return of gastrointestinal function, better pulmonary function, decreased postoperative pain, lower incidence of wound infection and shorter length of stay have all been proven in large randomised trials, systematic reviews and meta-analyses [3–5]. Obesity does have an adverse effect in conventional colorectal surgery on certain measures including operative time, blood loss, wound infections, fascial dehiscence, incisional hernias and anastomotic leaks in rectal anastomoses [6]. This negative impact is also seen in the laparoscopic approach to colorectal operations for benign and malignant disease with increased conversion rates and postoperative morbidity in the obese [7, 8].

Robotic surgery in the obese patient faces challenges, some common with laparoscopy and others unique to the robotic platform. Since most robotic colorectal operations begin as laparoscopic operations and a significant number are hybrid laparoscopic-robotic operations, problems with positioning, access and exposure are common and are well known [9].

Once the operative field is set up and the abdominal domain is created however, the unique aspects of the robotic platform including magnified optics, stable and very powerful retraction, reduced dependence on the assistant and extreme degrees of freedom level the playing field, making the obese individual the ideal candidate for the robotic approach especially the male patient with rectal cancer.

This chapter deals with the universal problems faced by the surgical team when dealing with the obese patient, the modification of surgical approaches, tips and tricks and the challenges faced when robotically handling the colon and rectum. Specific approaches and pearls for successful performance of right colectomy, left colectomy and total mesorectal excision (TME) as part of anterior and abdominoperineal resection for rectal cancer are dealt with in detail. Since the operative strategy varies only minimally between benign and malignant colorectal disease, no attempt is made to separate the two, and the reader is referred to specific chapters for information on disease-based approaches.

19.2 Definition of Obesity

Obesity is defined by the World Health Organization as a body mass index [BMI] $\geq 30 \, \mathrm{kg/m^2}$. By this measure, an estimated 35.7 % of the American population are obese. The age-adjusted prevalence of obesity was 35.5 % (95 % CI, 31.9–39.2 %) among adult men and 35.8 % (95 % CI, 34.0–37.7 %) among adult women in the 2009–2010 National Health and Nutrition Examination Survey (NHANES) [10]. This method has limitations as BMI assesses the entire body mass without differentiating between its components, namely, muscle, visceral fat, subcutaneous fat, bone and fluid. It does not differentiate those men with thick abdominal walls from those with excess omental/visceral fat. Waist-to-hip ratio (WHR) and waist circumference (WC) are other simple measurements to determine obesity. These measures, especially WHR, correlate better with an increase in visceral fat and a relative lack of gluteal muscle [11].

19.3 Preoperative Preparation

19.3.1 Medical Optimisation

Obese patients, especially the often elderly patients with colorectal cancer and diverticular disease, have multiple comorbid conditions including coronary artery disease, hypertension and type 2 diabetes, besides an increased risk of perioperative and postoperative deep vein thromboembolism [DVT] and death [12].

Extensive preoperative workup and optimisation are recommended. A simple but effective intervention is to operate patients scheduled for benign elective surgery only after they have lost a predefined amount of weight, which reduces perioperative morbidity and makes for easier surgery.

19.3.2 Bowel Preparation

Obesity is an independent predictor of inadequate bowel preparation and further reduces the working space in the peritoneal cavity due to increased visceral fat [13]. Adequate intensive bowel preparation, which produces flaccid collapsed bowels, increases the working space and facilitates layering of the bowel besides making it easier to use gravity-assisted exposure of the operative field. The standard bowel preparation regime consisting of a liquid diet for 24 h prior to surgery and use of bowel preparation with polyethylene glycol the evening prior may not adequately empty the bowels in the obese. The use of a low-residue diet for 8 days and polyethylene glycol preparation starting 2 days before operation has been used to great effect and should be utilised whenever possible [14].

19.3.3 Preventing Venous Thromboembolism

All patients with colorectal disease especially cancer are at increased risk of deep venous thromboembolism, especially when operated by the minimally invasive/robotic approach. The risk is exaggerated in the obese [15]. While preoperative prophylaxis with unfractionated intravenous or subcutaneous low-molecular-weight heparin is recommended, it is our policy to start prophylaxis the morning after surgery. The surgeons frequently rely on sequential compression boots, which are applied before anesthesia is induced and continue till patient discharge. The combination of mechanical compression and pharmacologic prophylaxis is more effective than either alone. Consideration is given to an inferior vena cava filter in patients at high risk for DVT [prior DVT, prior pulmonary embolism, BMI > 60 kg/m^2, hypercoagulable states].

19.3.4 Thoracic Epidural Analgesia

We routinely use epidural catheters for postoperative analgesia. Epidural analgesia leads to increased circulation in the lower extremities, reduced tendency for coagulation more efficient fibrinolysis and decreases blood loss due to permissive hypotension, thereby reducing transfusion requirements [16]. All these may explain the decrease in thromboembolic phenomena. Only patients undergoing robotic right colectomies do not have epidural catheters; we have not found added benefit over a combination of local anaesthetic infiltration and patient-controlled analgesia [PCA] in this group, and epidural analgesia does not lead to earlier return of bowel function in this group.

19.4 Surgical Considerations

19.4.1 Patient Positioning and Operating Room Setup

Standard operating tables accommodate patients with weights up to 450 lb; for heavier patients bariatric tables that can accommodate up to 1000 lb are recommended [MAQUET, Surgical Tables Inc., Steris, Magnatek]. The key to a successful robotic procedure is unfettered access for laparoscopic and robotic instruments, and the importance of positioning cannot be overemphasised. The patient needs to be rigidly immobilised to prevent sliding during position changes. The patient is positioned on a gel pad, which in turn is placed on a beanbag (Vac-Pac®, Olympic Medical Corporation, Seattle, WA, USA). The beanbag is a polyvinyl sleeve filled with polystyrene beads and uses a vacuum to force the beads

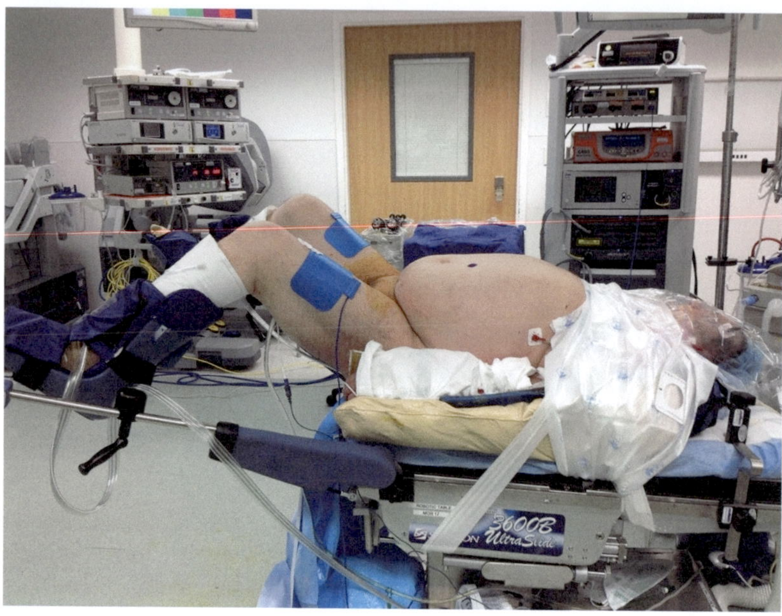

Fig. 19.1 Patient position and immobilisation for robotic rectal surgery (Lloyd-Davies position)

together, with atmospheric pressure keeping the beads in place, moulded to the patient's torso once the vacuum is connected. The right-sized beanbag covers the entire length of the patients' torso with adequate overlap on either side to support the arms and sufficient length to wrap over and immobilise the shoulders. Gel pads are further used to isolate the arms from the beanbag, cushion the wrists and protect all superficial nerves and bony prominences from damage. Foam packing is placed over the shoulders providing a tighter seal for the beanbag. 'C'-shaped padded orthopaedic shoulder supports prevent the patient form sliding upwards during steep Trendelenburg and do not increase the risk of brachial plexus injury. The use of rigid shoulder braces in the past led to brachial plexus injuries due to compression of the nerve between the clavicle and the ribs at the level of the scalene muscles [17]. Additional strapping across the chest is used to stabilise the patient during sideways tilt (Fig. 19.1).

For right colectomy, the patient is supine with arms tucked by the side. For left colon and rectal surgery, the modified lithotomy position of Lloyd-Davies is used, placing the buttocks at the edge of the table, with the legs in padded Allen stirrups and the hips minimally flexed to allow unrestricted movement of the robotic arms.

19.4.2 Positioning and Peripheral Neuropathy

Obesity increases the risk of postoperative peripheral neuropathy after minimally invasive colon and rectal surgery and is an independent risk factor despite adequate precautions; however, most neuropathy is temporary and self-limited, and the incidence is minimised with our approach as described above [18]. The overall incidence quoted in our paper is 2 % of all minimally invasive colorectal operations and 3.6 % in robotic operations (all were rectal operations performed in lithotomy). An analysis of our data showed that the side towards which the patient is tilted in the transverse plane suffers neurologic damage more frequently, specifically the left-sided nerve axis during right colectomy and the right-sided nerves during left colon operations. *The incidence theoretically should be minimised further by differential padding favouring the side towards which the patient is tilted.*

19.4.3 Access to the Peritoneal Cavity and Establishment of Pneumoperitoneum

Access to the peritoneal cavity is most rapid and effective in the obese and morbidly obese subjects with the Veress needle. Extra long needles (150 mm) as against the standard 120 mm are occasionally needed in the morbidly obese patient. We insert the Veress through a 2 mm stab incision through or just above the umbilicus after tenting up the tissues with two towel clips. The Palmer's point represents another site for Veress needle insertion in the morbidly obese as this location has less fat than the periumbilical area in these individuals. Optical trocar systems can also be used; Visiport (Covidien, Norwalk, CT) and Optiview (Ethicon Endo-surgery, Cincinnati, OH) are two FDA-approved commercially available devices which allow safe insertion under vision [19]. In patients who have prior surgeries especially midline incisions, we use the Palmer's point in the left subcostal region or place the first trocar by the optical method far out in the lateral quadrants. Once entry is established, we use a high-flow thermosufflator (Insuflow, Lexion Medical, St. Paul, MN, USA), which delivers CO_2 gas heated to 95 °F and 95 % relative humidity to rapidly establish pneumoperitoneum to 14–15 mmHg. The use of heated and humidified gas prevents hypothermia and tissue desiccation, which translates into less abdominal and shoulder pain [20]. The optical trocar is then placed either by enlarging the initial stab or in the location of choice through a separate incision. The use of two insufflation ports is recommended by bariatric surgeons in morbidly obese patients to maintain pneumoperitoneum, but we have never needed to use this method in our practice. The open Hasson technique is frequently difficult to perform in the morbidly obese, and it is even more difficult to achieve a tight fascial seal around the trocar and is the least preferred entry method in this group in our practice.

19.4.4 Trocar Positioning and Manipulation: Modification of Standard Trocar Position

Obesity alters the normal dimensions of the torso and alters spatial orientation of normal landmarks. Specifically, changes of torso length by 10–11 cm and torso girth by 12–13 cm are reported between underweight and obese patients [21]. Contrary to popular belief, the position of the umbilicus relative to the torso is not fixed. In normal-weight individuals, the umbilicus is located roughly halfway between the xiphoid and the pubic symphysis. With increasing BMI, the umbilicus shifts caudad (Fig. 19.2) [22]. Port positions based on the umbilical location may therefore be erroneous. A good rule of thumb is to use a 5 mm trocar to perform the abdominal survey and then place the additional robotic and assistant trocars under vision at the appropriate distance from the target anatomy rather than through defined premarked sites. When placing lateral ports for right and left colectomy, the ports should be placed at a defined distance usually 10–12 cm lateral to the optical trocar and not far lateral based on patient girth, so as to allow

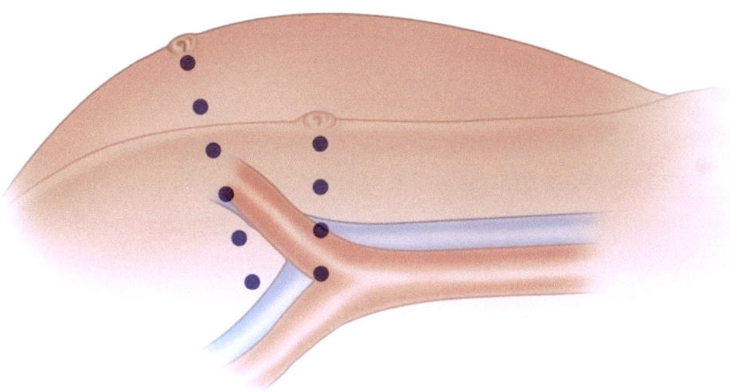

Fig. 19.2 Caudal shift of the umbilicus with increasing obesity

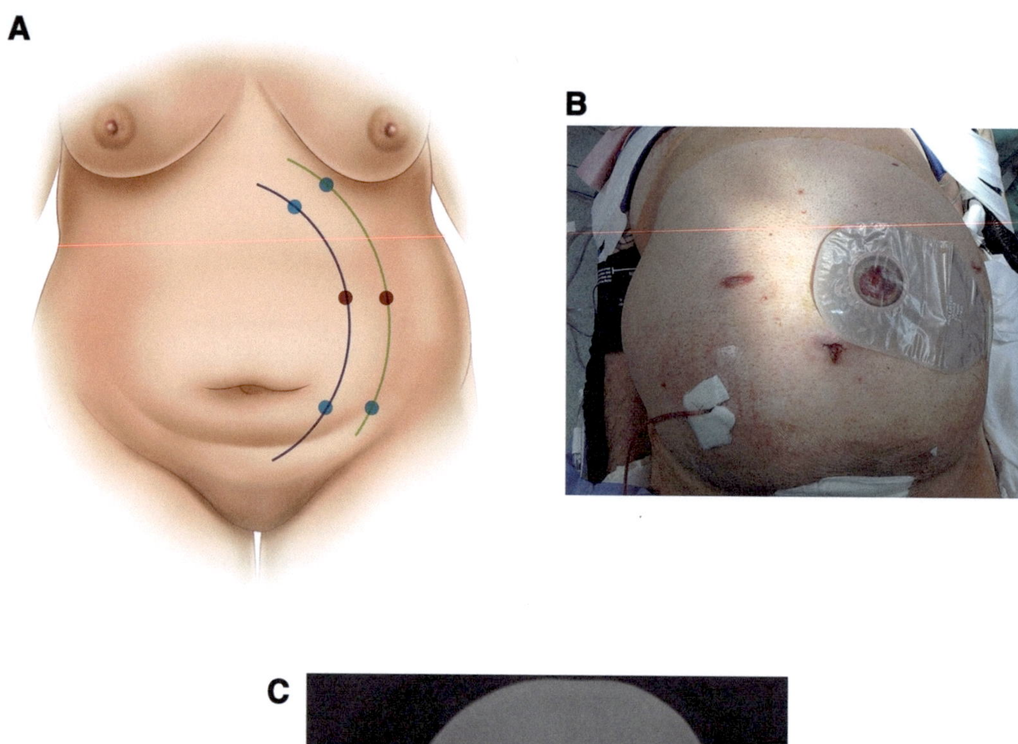

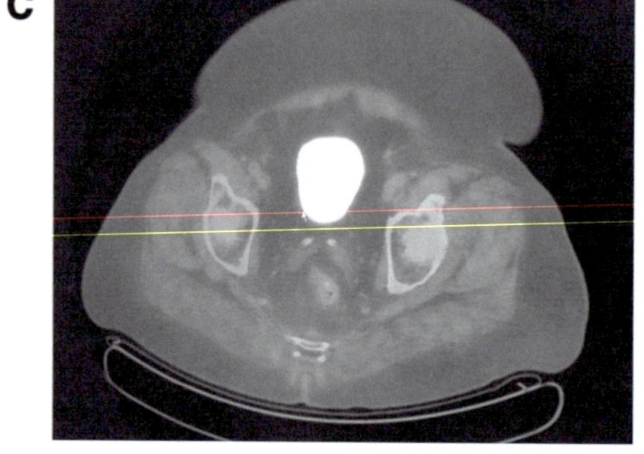

Fig. 19.3 (a) Correct [*purple line*] and incorrect [*green line*] port positions relative to the umbilicus for right colectomy. (b) Representative patient after robotic low APR showing clustering of ports in the middle of the torso representing the right location. (c) CT scan of the same patient showing small [normal torso] size despite morbid obesity with huge pannus

access to the colon on the opposite side. This is because the size of the actual muscular torso does not change much in most obese individuals, and placing the ports too far lateral leads to a tangential entry into the abdomen rather than the perpendicular entry which is desirable (Fig. 19.3a–c).

In low anterior resections, the entire trocar setup moves down closer to the pelvis to allow access to the low pelvis and the pelvic floor (Fig. 19.4a, b).

Length of the pelvis is also an important consideration and should be assessed in every patient by review of the CT scans. Tall obese males particularly may have a very long pelvis and we have encountered difficulties in reaching the pelvic floor with the robotic instruments with trocars in standard locations. In situations where the instruments don't reach the lower extremes of the pelvis, the robot is undocked, a fresh set of ports is placed closer to the target anatomy, redocking is performed and the procedure is continued. As experience grows, the trocars should be placed lower in the abdomen, thereby moving closer to the target anatomy.

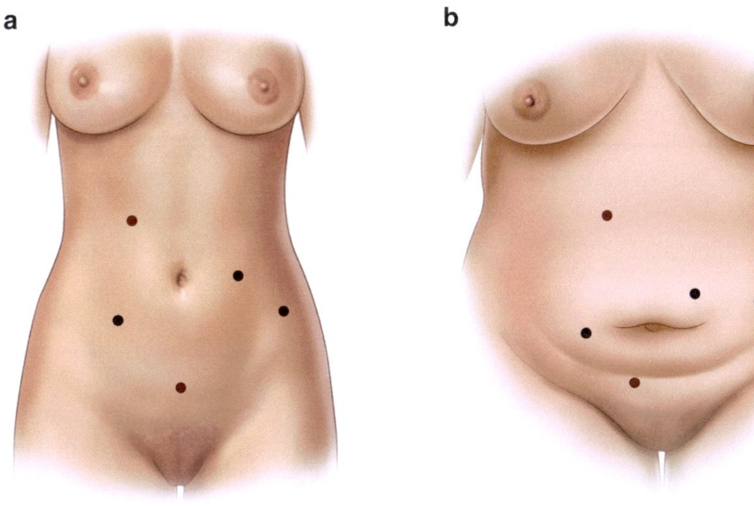

Fig. 19.4 Port positions in a normal (**a**) and obese individual (**b**) for robotic low anterior resection [note that ports are closer to the pelvis but are not related to umbilical position which moves caudally in the obese]

19.4.5 Robotic Docking

Docking the robot presents some unique challenges in the morbidly obese patient. A steep Trendelenburg position is often used in all colon and rectal operations (except during flexure mobilisation) to use gravity-aided exposure. The increase in abdominal wall fat leads to a massive increase in anteroposterior girth, and the robotic arms may not have sufficient space to clear the wall despite the table being dropped down to the lowest position (Fig. 19.5). A compromise with a slight decrease in head-down tilt with the assistant actively retracting the small bowel out of the field is often needed to physically allow the robot to reach the field. *The use of bariatric tables is useful because they allow a much steeper Trendelenburg tilt than with normal tables and their lowest height setting is as low as 25 in. as against the 32 in. standard.*

19.4.6 Creation of the Operative Field and Optimal Exposure

Gravity is the most important aid in exposure in robotic colorectal surgery especially in the obese. The use of steep Trendelenburg and right-down

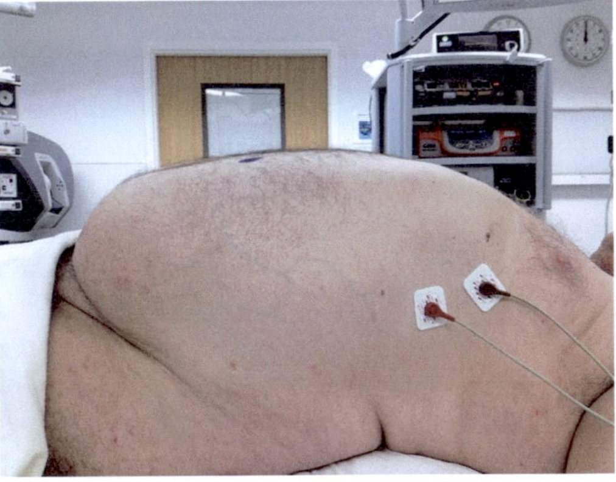

Fig. 19.5 Massive anteroposterior girth in the morbidly obese patient

tilt (low anterior resection and left colectomy) or left-down tilt (right colectomy) is indispensable. To allow the small bowel to fall away from the operative area, release of all adhesions is mandatory. The ligament of Treitz is always released for left-sided resections, to allow the small bowel to be packed into the right paracolic and supracolic compartments. Release of the omentum is often needed to allow space for the bowel to be thus placed. The use of radiopaque gauze as a sling over the small bowel to which it adheres is also a useful technique to keep the bowel in place. The fat-laden mesentery is prone to tearing, and it is often prudent to handle the bowel directly or with sweeping motions to deliver it out of the pelvis into the upper abdomen. The use of endoscopic paddles is recommended by some surgeons to retract the small bowel, but we have never found it necessary to do so.

19.4.7 Specimen Extraction and Anastomosis

Obese patients have an increased incidence of wound infections and fascial dehiscence leading to hernias. Careful consideration should be given to specimen extraction site and site for anastomosis when performed extracorporeally. The specimen tends to be bulky due to fat-laden mesocolon, giant epiploica and abundant fatty omentum in right colon specimens.

19.4.7.1 Right Colon

The preferred site for extraction and extracorporeal anastomosis is a supraumbilical incision incorporating the umbilical optical trocar with upward extension for 4–5 cm (adjusted to the specimen bulk). While intracorporeal anastomosis enables an unlimited choice of extraction sites, the benefits of this approach should be weighed against the dangers of manipulating the ileum with a thick friable and fat-laden mesentery with potential for devascularisation and bleeding. We strongly prefer extracorporeal anastomosis, as this is a safer approach given the increased risk of anastomotic leaks in obese patients. Even when extracorporeal anastomosis is planned, intracorporeal vessel ligation is preferable in obese patients; extracorporeal ligation can be remarkably difficult as the thickness of the abdominal pannus makes exteriorisation of the specimen difficult [23]. Obese patients often carry foreshortened mesentery and mesocolon, which are at increased risk of tearing at the time of bowel extraction. The bulky omentum needs to be detached completely before specimen extraction and extracted separately if resected for cancer. The supraumbilical region often has relatively less fat compared to the lower abdomen and is

therefore the preferred site for extraction. In a very select group of patients with low visceral obesity, with increasing surgeon experience, the intracorporeal method of reconstruction may be attempted. The Pfannenstiel incision is then the site of extraction.

19.4.7.2 Left Colon and Anterior Resection

For resections in the left colon and downwards, a suprapubic Pfannenstiel incision of 5 cm, placed 2–3 fingerbreadths above the upper border of the pubic symphysis, is our preferred method. The sheath is opened transversely, the muscles split in the midline and the peritoneum opened vertically. A commercially available wound protector (Alexis wound protector, Applied Medical, Rancho Santa Margarita, CA, USA) is placed to allow safe extraction without contaminating the abdominal wound. Our experience shows that the incidence of incisional hernia is nil after a Pfannenstiel incision compared to a 16 % rate for a vertical lower midline extraction site [24].

19.5 Specific Operative Procedures

19.5.1 Robotic Right Hemicolectomy

Conventionally, the robotic technique is ideally suited for medial-to-lateral dissection because its precise nature and dexterity enable the ileocolic pedicle to be skeletonised and dissected right down to the superior mesenteric vessels. In obese patients however the bulky mesocolon and large amount of fat around the pedicle make this approach difficult.

A modified approach: a caudal-to-cranial (inferior-to-superior) approach is safer and more effective. This involves incising the base of the ileocecal fold and allowing pneumodissection. Dissection then proceeds upwards towards the duodenum and laterally along the line of Toldt. In essence the direction of dissection is from inferolateral to superomedial (Fig. 19.6). Once the duodenum and head of the pancreas are separated

Fig. 19.6 Direction of dissection in right hemicolectomy; step 1: inferior to superior, step 2: medial to lateral

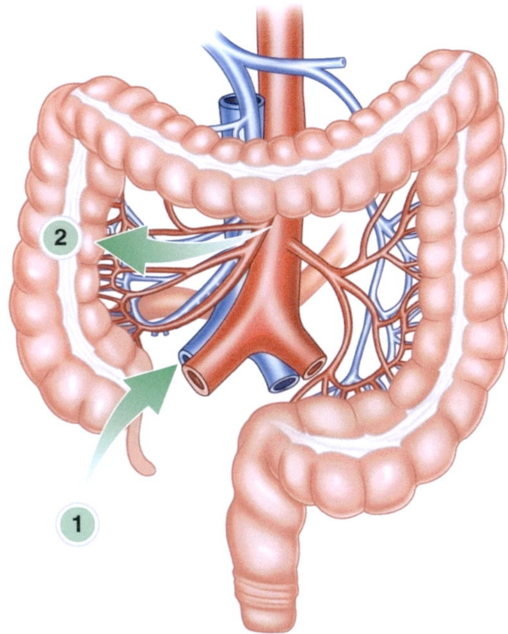

from the ascending mesocolon, the medial-to-lateral approach can be continued. The ileocecal junction is held upwards by the assistant and the peritoneum on either side of the pedicle is incised and the fat and nodes are swept laterally allowing a secure ligation and division of the ileocolic pedicle at its origin.

It should be noted that the ascending colon in the obese tends to be heavy and is difficult to retract and unfold using only the two robotic working arms. Rather than holding the peritoneal edge for retraction, the entire shaft of the fenestrated grasper should be placed parallel to the mesocolon so that it rests on it, thus enabling retraction of the entire colon and straightening it out (Fig. 19.7).

The supracolic dissection is best accomplished with the use of two robotic graspers, a bipolar fenestrated instrument in the left hypochondrial port and a Cadiere forceps in the left iliac fossa port for pulling the transverse colon downwards and the bulky greater omentum upwards. The assistant through the left flank port separates these structures, enters the lesser sac and takes down the hepatic flexure using an energy-sealing device. Our preference is for the Enseal device with straight jaws which functions as an atraumatic grasper, dissector and vessel sealer.

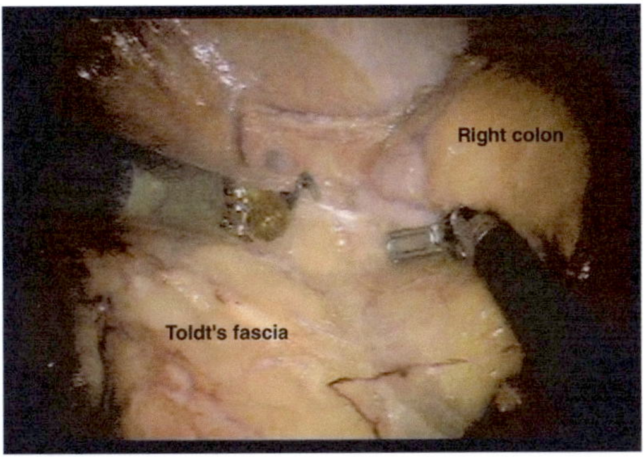

Fig. 19.7 Effective use of instrument shaft for colon retraction in robotic right hemicolectomy

Specimen extraction is facilitated by dividing the terminal ileum intracorporeally using the laparoscopic stapler through the left lower quadrant port. This manoeuvre allows the single limb of bowel to be exteriorised easily through a small supraumbilical incision. Prior to extraction the terminal ileum to be anastomosed should be held with the assistant's grasper so that it may be easily brought into the wound for anastomosis. Anastomosis is performed in the standard side-to-side functional end-to-end manner. In patients whose mesentery is short and thick, exteriorisation is difficult if not impossible. In this situation, the intracorporeal method using a laparoscopic stapler through one of the robotic ports as has been previously described is extremely useful [25].

19.5.2 Robotic Left Colectomy and Sigmoid Colectomy

Totally robotic approaches to the left colon and sigmoid are commonly performed for malignancy. These are difficult operations to perform due to the need for multiple cart positions, typically by the left shoulder and the left hip and the need for redocking even if a fixed left hip position is used [26, 27]. The one-cart (fit-it-all) position technique is rarely possible due to technical difficulties. The obese patient presents several unique anatomical features that make dissection difficult including:

1. Bulky, heavy and fat-laden omentum
2. Adhesions between the sigmoid mesocolon and the small bowel mesentery
3. Tortuous and heavy sigmoid and descending colon
4. Obscured origin of the inferior mesenteric artery (IMA) due to visceral fat
5. Higher chance of damage to the marginal artery due to lack of visualisation consequent to visceral adiposity
6. Friable peritoneum making it difficult to get a purchase on the specimen

In addition, the current generation of robotic graspers is not well suited to providing a secure but atraumatic hold on a bulky fat-laden mesentery or colon.

All of these make this operation difficult.

One trick is to use an umbilical tape or radiopaque gauze tied tightly around the colon after creating a mesocolic window as a handle, which can be grasped with the robotic graspers and used to manipulate the colon.

The standard approach involving an artery-first approach is modified to a vein-first approach. The inferior mesenteric vein (IMV) is usually not covered by fat, located as it is in the bare area between the middle colic and left colic territories. It is therefore easily visualised even in the most obese individual. Dissection and division of this vein allows access to the proper embryologic interface between Toldt's fascia and the mesocolon. The left colic artery is then skeletonised and divided [left colectomy] or preserved and used to develop the plane lateral to the superior rectal artery prior to its division [sigmoid colectomy]. Access to both sides of the inferior mesenteric artery (IMA)/superior rectal artery axis also allows visualisation of the autonomic nerves prior to division.

While the presence of large amounts of fat makes the dissection between Toldt's fascia and the mesocolon relatively easy compared to the patient with a low BMI, there may be considerable difficulty in entering the right plane. A combination of lateral-to-medial and medial-to-lateral approaches is often needed to complete the procedure. The plane is most easily entered cephalad underneath the IMV, and this is an additional advantage of the vein-first approach.

Bowel division and anastomosis are also more safely performed extracorporeally using a small midline or left upper quadrant incision for left colectomy and a Pfannenstiel incision for sigmoid resections.

19.5.3 Hybrid Laparoscopic-Robotic Low Anterior and Ultralow Anterior Resection

The hybrid approach uses laparoscopic dissection for vascular pedicle isolation and division, lymphadenectomy, left colon and sigmoid mobilisation and splenic flexure takedown. The robot is docked at the completion of these steps and is used only for TME. It is our preferred approach and increases the efficiency of the procedure besides reducing operative time as the robot is used only for the most critical and difficult part of the operation (Fig. 19.8) [28]. The total time is further reduced by a single docking of the robot [between the legs or by the left hip]. This approach is particularly beneficial in the obese as the left colon and sigmoid are bulky and fat laden, making manipulation with the robot time consuming and

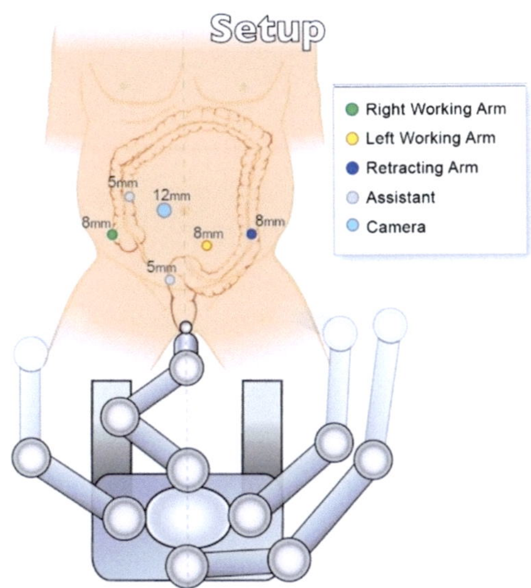

Fig. 19.8 Setup for hybrid robotic low anterior resection, single docking

tedious. In the morbidly obese, a hand-assisted approach in addition through a 7 cm suprapubic incision provides additional control and expedites this portion of the operation. The same incision is used for specimen extraction and anastomosis.

The totally robotic approach provides no additional benefit over the hybrid approach, and in fact in a comparison of the two approaches, Baik and colleagues found no difference in lymph nodes retrieved, distal or radial margin positivity between the two groups [29]. They did find that the length of stay for the hybrid robotic procedure was lower than the totally robotic operation (8.4±4.3 days hybrid, 10.8±7.3 days totally robotic procedure; $P<0.001$). In addition the complication rate was also lower in the hybrid group as compared to the totally robotic arm [16 % hybrid vs. 27.2 % robotic group]. Although this study was based on patients whose BMI was relatively low, it is expected that in the obese population the differences should be more pronounced.

19.5.4 Totally Robotic Low and Ultralow Anterior Resection

The left colon is mobilised in the standard fashion as for left colon and sigmoid resections. Mobilisation of the bowel is carried proximally up to the middle colic vessels; the entire bowel from the left of the middle colic vessels to just above the sacral promontory is freed from the retroperitoneum. The IMA is divided at its root 1 cm distal to the origin; this is accomplished safely with an endoscopic stapler or the energy device. The artery is often large, thick and atherosclerotic in these patients and the endoscopic stapler provides the most secure seal for these types of vessels. The mesocolon is divided up to the planned site of bowel transection either by the assistant using a laparoscopic vessel-sealing energy device or the robotic energy sealer.

The port positions for the pelvic component are as shown in Fig. 19.9. Arms 1 and 2 house a robotic monopolar hook and a bipolar fenestrated grasper, respectively. Arm 3 houses a prograsp forceps, which has a larger and longer jaw for better grip on the bowel/peritoneum for retraction. The assistant uses the right hypochondrial port for additional traction/countertraction with an atraumatic grasper and the suprapubic port for a suction-irrigation device. The sigmoid is divided as distally as possible in obese patients, which makes the stump easier to handle. In patients with a very bulky sigmoid-rectosigmoid component, additional traction is obtained as described before by tying the rectosigmoid and lymph node packet with an umbilical tape which can be used as a handle for retraction by the third robotic arm (Fig. 19.10).

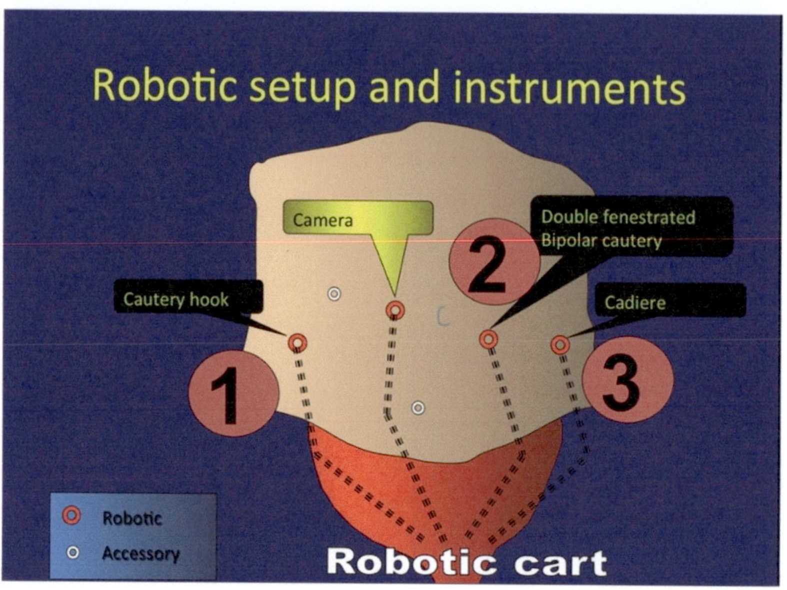

Fig. 19.9 Robotic port positions for rectal dissection

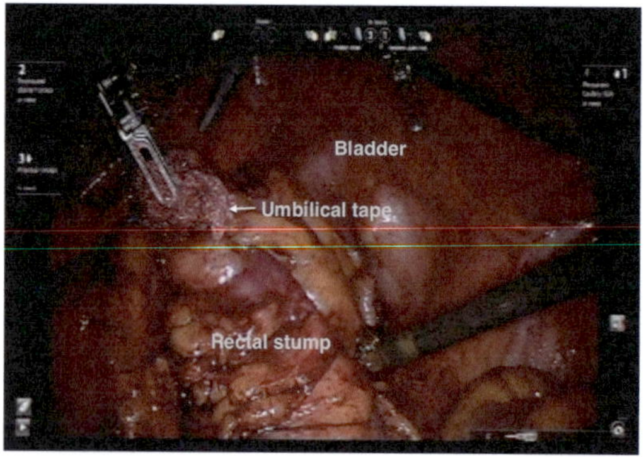

Fig. 19.10 Rectosigmoid suspension using an umbilical tape for traction

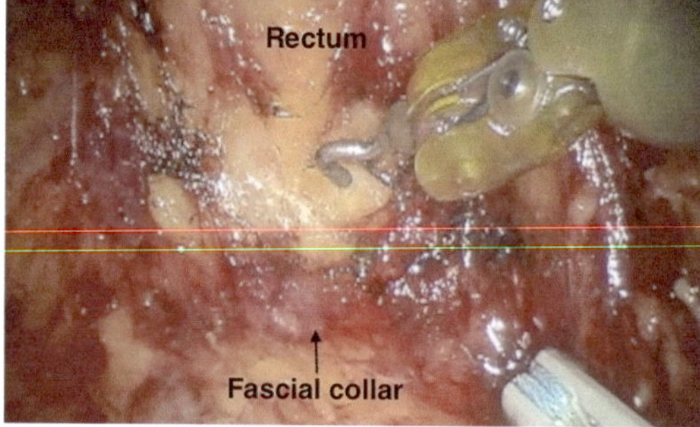

Fig. 19.11 Fascial collar around the upper rectum appreciated during commencement of robotic TME

The procedure commences by holding the bowel anteriorly and cranially under traction with arm 3. The avascular plane between the Toldt's fascia and the sigmoid mesocolon is entered just above the promontory, and dissection continues into the pelvis in the interval between the visceral and parietal fascia of the rectum. *It is critical to note that the Toldt's fascia slopes anteriorly and forms a collar around the posterior half of the rectosigmoid and incision of this collar* (Fig. 19.11) *is essential to enter the 'holy plane' described by Heald* [30]. In the obese patient, a large amount of presacral fat is encountered, and the distinction between the presacral and mesorectal fat and entry into the right plane may be tedious and time consuming. Once the 'holy plane' is entered, dissection continues caudally as far down as possible. The lateral peritoneal cuts are then taken and lateral dissection between the mesorectum and the endopelvic fascia carried out in standard fashion. Of note, a large amount of fat is encountered on the lateral pelvic wall in obese individuals again making the dissection difficult; the tendency is to go too far lateral in these patients (Fig. 19.12). *One tip is to start the anterior dissection at this point and connect the anterior and posterior planes at the mesorectal corners.* The mesorectum tends to be very fragile in the obese and very gentle traction is essential to avoid violation of and bleeding from the mesorectum. Our practice is to only grasp the peritoneal folds for traction and use the shaft of the instrument and the entire tip like a St. Mark's retractor for retraction allowing the rectum to rest on the instrument (Fig. 19.13a, b). The assistant is invaluable at this point, to provide a smoke-free field and lateral traction on the pelvic sidewall facilitating rapid and meticulous dissection.

During anterior dissection, the uterus in women and the bladder in men, which tend to be heavy and fatty, can be suspended out of the field by a 2-0 nylon stitch on a Keith needle passed through the anterior abdominal wall. The rectum tends to be bulky making anterior dissection challenging; switching to a 30° down scope and straightening and flattening the rectum by the assistant providing cranial and posterior traction (as one would with the fingers in open dissection) enable completion of this part of the procedure. We favour the hook cautery for pelvic dissection because it is more versatile than the monopolar shears, it can be used for precise dissection with the tip, for more rapid dissection using the large curved outer surface of the hook, and it is invaluable for preparing the rectal tube for anastomosis as the mesorectum can be hooked up and safely divided circumferentially.

Preparation of the rectal stump, division and anastomosis are as described elsewhere in the specific chapters. The only specific point is specimen extraction and anastomosis. These are best accomplished through a small Pfannenstiel incision, which allows a secure restoration of gastrointestinal continuity and prevents mishaps in this group of patients who are prone to complications. Natural orifice extraction (transrectal or transvaginal) is almost never possible due to large specimen size.

19.5.5 Totally Robotic Abdominoperineal Resection for Cancer

The pelvic floor is reached as described above for the sphincter-saving approach. The accepted standard of care now is to perform extralevator APR [ELAPR] to avoid circumferential resection margin positivity, mesorectal violation and iatro-

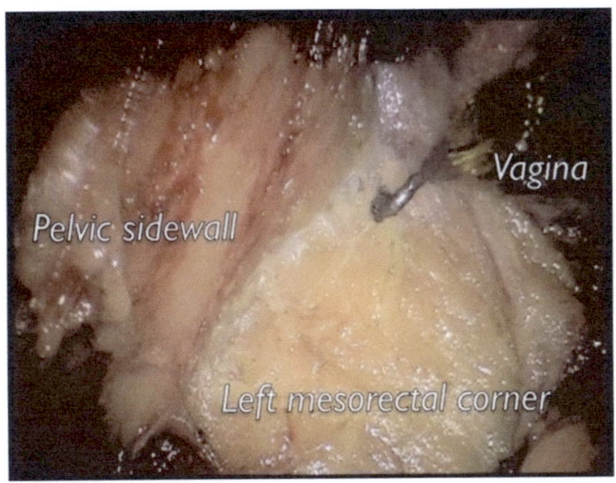

Fig. 19.12 Excessive endopelvic fat in the obese pelvis

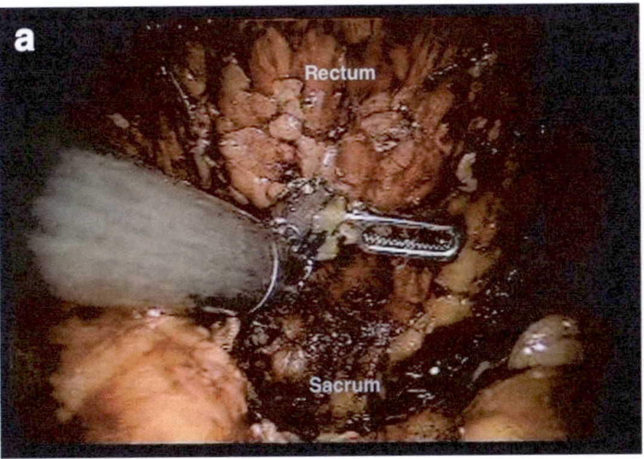

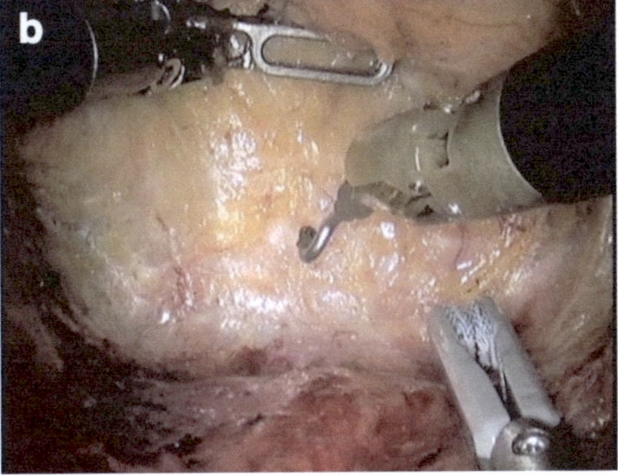

Fig. 19.13 (**a**) Use of bipolar forceps as a St. Mark's retractor for posterior dissection. (**b**) Use of fenestrated grasper/ Cadiere forceps as an effective retractor for lateral dissection

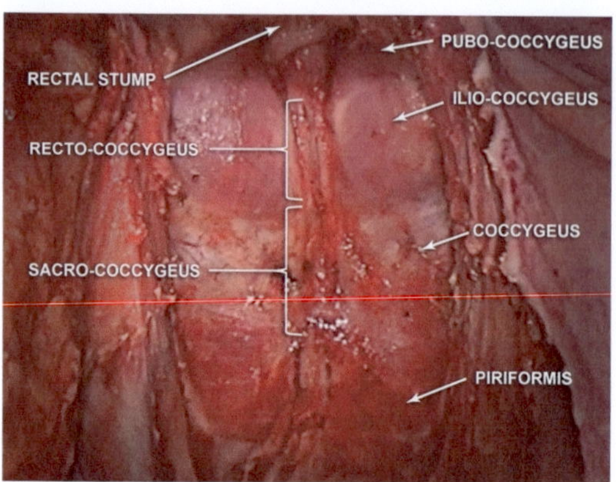

Fig. 19.14 Operative photograph of pelvic floor anatomy with the rectum removed

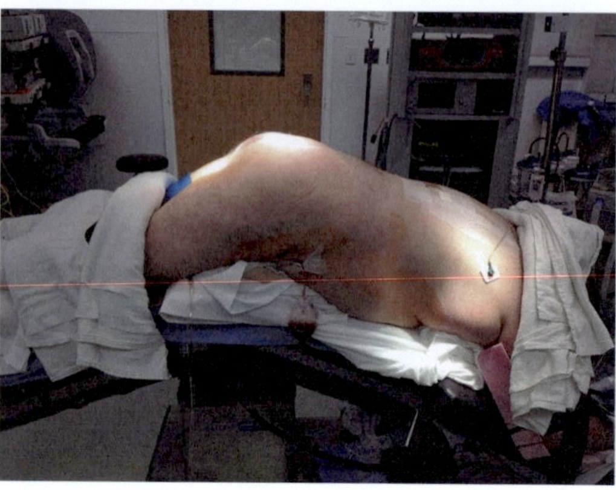

Fig. 19.15 Prone jackknife position for perineal dissection during APR

genic perforation. Our technique of controlled robotic cylindrical levator transection accomplished abdominally produces a wide cuff of tissue around the specimen and completes the essential oncologic steps transabdominally [31]. Entry into the ischiorectal fossa fat is performed by sequentially dividing portion of the puborectalis muscle and the iliococcygeus and coccygeus muscles, including the midline raphe at the level of coccygeal tip. The pelvic floor anatomy is as shown (Fig. 19.14). Anteriorly dissection in males is carried out as low as possible.

Stoma creation and omental pedicle flap harvest are accomplished laparoscopically after undocking the robot. The patient is then flipped to the prone position.

The importance of the prone jackknife position for perineal dissection in the obese patient cannot be overemphasised. It provides excellent exposure in the obese patient and converts the procedure into a 2-man operation unlike the lithotomy approach, which essentially is a 1-man operation due to space constraints (Fig. 19.15).

The final stages of anterior dissection and division of ischioanal fat are all that remain after a robotic cylindrical APR technique. Blind division of the levators as occurs in the open and laparoscopic approaches is avoided. Following specimen extraction, skin closure is never a problem in the obese due to lax and abundant perineal skin. The pelvic soft tissue defect however can be massive, and the use of an omental pedicle fat based on the left gastroepiploic vessels fills the dead space snugly and reduces perineal wound complications.

19.6 Postoperative Considerations

Care of the obese patient after colorectal surgery is as in standard laparoscopic operations. Specific points include:

1. Early ambulation
2. Aggressive chest physiotherapy
3. DVT prophylaxis with unfractionated heparin when an epidural is used and with LMWH in right colectomies where there is no role for epidural analgesia

19.7 Oncologic Outcomes in Obese Patients

The literature is remarkable for the absence of data comparing outcomes between obese and nonobese patients undergoing robotic colorectal operations for malignancy. We have accrued considerable experience in TME for rectal cancer in obese individuals, and our data (Prasad LM, Marecik SJ, Park JJ 2013, unpublished data) reveal equivalent perioperative and short-term and long-term oncologic outcomes between the

Table 19.1 Perioperative and short-term oncologic outcomes in an obese versus nonobese population undergoing robotic total mesorectal excision for rectal cancer

	Obese ($n=30$)	Nonobese ($n=72$)	P value
EBL [mL]	265.5 ± 211.3	188.14 ± 131.6	0.075^a
TME time [min]	110 ± 35.4	92.94 ± 37.8	0.03^a
OR time [min]	369.62 ± 73.2	327.4 ± 85.2	0.02^a
Hospital stay [days]	6.6 ± 2.6	6.8 ± 4.9	0.8^a
Conversions, n	3 (10)	2 (2.8)	0.15^b
CRM positivity, n	1 (3.3)	1 (1.39)	1.0^b
Lymph node harvest	12 ± 6.2	14.6 ± 7.8	0.08
Anastomotic leak, n	1 (3.3)	6 (8.3)	0.614^c

Prasad LM, Marecik SJ, Park JJ 2013, unpublished data

All values expressed as mean$\pm$SD except where indicated

EBL estimated blood loss, *TME* total mesorectal excision, *OR* operating room, *CRM* circumferential resection margin

[a]Student t test

[b]Fisher's exact test

[c]Pearson X^2

Table 19.2 Comparison of perioperative and clinicopathologic outcomes between obese males and females undergoing robotic-assisted total mesorectal excision for rectal cancers

Variable	Male ($n=18$)	Female ($n=15$)	P value
BMI (kg/m^2)	34.1 ± 3.3	33.3 ± 3.5	0.495
EBL (mL)	227.8 ± 148.7	210 ± 163.9	0.746
TME time (min)	110.2 ± 30.6	109.3 ± 40.5	0.947
LOS (days)	6.1 ± 2.4	6.7 ± 2.5	0.471
Conversions, n (%)	1 (5.6)	0	1.000
CRM positivity, n (%)	3 (16.7)	0	0.233
Node yield	14.4 ± 4.9	17.9 ± 9.1	0.233

Prasad LM, Marecik SJ, Park JJ 2013, unpublished data

All values expressed as mean$\pm$SD except where indicated

BMI body mass index, *EBL* estimated blood loss, *TME* total mesorectal excision, *LOS* length of stay, *CRM* circumferential resection margin

two cohorts (Table 19.1). Operative times are expectedly higher and blood loss more in the obese subgroup, but all other parameters are similar. Conversion rates are also negligible compared to the 44 % quoted by some authors, when laparoscopic TME is performed in the obese. The mean BMI at which conversion occurs is also higher in robotic rectal surgery (41.5–44) compared to that in laparoscopy [7]. Comparison of a cohort of obese patients with respect to outcomes between males and females also revealed no difference; this is surprising given the fact that the female pelvis is wider and much easier to operate in, especially robotically (Table 19.2). The implication is that the robot levels the playing field in the patient with rectal cancer irrespective of location, BMI, sex and prior chemoradiation. In essence this technology abrogates the negative influence and connotations of obesity in the minimally invasive approach to rectal cancers.

19.8 Conclusions

Robotic surgery is technically feasible and safe in the obese patient and can be used for the entire spectrum of pathologies and at all sites. Problems with patient optimisation, positioning, access and creation of the abdominal domain are the norm, and the use of standard protocols developed for laparoscopic surgery is to be incorporated. The use of laparoscopy either in its pure form or as a hand-assisted approach is encouraged in the morbidly obese patient to expedite the operation as part of the hybrid approach especially in the operation for rectal cancers. Considerable experience must be accrued in robotic surgery before venturing into the obese patient robotically. The greatest benefit of this technology is in the management of low rectal cancers in the obese male pelvis. In these situations the robot neutralises the difference between the obese and the nonobese patients and levels the playing field.

References

1. Jayne DG, Thorpe HC, Copeland J, et al. Five-year follow-up of the Medical Research Council CLASICC trial of laparoscopically assisted versus open surgery for colorectal cancer. Br J Surg. 2010;97:1638–45.

2. Fleshman J, Sargent DJ, Green E, et al. Laparoscopic colectomy for cancer is not inferior to open surgery based on 5-year data from the COST Study Group trial. Ann Surg. 2007;246:655–62.

3. Guillou PJ, Quirke P, Thorpe H, et al. Short-term endpoints of conventional versus laparoscopic-assisted surgery in patients with colorectal cancer (MRC CLASICC trial): multicentre randomised controlled trial. Lancet. 2005;365:1718–26.

4. Abraham NS, Young JM, Solomon MJ. Meta-analysis of short-term outcomes after laparoscopic resection for colorectal cancer. Br J Surg. 2004;91:1111–24.

5. Schwenk W, Haase O, Neudecker J, et al. Short term benefits for laparoscopic colorectal resection. Cochrane Database Syst Rev. 2005;(3):CD003145.

6. Gendall KA, Raniga S, Kennedy R, Frizelle FA. The impact of obesity on outcome after major colorectal surgery. Dis Colon Rectum. 2007;50:2223–37.

7. Singh A, Girivasan M, Pawa N, et al. Laparoscopic colorectal cancer surgery in obese patients. Colorectal Dis. 2011;13:878–83.

8. Scheidbach H, Benedix F, Hügel O, et al. Laparoscopic approach to colorectal procedures in the obese patient: risk factor or benefit? Obes Surg. 2008;18:66–70.

9. Makino T, Shukla PJ, Samuels JD, Rubino F, Milsom JW. Identifying specific surgical tools and methods for laparoscopic colorectal operations in obese patients. J Gastrointest Surg. 2012;16:2304–11.

10. Flegal KM, Carroll MD, Kit BK, Ogden CL. Prevalence of obesity and trends in the distribution of body mass index among US adults, 1999-2010. JAMA. 2012;307:491–7.

11. Moyad MA. Current methods used for defining, measuring and treating obesity. Semin Urol Oncol. 2001;19:247–52.

12. Patel NM, Patel MS. Medical complications of obesity and optimization of the obese patient for colorectal surgery. Clin Colon Rectal Surg. 2011;24:211–21.

13. Borg BB, Gupta NK, Zuckerman GR, Banerjee B, Gyawali CP. Impact of obesity on bowel preparation for colonoscopy. Clin Gastroenterol Hepatol. 2009;7:670–5.

14. Leroy J, Ananian P, Rubino F, Claudon B, Mutter D, Marescaux J. The impact of obesity on technical feasibility and postoperative outcomes of laparoscopic left colectomy. Ann Surg. 2005;241:69–76.

15. Kuruba R, Koche LS, Murr MM. Preoperative assessment and perioperative care of patients undergoing bariatric surgery. Med Clin North Am. 2007;91(3):339–51. 3.

16. Modig J. Influence of regional anesthesia, local anesthetics, and sympathicomimetics on the pathophysiology of deep vein thrombosis. Act Chir Scand Suppl. 1989;550:119–24.

17. Winfree CJ, Kline DG. Intraoperative positioning nerve injuries. Surg Neurol. 2005;63:5–18.

18. Velchuru VR, Domajnko B, deSouza A, Marecik S, Prasad LM, Park JJ, Abcarian H. Obesity increases the risk of postoperative peripheral neuropathy after minimally invasive colon and rectal surgery. Dis Colon Rectum. 2014;57(2):187–93.

19. Sabeti N, Tarnoff M, Kim J, Shikora S. Primary midline peritoneal access with optical trocar is safe and effective in morbidly obese patients. Surg Obes Relat Dis. 2009;5:610–4.

20. Farley D, Greenlee S, Larson D, Harrington J. Double-blind, prospective, randomized study of warmed, humidified carbon dioxide insufflation vs standard carbon dioxide for patients undergoing laparoscopic cholecystectomy. Arch Surg. 2004;139:739–44.

21. Ambardar S, Cabot J, Cekic V, Baxter K, Arnell TD, Forde KA, Nihalani A, Whelan RL. Abdominal wall dimensions and umbilical position vary widely with BMI and should be taken into account when choosing port locations. Surg Endosc. 2009;23:1995–2000.

22. Hurd WW, Bude RO, DeLancey JO, Pearl ML. The relationship of the umbilicus to the aortic bifurcation: implications for laparoscopic technique. Obstet Gynecol. 1992;80:48–51.

23. Martin ST, Stocchi L. Laparoscopic colorectal resection in the obese patient. Clin Colon Rectal Surg. 2011;24:263–73.

24. DeSouza A, Domajnko B, Park J, Marecik S, Prasad L, Abcarian H. Incisional hernia, midline versus low transverse incision: what is the ideal incision for specimen extraction and hand-assisted laparoscopy? Surg Endosc. 2011;25:1031–6.

25. Park SY, Choi GS, Park JS, Kim HJ, Choi WH, Ryuk JP. Robot-assisted right colectomy with lymphadenectomy and intracorporeal anastomosis for colon cancer: technical considerations. Surg Laparosc Endosc Percutan Tech. 2012;22(5):e271–6.

26. Choi DJ, Kim SH, Lee PJ, et al. Single stage totally robotic dissection for rectal cancer surgery: technique and short term outcome in 50 consecutive patients. Dis Colon Rectum. 2009;52:1824–30.

27. Park YA, Kim JM, Kim SA, et al. Totally robotic surgery for rectal cancer: from splenic flexure to floor in one setup. Surg Endosc. 2009;24:715–20.

28. Zawadzki M, Velchuru VR, Albalawi SA, Park JJ, Marecik S, Prasad LM. Is hybrid robotic laparoscopic assistance the ideal approach for restorative rectal cancer dissection? Colorectal Dis. 2013;15:1026–32.

29. Baik SH, Kim NK, Lim DR, Hur H, Min BS, Lee KY. Oncologic outcomes and perioperative clinico-pathologic results after robot-assisted tumor-specific mesorectal excision for rectal cancer. Ann Surg Oncol. 2013;20:2625–32.

30. MacFarlane JK, Ryall RD, Heald RJ. Mesorectal excision for rectal cancer. Lancet. 1993;341:457–60.

31. Marecik SJ, Zawadzki M, Desouza AL, Park JJ, Abcarian H, Prasad LM. Robotic cylindrical abdominoperineal resection with transabdominal levator transection. Dis Colon Rectum. 2011;54:1320–5.

Robotic Use in Inflammatory Bowel Disease

20

Konstantin Umanskiy

Abstract

Robotic surgical approach for patients with inflammatory bowel disease (IBD) provides several potential advantages, particularly to the surgeons who are early in their robotic learning curve. Unlike the operations for malignant tumors with strict requirements for precise oncologic resection such as high ligation of the mesenteric vessels or total mesorectal excision, the operations for IBD allow some leeway for the surgeon who is just embarking on adaptation of the robotic technique. On the other hand, operations for IBD could be complex and technically challenging due to inflammation in the operative field resulting in oozing or bleeding; the tissues may be more friable due to preoperative use of steroids or biologics, and the dissection planes can be more difficult to define. Nevertheless, robotic surgery for IBD has several advantages to the patients, particularly those requiring low pelvic dissection for an ileal pouch-anal anastomosis (IPAA) procedure or patients with Crohn's disease requiring proctectomy. This chapter will focus primarily on technique of low pelvic dissection where robotic advantages are the most pronounced.

Keywords

Robotic surgery • Inflammatory bowel disease • Crohn's disease • Ulcerative Colitis • Proctectomy • J-pouch

Electronic supplementary material: The online version of this chapter (doi: 10.1007/978-3-319-09120-4_20) contains supplementary material, which is available to authorized users. Videos can also be accessed at http://link.springer.com/book/10.1007/978-3-319-09120-4_ 20.

K. Umanskiy, M.D. (✉)
Department of Surgery, University of Chicago, Chicago, IL, USA
e-mail: kumanskiy@surgery.bsd.uchicago.edu

20.1 Introduction

The application of a robotic platform to minimally invasive surgery in inflammatory bowel disease (IBD) continues to evolve. The most well-established minimally invasive surgical operations in colonic and terminal ileal IBD such as segmental colectomy and total abdominal colectomy have also been adapted for the robotic approach [1, 2] and are covered elsewhere in this book. In contrast, the technique of laparoscopic proctectomy for J-pouch or completion proctectomy for Crohn's disease has been slow to gain acceptance largely due to technical difficulties from exposure and handling of the rectum within the confines of a deep and often narrow pelvis. Robotic surgery provides unique advantages to overcome these limitations and, therefore, serves as a valid alternative to the laparoscopic technique in approaching the patients requiring proctectomy in IBD. While adherence to principles of total mesorectal excision (TME) is not required in benign disease, this technique is preferred because it allows dissection in the relatively bloodless plane. Our group has previously reported on the benefit of the staged approach in patients who require a restorative proctocolectomy for Ulcerative Colitis (UC) or total proctocolectomy in Crohn's disease [3]. In our practice, we advise patients with severe UC or Crohn's disease to undergo proctectomy following the recovery period after a laparoscopic total abdominal colectomy. In patients who are otherwise candidates for total proctocolectomy, the procedure is done as a hybrid approach with the total abdominal colectomy performed laparoscopically, and the proctectomy is performed using the robotic technique. We have previously reported our experience with robotic proctectomy (Video 20.1) for either a J-pouch or completion proctectomy in Crohn's disease [4]. We noted similar functional and postoperative outcomes between laparoscopic and approaches with an added benefit of robotic surgery providing improved ergonomics for the surgeon and precision of dissection within the pelvis.

The goal of this chapter is to outline the steps of the room setup and operative steps in low pelvic dissection for IBD. While the proctectomy technique for J-pouch compared to completion proctectomy in Crohn's disease are mostly similar, a few differences between the port placement will be outlined within this chapter.

20.2 Indications for Robotic Proctectomy in IBD

Almost all patients in our practice undergo laparoscopic or conventional open total abdominal colectomy prior to being considered for proctectomy. Separating these two procedures is important in improving the patient's physiological reserve prior to undergoing proctectomy, which is a technically demanding and physiologically taxing procedure. Moreover, proctectomy should always be done as an elective procedure with careful preoperative planning, counseling, and understanding of patient's wishes and expectations. Since almost all of our patients undergo total abdominal colectomy with either laparoscopic or laparoscopic hand-assisted approach, we encounter little or no adhesions within the abdominal cavity and, therefore, find it rather straightforward to reenter the abdomen and establish the pneumoperitoneum at the time of robotic proctectomy. Another advantage of separating the colectomy and proctectomy into two different operations is to allow the surgeon to perform the robotic proctectomy, the operation as an initial step of an operation. It may be ill-advised to perform minimally invasive proctocolectomy with robotic proctectomy as a single procedure, especially early in one's robotic practice. The surgeons may find themselves docking the robot several hours into the operation when they may be tired and frustrated while dealing with other challenging aspects of the operation leading to proctectomy. In order to provide operative flexibility and a backup in case of emergency, we always set up our robotic cases for laparoscopic-robotic hybrid approach. While this in some way clutters the operative field, we find a hybrid approach to be the most effective and safest way in complex situations. Additionally, bedside assistants who in most institutions are surgical residents may not be as familiar with robotic equipment but are quite comfortable with the use of laparoscopic instruments and equipment.

The indications to perform restorative proctectomy with J-pouch or completion proctectomy have been extensively studied and reported [5]. Any patient who is physiologically fit and does not have contraindications to a minimally invasive approach is considered to be a candidate for robotic proctectomy. While there are no clearly described advantages to robotic rectal dissection, we find this technique to be more accurate than the laparoscopic or conventional open technique because it allows better visualization and precise dissection, especially around the superior hypogastric nerves and anteriorly at the level of the seminal vesicles and prostate and within the rectovaginal septum. Since most of our patients who undergo the pouch procedure are young, there are always concerns that pouch procedures or proctectomy in Crohn's disease will negatively affect fecundity [6]. This could be in large part due to the handling of the pelvic organs during the conventional dissection. We speculate that minimizing contact or gentle and careful manipulation only when absolutely necessary of the uterus, fallopian tubes, and ovaries as we tend to do during robotic approach may result in improved fecundity.

The ultimate measure of a satisfactory outcome in a patient who undergoes J-pouch procedure is an excellent pouch function with complete continence and a low degree of inflammation in the remaining rectal cuff [5]. This is achieved by a precisely performed low pelvic dissection, which enables a surgeon to transect the diseased rectum as close to the levators as possible. The robotic approach is ideally suited to work within the deep pelvis where accurate dissection, especially anteriorly, is critical to achieve low dissection of the rectum. A clear advantage of robotics as compared to laparoscopy can be seen during the final stages of pelvic dissection. In laparoscopy, one can struggle with the degradation of motion as the dissection advances deep into the pelvis—exactly at the time where the most accurate and controlled dissection is needed. With the robotic approach, the accuracy of the dissection remains precise regardless of the depth of the dissection. In fact, surgeons can scale the movements down to improve the accuracy of the dissection as one advances deeper into pelvis and begins to work between the rectum and prostate or in the rectovaginal septum.

20.3 Procedure for Robotic Proctectomy

20.3.1 Room Setup

- The room setup will vary based on individual institutions and provider preferences. Our recommendation is to use a spacious room that will accommodate both robotic and laparoscopic equipment.
  - We recommend placing laparoscopic equipment on one side (at our institution patient's right side) and robotic vision tower on the opposite side (patient's left side).
  - We prefer to dock the robotic patient cart between the patient's legs.
- One or two assistants, depending on availability, can assist from both left and right sides of the patient.

20.3.2 Patient Positioning

- Modified lithotomy in Yellofins® stirrups position is preferred. Patient's buttocks should be slightly hanging off the table. The patient's knees are almost fully extended with thighs parallel to the floor.
- Both upper extremities are tucked alongside the patient's body using a draw sheet. We find this to be sufficient to secure the patient to the table. We do not routinely tape the patient to the table unless the patient is obese or we anticipate the need for significant tilting.

20.3.2.1 Port Placement
- We begin by inserting a 12 mm port supraumbilically (Fig. 20.1). This is done by dissecting the base of the umbilicus and incising the fascia just at the base of the umbilicus under direct visualization. We use a 12 mm bladeless trocar that can be easily grasped by the robotic camera clamp.

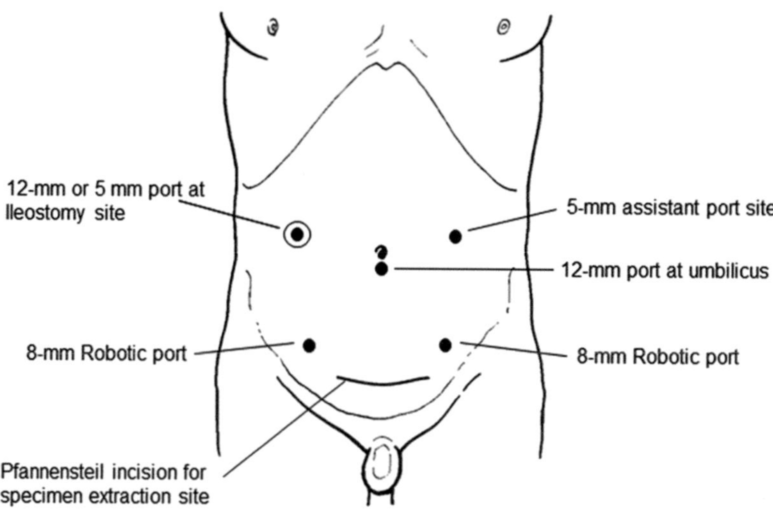

Fig. 20.1 Robotic IPAA port placement diagram. 12 mm camera port can be placed supra- or infraumbilically. Right upper quadrant port can be placed either through the ileostomy opening for IPAA or next to the ileostomy for completion proctectomy

- Initially we begin with laparoscopic approach using 10 mm 30° laparoscope.
- Two 8 mm robotic cannulas are placed 8 cm caudally to the umbilical port site approximately along the mid-clavicular line.
- Two 5 mm ports to be used by the assistants are placed in the left and right upper quadrants.
  - In case of the proctectomy for J-pouch procedure, we initially begin with the takedown of end ileostomy (almost all of our patients have previously undergone laparoscopic total abdominal colectomy). Through the stoma opening, we place a 12 mm balloon tipped port. The remainder of the ports are placed as indicated above.
  - In case of a completion proctectomy for Crohn's disease, care must be taken to avoid injury to the ileostomy while placing the ports.
- It is important not to place robotic cannulas too laterally as the range of motion of robotic instruments will be limited due to high likelihood of their collision with pelvic sidewall as rectal dissection advances into deep pelvis.
- Occasionally, the positions of robotic cannulas have to be adjusted caudally or cephalad to assure that the instrument will reach into the deep pelvis. Prior to inserting the robotic cannula, the surgeon can place a robotic instrument over the patient's abdomen to assess whether the ports are at an optimal distance from the final point of dissection within the deep pelvis.

20.4 Initial Laparoscopic Dissection

- We begin by laparoscopic surveillance of the abdominal cavity and adhesiolysis if necessary.
- In thin patients, left ureter can often be visualized through the peritoneum. If the left ureter is not clearly visible, the peritoneum over right pararectal sulcus is incised and the plane advancing from right to left is developed within the bloodless plane just posterior to the superior hemorrhoidal artery. The left ureter can be identified along the pelvic sidewall using this technique, which is similar to the medial-to-lateral approach used for initial dissection during low anterior resection.
- Once the left ureter is identified and protected, the superior hemorrhoidal artery is ligated and divided with a bipolar energy device.
- In case of J-pouch procedure, we would also elongate the mesentery of the distal ileum using a laparoscopic technique to assure sufficient reach of the J-pouch.

- The uterus is retracted anteriorly by suspending it with sutures using a Keith needle placed through its fundus and brought through the anterior abdominal wall.
- Following that, the robot can be docked.

20.4.1 Docking the Patient-Side Cart

- The patient is placed in approximately 30° Trendelenburg position.
- The robotic patient's cart is docked between the legs.
  - We begin with 30° down robotic scope placed through the umbilical port. The use of the 30° down robotic scope allows for better visualization of the pelvic structures located posteriorly within the pelvis, particularly superior hypogastric nerve trunks as we advance over sacral promontory. As dissection advances deeper into the pelvis, we switch to 0° scope.

20.4.1.1 Instrument Selection

- For a right-hand instrument, we use a monopolar hook cautery.
- For a left-hand instrument, we use a bipolar single fenestrated grasper.
  - By limiting the number of instruments to only two, we aim to provide simplicity and avoid frequent swapping of the instruments. This also helps to contain the cost of the robotic segment of the operation.
  - We prefer not to use the third robotic arm as retraction provided by an assistant is more dynamic and allows more active involvement of a trainee in the case. However, if no appropriate assistant is available, a fourth arm can be used with the double fenestrated bowel grasper placed through the left upper quadrant port.
  - We routinely use normal scaling of robotic masters during the initial segments of the operation and occasionally switch to fine scaling for deep pelvic dissection in the rectovaginal and recto-prostatic plane.
- The assistant grasps the rectum with the bowel grasper from the left upper quadrant port and retracted anteriorly and cephalad. Either the same assistant or a different assistant uses laparoscopic suction inserted through the right upper quadrant port to help with smoke evacuation and gentle retraction if needed.
- We use heated CO_2 insufflation, which helps to decrease the scope fogging.

20.4.2 Posterior Dissection

- Rectal dissection begins in posterior plane. We prefer the TME plane because it provides a relatively bloodless plane of dissection and creates an anatomical reference point from which lateral and interior dissection can proceed.
- With an assistant retracting the rectum anteriorly and cephalad, the robotic single fenestrated grasper retracts the posterior aspect of the mesorectum anteriorly and slightly caudally. When performed correctly, the surgeon can visualize a "cotton candy"-like areolar tissue between the fascia propria of the rectum and presacral fascia. While applying continued traction with the grasper, the hook cautery is used to divide the tissue in a U-shaped fashion. The dissection is taken to the level of Waldeyer's fascia. Care must be taken to follow the TME plane of dissection anteriorly as one advances deeper in the pelvis. Failure to do that may result in troublesome bleeding from the presacral veins.
- Pigazzi [7] has proposed a variation of a posterior dissection technique as it applies to the robotic approach. In this technique, the dissection posteriorly proceeds in an oblique fashion including the division of the tissue along the right lateral stalk curving posteriorly and to the left. This approach allows excellent exposure of the pelvis since the surgeon is no longer "working in the hole" of straight posterior dissection. By carrying this dissection slightly to the left within the TME plane, it helps to provide an initial dissection of the left lateral aspect where anatomical relationships of the mesorectum and the left ureter could be more challenging.

20.4.3 Lateral Dissection and Division of Lateral Stalks

- The lateral dissection proceeds initially on the right side where the surgeon has a safer plane of dissection.
- Retraction by a robotic grasper is achieved by angling it in approximately 90° to create a retracting a "hockey stick."
- A monopolar hook moves from posterior to anterior in a deliberate pace while applying current. It is important to control all vessels, even the ones that appear to be only mildly oozing. Failure to do so may result in the field becoming bloody and dark.
- If one encounters a vessel (middle rectal artery or vein), it must be coagulated using a bipolar grasper while retracting the mesorectum with the hook. After the vessel is coagulated, it can be divided with hook cautery.
- While advancing lateral dissection, the surgeon must check the progress in relation to the anterior aspect visualizing the cul-de-sac or prostate in order to avoid carrying the dissection past the desired anterior plane.
- The left lateral side is dissected by dividing the peritoneum over the left pararectal sulcus. The left ureter must be visualized during this step. If the right and posterior dissection was performed correctly, the only structures that need to be divided are a layer of peritoneum and a small amount of remaining lateral stalks.

20.4.4 Anterior Dissection

- As the dissection advances anteriorly, the right and left lateral peritoneal incisions that are created during lateral dissection at this point are connected in front of the rectum.
- At this stage in operation, with the switch to a 0° scope and change of the retraction of the rectum from anterior and cephalad to posterior and cephalad, the rectum is pulled straight out of the pelvis. Because the posterior dissection has now released the mesorectum, the rectum can be easily stretched placing under tension the anterior plane of dissection.

- The surgeon needs to identify a bloodless areolar plane anteriorly. This can be done by gently pressing the rectum posteriorly, thus performing a blunt dissection. Once the correct plane has been identified and the initial anterior dissection has begun, the attention is once again turned to the lateral and posterior dissection.

20.4.5 Circumferential Dissection of the Rectum

- The unique aspect of the pelvic dissection for a J-pouch procedure is the requirement for mobilization of the rectum to the level of pelvic floor and occasionally performing some dissection within the levator muscle complex. This is done in order to achieve a very short rectal cuff of the remaining rectum in order to minimize the chance of inflammation referred to as "cuffitis."
- As the surgeon advances towards the pelvic floor, the dissection alternates between the posterior, lateral, and interior planes as the tissue tension changes based on dissection performed. For example, in order to obtain sufficient tension on the tissue to perform additional posterior dissection, the surgeon may need to dissect the anterior and lateral aspects first. Once this is accomplished, the posterior plane of dissection presents itself better and can be easily divided.
- One of the signs that the dissection is at the level of pelvic floor is observation of *levator ani* skeletal muscle fibers that contract upon contact with electrocautery and the tapering of the mesorectum. As it narrows at the level of pelvic floor, the rectum can be carefully grasped with a robotic grasper and retracted to obtain the necessary tension to provide dissection.
- An assistant may need to perform a limited rectal exam to assess the level of dissection. Preferably the dissection should continue to as low as 2–3 cm from anal verge.
- Once full circumferential dissection is complete, the robot is undocked.

20.4.6 Rectal Transection and J-Pouch Anastomosis

- Despite advances in the laparoscopic and robotic stapling technology, we have not found a satisfactory stapler to perform an intra-corporeal rectal transection. We prefer to make a limited Pfannenstiel incision in order to use a handheld stapler.
  - Some surgeons may prefer to use a laparoscopic stapler. In order to achieve a low transection, the smallest length cartridge should be used. Because a single laparoscopic stapler fire is unlikely to completely transect the rectum, it is important to avoid overlapping or crossing the staple lines as multiple stapler fires are performed.
- We encourage those surgeons who are just embarking on robotic proctectomy for J-pouch to consider making the small Pfannenstiel incision at the beginning of the robotic segment of the operation and cover it with a gel port. This will provide an additional level of safety should an emergency occur. A surgeon can rapidly enter the abdomen with the hand and compress a bleeding vessel or place laparotomy pads to control hemorrhage.
- For completion proctectomy in Crohn's disease, the rectum is removed through the perineal incision via an intersphincteric dissection.

20.5 The Evidence for Robotic Use in IBD

There is a relative paucity of literature on robotic surgery for IBD. While in personal communications, most robotic colorectal surgeons endorse performing rectal dissection for IBD, most have not accumulated sufficient series to report in literature. Our group has reported on the initial series of patients with Crohn's disease and UC who underwent restorative proctectomy with the J-pouch or completion proctectomy [4]. This group of patients was compared to a laparoscopic cohort via case match. We demonstrated the equivalent outcomes between laparoscopic and robotic groups. The robotic approach was shown to be safe and effective and importantly resulting in similar functional outcomes and pouch function. The robotic procedures, however, were longer compared to laparoscopic ones. It is reasonable to anticipate that robotic time will improve with experience, which was demonstrated by Byrn at al. [8] . Even though this paper did not have a comparison group, the authors demonstrated that their operative time and cost have improved over time. This cohort included only 18 patients with IBD out of 51 patients in the study. Two other smaller studies by Pedraza [9] and McLemore [10] demonstrated their groups' initial experiences with robotic surgery for IBD. All of the available studies addressed only proctectomy for IBD.

20.6 Conclusions

The greatest benefit of robotic surgery for IBD appears to be related to proctectomy for Crohn's disease or restorative proctectomy with J-pouch for UC. As in many other robotic applications, the benefit of robotic surgery is greatest in the confines of a deep, narrow pelvis where low pelvic dissection with precise tissue handling is required. While rectal dissection in IBD may be in many aspects similar to TME for cancer, the unique aspect of distal dissection and the need of carrying the dissection to the level of the levators make the robotic approach particularly advantageous. We find that completion proctectomy for Crohn's disease is an ideal case with which to begin the learning curve of robotic proctectomy. On the other hand, robotic dissection for IPAA is a higher stakes procedure, where even minor injury to the distal rectum can result in significant intraoperative challenges.

20.7 Key Points

- The robotic approach to the patient with IBD should be based on the same principles as in laparoscopic or conventional surgery—the robotic approach, however, requires additional equipment, a larger room, a more complex setup, and a learning curve for the surgeon, assistants, and operating room staff.

- Most of the robotic procedures in IBD are performed using laparoscopic-robotic hybrid approach. Port placement and patient positioning should satisfy all of the steps of both laparoscopic and robotic segments of the operation in order to improve ergonomics and avoid collisions with the robotic arms.
- Stay consistent! The operating team and bedside assistants will work best if you have little variation from case to case in regard to case progression, use of instruments, and changes in patient positioning.
- Have all appropriate equipment and staff education in the event of an unexpected outcome or an emergency. The surgeon needs to have ability to re-scrub quickly if the bedside assistants have difficulty managing robotic patient cart at the bedside.

References

1. Marcello PW, Milsom JW, Wong SK, Brady K, Goormastic M, Fazio VW. Laparoscopic total colectomy for acute colitis: a case-control study. Dis Colon Rectum. 2001;44(10):1441–5.
2. Milsom JW, Lavery IC, Bohm B, Fazio VW. Laparoscopically-assisted ileocolectomy in Crohn's disease. Surg Laparosc Endosc. 1993;3(2):77–80.
3. Pandey S, Luther G, Umanskiy K, Malhotra G, Rubin MA, Hurst RD, et al. Minimally invasive pouch surgery for ulcerative colitis: is there a benefit in staging? Dis Colon Rectum. 2011;54(3):306–10.
4. Miller AT, Berian JR, Rubin M, Hurst RD, Fichera A, Umanskiy K. Robotic-assisted proctectomy for inflammatory bowel disease: a case-matched comparison of laparoscopic and robotic technique. J Gastrointest Surg. 2012;16(3):587–94.
5. Michelassi F, Lee J, Rubin M, Fichera A, Kasza K, Karrison T, et al. Long-term functional results after ileal pouch anal restorative proctocolectomy for ulcerative colitis: a prospective observational study. Ann Surg. 2003;238(3):433–41. discussion 42-5. PMCID: 1422709.
6. Rink AD, Radinski I, Vestweber KH. Does mesorectal preservation protect the ileoanal anastomosis after restorative proctocolectomy? J Gastrointest Surg. 2009;13(1):120–8.
7. Pigazzi A, Ellenhorn JD, Ballantyne GH, Paz IB. Robotic-assisted laparoscopic low anterior resection with total mesorectal excision for rectal cancer. Surg Endosc. 2006;20(10):1521–5.
8. Byrn JC, Hrabe JE, Charlton ME. An initial experience with 85 consecutive robotic-assisted rectal dissections: improved operating times and lower costs with experience. Surg Endosc. 2014;28(11):3101–7.
9. Pedraza R, Patel CB, Ramos-Valadez DI, Haas EM. Robotic-assisted laparoscopic surgery for restorative proctocolectomy with ileal J-pouch-anal anastomosis. Minim Invasive Ther Allied Technol. 2011;20(4):234–9.
10. McLemore EC, Cullen J, Horgan S, Talamini MA, Ramamoorthy S. Robotic-assisted laparoscopic stage II restorative proctectomy for toxic ulcerative colitis. Int J Med Robot. 2012;8(2):178–83.

Robotic Training

Elizabeth McKeown and Amir Loucas Bastawrous

Abstract

Robotic surgery requires a complex set of skills not entirely scalable from laparoscopic or open surgery. While some of the robotic maneuvers are more natural than matched traditional laparoscopic steps, the platform, surgical conduct, and planning are foreign to most surgeons. This is evident in the long learning curve to achieve technical proficiency. To facilitate learning, a graded approach has shown promise to efficiently ramp up to safe operations.

Keywords

Robotic surgery • Training • Simulation • Resident training • Evaluation

21.1 Introduction

When new technologies or medical devices are introduced into clinical medicine, there is an initial period during which practitioners learn to use them. For relatively simple devices or those that are iterative advancements of established products, this training period may last as little as a few minutes. However, for more complicated devices, those that are associated with high risk or those that are entirely new platforms, the training of clinicians becomes more complicated. These latter situations, among which robotic surgery utilizing the Intuitive Surgical da Vinci® system (Intuitive Surgical, Sunnyvale, CA) clearly includes, require comprehensive education of the end users. Efficient instruction utilizes an established curriculum and pathway to competency and will differ depending on the students' level of prior experience. See Tables 21.1 and 21.2 [1–3].

21.2 Components of Robotic Training

While there are not yet consistent and enforceable regulations to robotics training, there are guidelines published by Intuitive Surgical, Inc.,

E. McKeown, M.D.
Swedish Colon and Rectal Clinic, 1101 Madison, Suite 510, Seattle, WA 98104, USA
e-mail: Bastawrous@gmail.com

A.L. Bastawrous, M.D., M.B.A. (✉)
Department of Surgery, Swedish Cancer Institute, Seattle, WA, USA
e-mail: Amir.bastawrous@swedish.org

© Springer International Publishing Switzerland 2015
H. Ross et al. (eds.), *Robotic Approaches to Colorectal Surgery*,
DOI 10.1007/978-3-319-09120-4_21

Table 21.1 Differences between training residents, fellows, and attending surgeons

	Resident	Colorectal resident (Fellow)	Attending
Laparoscopic experience	Hurdle	Advantage	Advantage[a]
Diversity of cases available	Advantage	Hurdle	Hurdle
Time and income investment	Advantage	Advantage	Hurdle
Interest and acceptance of robotics	Advantage	Advantage	Advantage[a]
Available mentor	Advantage	Advantage[a]	Hurdle
Understand anatomy, tissue dynamics and general surgical principles	Hurdle	Advantage	Advantage
Access to patients and training	Hurdle	Advantage[a]	Advantage
Available robot	Hurdle	Advantage[a]	Advantage[a]
Available of skilled trainers or proctors	Hurdle	Advantage[a]	Hurdle
Sufficient time to learn the technology	Advantage	Hurdle if naïve entering fellowship	Hurdle

[a]In the proper setting with a motivated and experienced team, these are advantages

Table 21.2 Components of robotics training

	Resident	Fellow	Attending
Online modules	X	X	X
Video review of complete cases	X	X	X
Dry lab on inanimate models	X	X	X
Animal lab	+/−	+/−	X
Cadaver lab	+/−	+/−	X
Simulation	X	X	X
Bedside assist	X	X	+/−
Proctored cases	−	−	X
Dual console	X	X	+/−

surgical journals, and professional societies. The disadvantages of colorectal surgery has had to date as a specialty in adopting robotic surgery have been a lack of appropriate tools, more variability to surgical procedures and more complex and higher risk operations. But robotic colorectal surgery has the advantage of following robotic urology and gynecology in acceptance and penetration. This allows colorectal surgeons to benefit from the experiences of these other specialties with regard to what works in robotic training.

21.3 Simulator

Training includes time on a simulation console. The digital nature of robotic surgery has lent itself to the development of robust simulation opportunities utilizing the robotic surgical console as they would in the real world. Skill exercises have been identified to facilitate efficient learning of the da Vinci Surgical System and specific skills such as intracorporeal knot tying (Fig. 21.1). These exercises can be performed an unlimited number of times with scores assigned to the trainee with each attempt. This provides immediate feedback, assists with goal setting, and provides an opportunity to compare one trainee with another. There is also the added incentive for the trainee to compete with other users. The opportunity to practice prior to an actual operation helps the trainee as well as the established surgeon. Studies have shown a shortening of the learning curve with the use of the robotic simulator.

A systematic review of all available simulators was performed; though there are too few studies to make valid conclusions about which is the best, one group found that all simulators functioned to train surgeons well before performing in vivo robotic resections [4]. A training metric, the Robotic Skills Assessment Score (RSA-Score), was validated in 2013 in order to score practitioners based on skill [5]. Safety, critical error, economy, bimanual dexterity, and time management were the parameters measured.

A multi-institutional "Fundamental Skills of Robotic Surgery" (FSRS) is a simulation curriculum based on the da Vinci robotic system that has been developed and is in use. It has been validated and shows significant improvement in basic

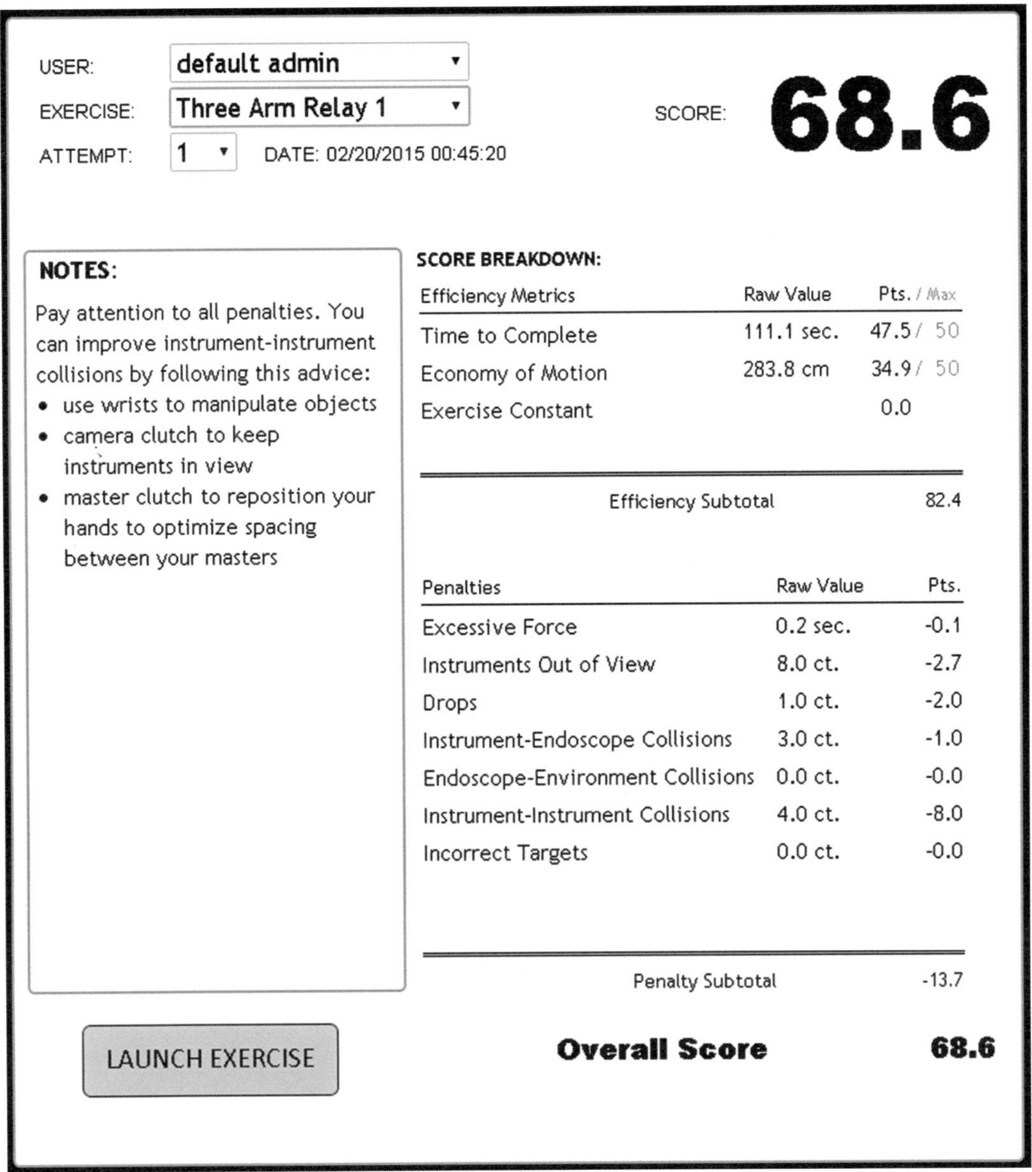

SCORE BREAKDOWN:		
Efficiency Metrics	Raw Value	Pts. / Max
Time to Complete	111.1 sec.	47.5 / 50
Economy of Motion	283.8 cm	34.9 / 50
Exercise Constant		0.0
Efficiency Subtotal		82.4
Penalties	Raw Value	Pts.
Excessive Force	0.2 sec.	-0.1
Instruments Out of View	8.0 ct.	-2.7
Drops	1.0 ct.	-2.0
Instrument-Endoscope Collisions	3.0 ct.	-1.0
Endoscope-Environment Collisions	0.0 ct.	-0.0
Instrument-Instrument Collisions	4.0 ct.	-8.0
Incorrect Targets	0.0 ct.	-0.0
Penalty Subtotal		-13.7
Overall Score		**68.6**

Fig. 21.1 Simulator skill assessment. *Intuitive Surgical, Inc., Sunnyvale, CA*

robotic skills across specialties [6]. Another group uses deconstructed skills (i.e., docking, positioning, blunt dissection, retraction) in a 23-item training program for their robotic novices [7]. The Hasbro® Game, *Operation* has been used as a more lighthearted and accessible bridge between simulation and in vivo surgery [8].

21.4 Pathways and Evaluation

Pathways to training create a necessary structure to learning. Intuitive Surgical has published suggested pathways to robotic training for operating surgeons, bedside assist, and the operating room staff (Fig. 21.2). Pathways are also being developed

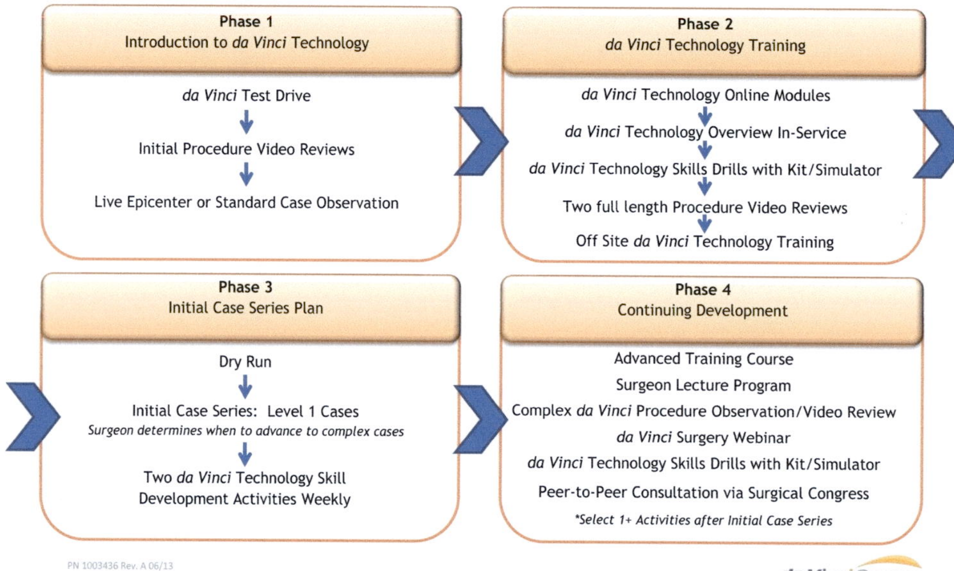

Fig. 21.2 da Vinci® Training Pathway for Surgeons. *Intuitive Surgical, Inc., Sunnyvale, CA*

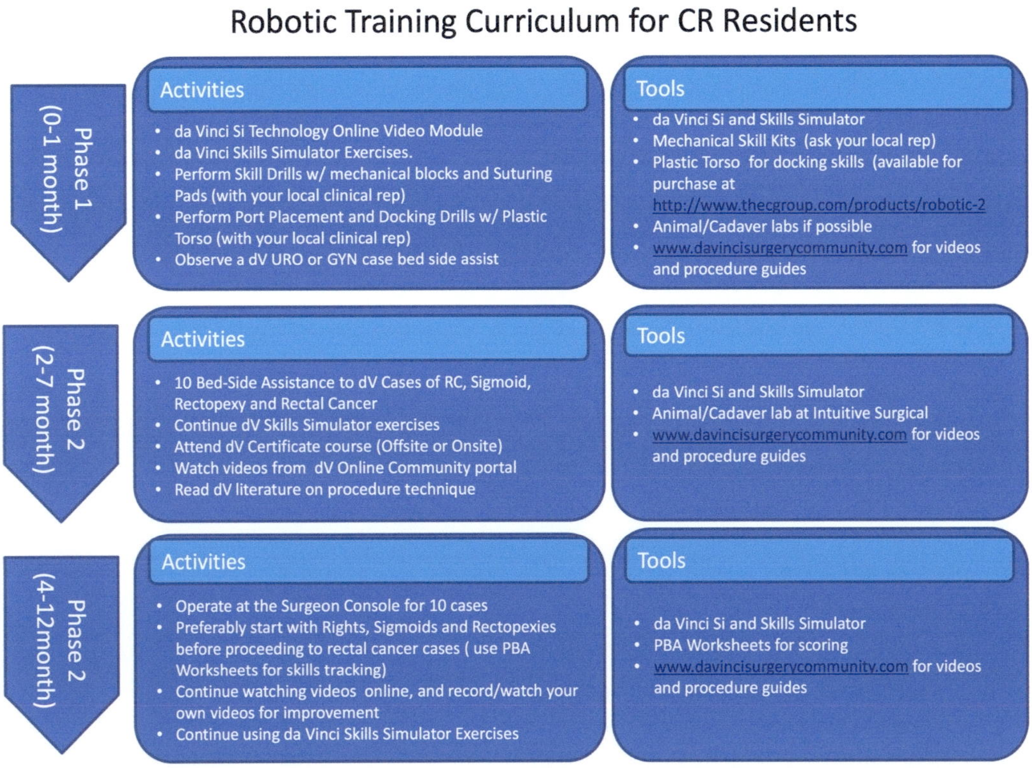

Robotic Training Curriculum for CR Residents

Phase 1 (0-1 month)

Activities
- da Vinci Si Technology Online Video Module
- da Vinci Skills Simulator Exercises.
- Perform Skill Drills w/ mechanical blocks and Suturing Pads (with your local clinical rep)
- Perform Port Placement and Docking Drills w/ Plastic Torso (with your local clinical rep)
- Observe a dV URO or GYN case bed side assist

Tools
- da Vinci Si and Skills Simulator
- Mechanical Skill Kits (ask your local rep)
- Plastic Torso for docking skills (available for purchase at http://www.thecgroup.com/products/robotic-2
- Animal/Cadaver labs if possible
- www.davincisurgerycommunity.com for videos and procedure guides

Phase 2 (2-7 month)

Activities
- 10 Bed-Side Assistance to dV Cases of RC, Sigmoid, Rectopexy and Rectal Cancer
- Continue dV Skills Simulator exercises
- Attend dV Certificate course (Offsite or Onsite)
- Watch videos from dV Online Community portal
- Read dV literature on procedure technique

Tools
- da Vinci Si and Skills Simulator
- Animal/Cadaver lab at Intuitive Surgical
- www.davincisurgerycommunity.com for videos and procedure guides

Phase 2 (4-12month)

Activities
- Operate at the Surgeon Console for 10 cases
- Preferably start with Rights, Sigmoids and Rectopexies before proceeding to rectal cancer cases (use PBA Worksheets for skills tracking)
- Continue watching videos online, and record/watch your own videos for improvement
- Continue using da Vinci Skills Simulator Exercises

Tools
- da Vinci Si and Skills Simulator
- PBA Worksheets for scoring
- www.davincisurgerycommunity.com for videos and procedure guides

Fig. 21.3 Colorectal robotic training curriculum

specifically for colorectal residents (Fig. 21.3). The use of pathways is important not only for guidance but also for identifying areas of deficiency that need further improvement. They also establish a framework for evaluation of the trainee. Assessment tools have also been created with which a trainer can appraise and grade the trainee, thus providing necessary feedback (Fig. 21.4).

21.5 Established Surgeons

Once robotic technology is fully pervasive in surgical training, there will no longer be a need to train established surgeons. If robotics follows the timeline of the experience with laparoscopic surgery (arguably simpler and indisputably less expensive technology), that time will need 10–20 years or more until surgical residents universally graduate with consistent proficiency in robotic surgery. Until that time, there will continue to be a need to teach surgeons who have already completed residency.

Hurdles to Training Graduated Surgeons
- Variable laparoscopic experience
- Diversity of cases limits opportunity to standardize techniques
- Time and income investment
- Lack of interest or acceptance ("if it ain't broke, don't fix it" mentality)
- Don't see or don't believe the benefits outweigh the costs
- Usually don't have active mentor

Advantages to Training Graduated Surgeons
- Laparoscopic experience, tissue dynamics
- Those who decide to learn robotics are typically motivated
- Already understand anatomy, surgical principles
- Have access to patients

Procedure-Based Assessment Tool for Robotic Right Hemicolectomy

ID number of patient

Date of Surgery   Diagnosis

Trainer   Trainee

Detailing	Y/N/NA	Needs further improvement	Plan of action
Consent from the patient (described the pros and cons of the robotic procedure including complications)			
Demonstrate understanding of the pre-operative investigations and the management of the case			
Appropriate prepping and positioning of the patient			
Understands port placements and places ports safely			
Ensures safe Robotic set up and understands the instrumentation			
Performs Safe assistance			
Console experience			
Identifies anatomy and the pathology appropriately			
Handles the tissue without excessive force			
Utilizes the robotic arms ergonomically			
Collision of robotic arms and instrumentation			
Follows previously identified protocol			
Division of the lateral peritoneal attachments			
Division of the gastrocolic ligaments			
Medial to lateral dissection			
Mobilization of the hepatic flexure			
Identifies ileocolic vessels and plane of dissection			
Performs Safe vascular pedicle transection			
Follows good surgical principles for a safe anastomosis			
Closes the abdominal wound appropriately			
Documents orders and operative note correctly			

Complexity of the case: Simple/   Difficult/Very difficult

Learning Outcomes/Comments-

Signature of the trainee..................Signature of the trainer.....................................

Fig. 21.4 Colorectal resident assessment tools

21.6 Surgeons in Training

21.6.1 Residents

Teaching robotic naïve trainees has some benefits when compared to surgeons in practice, but carries with it its own challenges. Residents are still learning the science of surgery, the steps to an operation open and operative anatomy. They also usually lack laparoscopic skills of depth perception, tactile response of tissue to handling, and unique advantages and limitations of laparoscopy. In many ways, they are more receptive to learning because they have not yet had their surgical experience swayed to one approach versus another. Surgical training in the United States has the advantage of time in that compared to established surgeons and fellows, residents have 5 or more years to develop their robotic skills in parallel with their open, endoscopic, and laparoscopic abilities.

Lessons for training residents can be learned from Gynecology and Urology training programs that adopted robotic training years before General Surgery. Gynecologic oncology fellowships looked at the two measures of adequacy of training by the end of fellowship; that is, operative times and lymph node retrieval counts [9]. They found that, after 4 years with a robot at their institution, and with increasing instances of the fellow being the primary surgeon at the console, the fellows' times and nodal counts equaled those of the staff. Transitioning from residency to practice poses another challenge. In the urology literature, robotic prostatectomies are among the most frequent operation currently performed. One surgeon examined the outcomes of his first 100 prostatectomies, in training and beyond, and concluded that the mentorship model in teaching and early exposure to the console are the keys to success [10].

21.6.1.1 Hurdles to Training Residents
- Cost of the technology (up to $2 million) creates slower program adoption
- Lack of robotic surgeons as trainers
- Those surgeons with robotic training are still early in a long learning curve
- Consistent curricula for resident training
- Diversity of types of cases

21.6.1.2 Advantages to Training Residents
- No bad habits
- Have time to learn
- Can learn a variety of surgical procedures
- Have access to direct and continuous mentor

21.6.2 Colorectal Residents (Fellows)

Teaching advanced residents (colorectal fellows) is a unique hybridization of teaching residents and of training established surgeons. Advanced trainees have some of the advantages and disadvantages of each. Unless they are in a dedicated robotics fellowship, these individuals typically have 1 year to learn robotics in addition to other techniques. In colorectal surgery, for example, an incoming colorectal advanced resident will need to become proficient in colonoscopy, office proctology, laparoscopic colon and rectal surgery, open surgery, and a multitude of operations for anorectal disorders, all this in 1 year. Adding robotics means something else may have to be given up, particularly in the era of limited duty hours.

21.6.2.1 Hurdles to Training Colorectal Residents (Fellows)
- Cost of the technology (~$2 million) creates slower program adoption
- Lack of robotic surgeons as trainers
- Lack of robotics training in residency
- Those surgeons with robotic training are still early in a long learning curve and may be unwilling or unable to pass the case onto a trainee
- Diversity of types of cases
- No bad habits
- Have time to learn

21.6.2.2 Advantages to Training Colorectal Residents (Fellows)

- Can perfect a limited number of surgical procedures
- Have access to direct and continuous mentor
- Consistent curricula for training

Robotic training is only now beginning to be integrated into colorectal fellowship. Both manual dexterity and integration into the robotic system are components of becoming comfortable with robotically assisted surgery, and both must be evaluated and improved as part of a training program. As a measure of manual dexterity as opposed to simulation, one urology training program has their residents perform a series of five tasks in an open fashion, laparoscopically, and robotically. They found universally improved surgical technique while open, followed by robotic and then laparoscopic. This institution found that the two tasks that best measured competency were suture and knot tying and threading rings, and so as a result they have increased the focus on these metrics early in training [1]. Importantly, the da Vinci robot overcomes handedness for those surgeons who are less dexterous with their nondominant hand [2]. There are also data to suggest that the steep learning curve found in the transition from open surgery to laparoscopic surgery does not exist in the transition from laparoscopic to robotic-assisted surgery, which may improve those mid-level residents' transition to the console [3].

21.7 Team Training

Despite the unparalleled control that the da Vinci Surgical System affords the minimally invasive surgeon, the complexity of the technology requires a team to be able to operate efficiently and safely. So training of the operating room staff and bedside assist are critical components. Establish and train a consistent team, perform dry runs and document preferences and operative steps to minimize unnecessary variability and maintain a high level of operative quality (See Fig. 21.5).

21.8 Credentialing and Maintenance of Skills

Credentialing has not yet been standardized. The requirements for robotics privileging and maintenance of privileges are widely variable between regions, institutions, and specialties. Some institutions require at least 20 robotic cases per year to maintain robotic privileges while others in the same region may require as few as 10. With time, guidance from national guidelines or regulatory agencies and evidence publication, these differences should disappear.

There is excellent data from Tacoma, Washington, that demonstrates that those surgeons who perform <20 cases per year robotically have worse outcomes, with increased blood loss and longer operative times, than those higher volume surgeon [11]. Though there are no hard and fast rules for low volume surgeons, guidelines suggest that surgeons should perform at least 1–2 robotic cases per month to keep up their skillset [12].

Specifically in regard to colorectal surgery, Jiminez-Rodriguez et al. examined forty-three cases performed by the fellow. They found that the first 9–11 cases consisted of learning technique, the next 12 cases represent consolidation and increased competence, and the final 20 cases represent the "mastery" phase of learning the robot [13]. Bokhari et al. also found this to be true in their study in the learning curve for robot-assisted cases [14]. Interestingly, one attending surgeon who was fairly laparoscopically naïve (13 cases) was able to gain proficiency on the robot within 20 cases for total mesorectal excision without an increase in complications [15]. Another study suggests that the use of the robot may decrease the steep learning curve associated with laparoscopic TME [16].

21.9 Key Points

Robotics training tactics will vary depending on the experience of the trainee.

Components of teaching of robotic surgical skills:

- Online modules
- Video review of cases

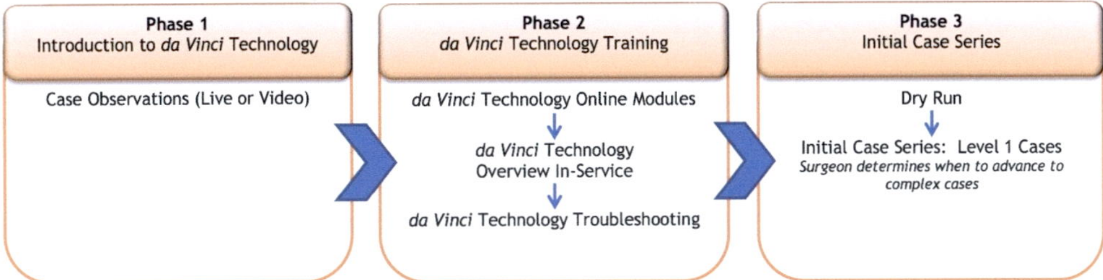

Fig. 21.5 da Vinci® training pathway for operating room team. *Intuitive Surgical, Inc., Sunnyvale, CA*

- In person dry lab on models
- Simulation
- Observation of cases in person
- Bedside assist
- Proctored cases
- Dual console

Objective assessment of results and outcomes are important aspects of quality assessment.

After initial experience, it is helpful to also revisit training in an advanced course or CME activity.

References

1. Menhadji A, Abdelshehid C, Osann K, et al. Tracking and assessment of technical skills acquisition among urology residents for open, laparoscopic, and robotic skills over 4 years: is there a trend? J Endourol. 2013;27(6):783–9.

2. Mucksavage P, Kerbl DC, Lee JY. The da Vinci(®) surgical system overcomes innate hand dominance. J Endourol. 2011;25(8):1385–8.

3. Stolzenburg JU, Qazi HA, Holze S, et al. Evaluating the learning curve of experienced laparoscopic surgeons in robot-assisted radical prostatectomy. J Endourol. 2013;27(1):80–5.

4. Abboudi H, Khan MS, Aboumarzouk O, et al. Current status of validation for robotic surgery simulators—a systematic review. BJU Int. 2013;111(2):194–205.

5. Chowriappa AJ, Shi Y, Raza SJ, et al. Development and validation of a composite scoring system for robot-assisted surgical training—the Robotic Skills Assessment Score. J Surg Res. 2013;185(2):561–9.

6. Stegemann AP, Ahmed K, Syed JR, et al. Fundamental skills of robotic surgery: a multi-institutional randomized controlled trial for validation of a simulation-based curriculum. Urology. 2013;81(4):767–74.

7. Dulan G, Rege RV, Hogg DC, et al. Developing a comprehensive, proficiency-based training program for robotic surgery. Surgery. 2012;152(3):477–88.

8. Falcone JL. Don't touch the sides: a fun and novel system for using Operation(®) for practicing open and robotic surgical skills. Am Surg. 2013;79(5):547–9.

9. Soliman PT, Iglesias D, Munsell MF, et al. Successful incorporation of robotic surgery into gynecologic oncology fellowship training. Gynecol Oncol. 2013;131(3):730–3.

10. Thiel DD, Chavez M, Brisson TE. Transition from resident robotic training program to clinical practice: robotic-assisted radical prostatectomy benchmark for perioperative safety. J Laparoendosc Adv Surg Tech A. 2013;23(6):516–20.

11. Lenihan Jr JP. Navigating credentialing, privileging, and learning curves in robotics with an evidence and experienced-based approach. Clin Obstet Gynecol. 2011;54(3):382–90.

12. Ben-Or S, Nifong LW, Chitwood Jr WR. Robotic surgical training. Cancer J. 2013;19(2):120–3.

13. Jimenez-Rodriguez RM, Diaz-Pavon JM, de la Portilla de Juan F, Prendes-Sillero E, Dussort HC, Padillo J. Learning curve for robotic-assisted laparoscopic rectal cancer surgery. Int J Colorectal Dis. 2013;28(6):815–21.

14. Bokhari MB, Patel CB, Ramos-Valadez DI, Ragupathi M, Haas EM. Learning curve for robotic-assisted laparoscopic colorectal surgery. Surg Endosc. 2011; 25(3):855–60.

15. Kim YW, Lee HM, Kim NK, Min BS, Lee KY. The learning curve for robot-assisted total mesorectal excision for rectal cancer. Surg Laparosc Endosc Percutan Tech. 2012;22(5):400–5.

16. Akmal Y, Baek JH, McKenzie S, Garcia-Aguilar J, Pigazzi A. Robot-assisted total mesorectal excision: is there a learning curve? Surg Endosc. 2012;26(9): 2471–6.

Cost and Outcomes in Robotic-Assisted Laparoscopic Surgery

22

Maher Ghanem, Anthony J. Senagore, and Samuel Shaheen

Abstract

The modern era of advanced laparoscopic surgery is the direct result of the disruptive work of Prof. Dr. Erich Mühe with laparoscopic cholecystectomy in 1985 (Reynolds Jr, JSLS 5(1):89–94, 2001). Since his original work in the field of minimally invasive surgery has incorporated diverse and aggressive refinements of instrumentation and techniques for many operative indications (Reynolds Jr, JSLS 5(1):89–94, 2001). These efforts at reducing surgical stress while improving cosmesis have included reductions in port size/number, altered extraction sites, attempts at hand assistance, and ultimately single port access (Bucher et al., Br J Surg 98(12):1695–1702, 2011). The ultimate goal of all these innovations is to provide our patients with high quality surgical care while maintaining high value.

Keywords

Cost • Robotic surgery • Laparoscopic surgery • Outcomes • Colorectal surgery

The modern era of advanced laparoscopic surgery is the direct result of the disruptive work of Prof. Dr. Erich Mühe with laparoscopic cholecystectomy in 1985 [1]. Since his original work in the field of minimally invasive surgery has incorporated diverse and aggressive refinements of instrumentation and techniques for many operative indications [1]. These efforts at reducing surgical stress while improving cosmesis have included reductions in port size/number, altered extraction sites, attempts at hand assistance, and ultimately single port access [2]. The ultimate goal of all these innovations is to provide our patients with high quality surgical care while maintaining high value.

Robotic-assisted laparoscopic surgery has been the most recent attempt to further refine minimally invasive procedures. The device features EndoWrist instruments, providing seven

M. Ghanem, M.D. (✉) • A.J. Senagore, M.D., M.S., M.B.A. • S. Shaheen, M.D.
Department of Surgery, Central Michigan University (CMU) College of Medicine, 912 S. Washington Avenue, Saginaw, MI 48601, USA
e-mail: maher.ghanem@cmich.edu

degrees of freedom for instrument movement and tremor filtering. It allows surgeons to be in a seated posture for long operation tolerance and permits three-dimensional imaging, real-time radiographic correlation, and easy suture maneuvering [3, 4]. Hyung suggested that the application of robotic technology for general surgery is technically feasible and safe, improves dexterity, allows for better visualization, and attains a high level of precision [5]. However, the widespread adoption is limited by the absence of tactile sensation and the extremely high cost for acquisition and utilization of the technology [5]. The recent appearance in the market of three-dimensional laparoscopic cameras at substantially lower costs further erodes the potential benefits of the robotic platform.

Robotic-assisted laparoscopic surgery has been adopted to perform many general surgical procedures including cholecystectomy, Nissen fundoplication, Heller myotomy, and Roux-en-Y gastric bypass. More recently, colorectal procedures [5, 6] are being incorporated into an ever-growing number of robotic-assisted indications. The da Vinci robot is postulated to provide improved visualization due to incorporation of the three-dimensional viewing system, mitigate surgeon tremor and improve ergonomics [7]. The available data from robotic-assisted laparoscopic procedures, confirms that the majority of patient outcome benefits associated with laparoscopic surgery are maintained, albeit consistently at higher costs.

Robotic-assisted procedures have been widely adopted in urology and increasingly in gynecologic surgery, due to the shorter learning curve for advanced suturing compared to conventional laparoscopy. This is especially true in confined spaces due to the added articulation and the three-dimensional visualization. One of the limitations of conventional laparoscopic surgery results from working with long instruments through a fixed entry point on the surface of the body while watching a screen. This leads to reduced tactile feedback, diminished fine motor control, tremor amplification, and difficult hand–eye coordination [8]. There have been only limited assessments of the recently available three-dimensional laparoscopes; however, the improved visualization contributes significantly to suturing skills compared to traditional two-dimensional optics.

Although both laparoscopic prostatectomy and hysterectomy were described in the 1990s, the percentage of prostatectomies and hysterectomies performed laparoscopically was insignificant until the advent of the surgical robotics. This delay in the adoption of minimally invasive techniques in these two very common pelvic surgeries is directly related to their degree of technical difficulty associated with conventional laparoscopy, especially with laparoscopic intracorporeal suturing. However, it is possible to master the requisite laparoscopic skills without robotic assistance. Therefore, it is imperative that rigorous assessment of cost efficiency and possible reduction in learning curve associated with robotic surgery is performed before widespread adoption of robotics is recommended.

There are significant financial obstacles to universal adoption of robotic-assisted laparoscopic surgery: high cost of the robotic platform, disposable instruments, and annual service contracts. The robotic systems are sold to hospitals for a cost of $1.0–$2.3 million, depending on the model. Mandatory annual service agreements range from $100,000 to $170,000 per year. There are also significant costs related to mandatory training at the manufacturer's facility ($3–4000) and the often required proctoring by an outside surgeon for 3–5 cases ($3000 per session). While the acquisition cost of the da Vinci robotic system is compelling ($1.2–2.4 million), the cost could be offset by the institution if other sources of cost savings can be achieved. However, robotic surgery requires significant costs for disposable or limited use instruments (e.g., shears, needle drivers, graspers, forceps) at a cost of approximately US$1–2000 per instrument every 10 surgeries [9]. These costs are generally higher when compared to the mostly reusable instruments in standard laparoscopic surgery. The available literature suggests that robotic surgery takes consistently longer than open or laparoscopic surgery, thus there is no cost savings in operating room or anesthesia time. This leaves the only potential for cost savings in a decreased length of hospital stay when compared to open. Other limitations to robotic-assisted laparoscopic surgery include the lack of tactile feedback [10], the large and cumbersome footprint of the robot, the fixed positioning of the operating table after the robot has been docked, the longer operative time compared to open surgery, and the limited outcomes data.

Several cost comparison studies have evaluated the relative cost drivers of robotic surgery versus open surgery. The largest cost comparison study was recently published in European Urology by Bolenz et al. [9]. The study compared operating costs (not including maintenance and equipment purchase) of robotic (RALP), laparoscopic (LRP), and open radical prostatectomy (ORP) for prostate cancer in a sample of 643 consecutive patients. Results showed that the cost of RALP was 50 % higher than the cost of ORP even before the cost of purchasing and maintaining the robot was factored in to the calculations. The median cost for the RALP was $6752, followed by LRP at $5687 and RRP at $4437 (all adjusted to 2007 US dollars). RALP had higher surgical supply costs and higher OR cost due to increased average length of procedure. The one cost benefit for RALP was the shorter average length of hospital stay (1 day) relative to LRP and ORP (2 days). However, the shorter RALP hospital stay relative to LRP and ORP did not make up for the RALP higher operating costs, even before considering the additional cost for the purchase and maintenance of the robot. It is also unclear if the all study groups followed the same postoperative plan because both RALP and LRP groups' patients should have had the same minimally invasive advantage. The additional cost for the purchase and maintenance of the robot ($340,000 per year when amortized over a presumed 7 years life of the robot) would add an additional $2698 per patient undergoing a RALP (assuming 126 cases per year) [9].

A similar cost comparison study was recently completed for robotic versus open radical cystectomy for bladder cancer at the University of North Carolina at Chapel Hill. In this study, the 20 most recent cases of robotic cystectomy were compared with the 20 most recent cases of open cystectomy. The total cost (including base OR costs, OR disposable equipment costs, amortized purchase cost of the robot distributed over 5 years, and yearly maintenance costs) of the robotic radical cystectomy was $1640 more than the open radical cystectomy ($16,248 versus $14,608). In the breakdown of the costs, the majority of the difference came from the higher mean fixed OR costs for robotic cases (OR disposable equipment costs, amortized purchase cost, and yearly maintenance cost distributed over 288 cases per year). The OR variable costs were also slightly higher for the robotic cystectomy due to the increased length of these cases.

Similar to the robotic prostatectomy cost data, there was some cost savings due to a shorter postoperative stay as well as a lower frequency of postoperative transfusion after open cystectomy. While these savings were not enough to overcome the increased OR costs of the robotic cystectomy, the cost differential of $1640 per surgery was much closer than the robotic prostatectomy cost study [11].

The field of robotic-assisted laparoscopic surgery is being actively assessed for a variety of applications as demonstrated by the rapid growth and dissemination of the applications for the approach. Yet with the rising cost of health care becoming a critical element in the assessment of value-based health care, one cannot dismiss the need for cost efficiency. At this point in time, the only argument in favor of robotic-assisted laparoscopy from the cost perspective is the reduction in length of stay compared to open surgery. This creates a very high bar when the technology must compete against established laparoscopic procedures performed by trained and highly skilled laparoscopic surgeons. This contention was eloquently presented in a recent review by Satava [12] where the entire cost benefit or adopting robotics was based upon the ability of an institution to create capacity for other sources of revenue generation by other surgical admissions. Under no scenario assessed, did the robotic platform create positive cash flow for the facility.

22.1 Cholecystectomy

Recently, Intuitive Surgical launched an elegant single-incision platform for cholecystectomy designed to resolve many of the technical limitations associated with the single port approach performed with two-dimensional conventional laparoscopy and the frequent need to cross hands. Although the technology is truly groundbreaking, the limited potential benefits associated with single port vs. multiport laparoscopic colectomy (quote the PRCT multicenter trial) coupled with the limited reimbursement for the procedure raises significant concerns regarding the sustainability of the procedure. Unfortunately, these kinds of economic assessments are unavailable at this time.

According to Lucas et al., single-incision surgery when compared to multi-port cholecystectomy was associated with better cosmesis. Patient preference based on cosmesis was more prominent for females, patients younger than 50 years old, and for benign surgical indications. It is interesting that the authors did not query whether patients were willing to pay the additional cost [13]. This concept warrants further assessment because a da Vinci cholecystectomy has higher variable costs compared to an outpatient laparoscopic cholecystectomy ($2383 vs. $1926 per case). As with the Satava analysis, it is unclear that a hospital may be able to offset the added variable cost per robotic single-site cholecystectomy procedure based solely on cost shifting to a more favorable payer mix.

22.2 Colorectal Surgery

There has been a steady increase in reports regarding the role of robotic-assisted laparoscopic colectomy since the initial report in 2001, albeit few data directly comparing conventional to robot-assisted colectomy. There is some data comparing the two techniques in proctectomy, including an ongoing randomized multicenter trial for rectal cancer [14, 15]. In general, the data have supported the feasibility of total mesorectal dissection and suggested a variety of robotic benefits related to the attributes of multiple degrees of freedom and improved three-dimensional imaging. Despite the limited clinical evidence supporting robotic-assisted colectomy, Tyler et al. found a trend toward increased use during the 15-month study period [16]. The authors found no difference in overall morbidity rates between robot-assisted colectomy and conventional laparoscopic colectomy. However, the robotic approach was associated with an increased rate of ostomy a bias in case selection with either greater use in distal resections or less comfort leaving unprotected anastomoses. The operative times were also significantly longer with the robotic approach and are consistent with several other reports. The other consistent theme in this report was an increase in cost, on average, of $3424 per colectomy over the laparoscopic approach. Similarly, a review by Fung et al. of 15 available high quality studies comparing conventional laparoscopic and robotic-assisted laparoscopic colorectal surgery confirmed a longer operative time and total cost [17].

Huettner et al. presented 70 consecutive robotic-assisted laparoscopic colectomies over 5 years. The component operative times for right colectomies were: port setup time 33.6 ± 12.1 (20–64) min, robotic time 147.2 ± 44.4 (53–306) min, and total case time 221.3 ± 43.7 min. The median LOS was 3 (2–27) days. Times for the sigmoid colectomies were: port setup time 30.0 ± 9.8 (10–57) min, robotic time 101.8 ± 25.3 (67–165) min, and total case time 228.4 ± 40.5 (147–323) min. The median LOS was 4 (2–27) days. This was accomplished with a conversion rate of 11 %. The authors concluded that the approach was feasible and appeared safe without providing comparative outcomes to standard laparoscopy [18].

Deutsch et al. provided one of the largest retrospective analyses of 171 patients who underwent robotic and laparoscopic colectomies (79 and 92, respectively). The results indicated no statistical difference in length of stay, time to return of bowel function, and time to discontinuation of patient-controlled analgesia between robotic and laparoscopic left and right colectomies. They did report some of the best data on operating time for laparoscopic versus robotic-assisted as the differences were not clinically relevant (140 min vs. 135 min for right colectomy; 168 min vs. 203 min for left colectomy). The authors did not assess cost [19].

de Souza et al. compared 40 robot-assisted right hemicolectomies to 135 laparoscopic right hemicolectomies performed by a group of highly skilled laparoscopic surgeons at a single institution [20]. There were no significant differences in surgical quality measures or short-term clinical outcomes. Unlike the Deutsch data mentioned earlier, the operative time was significantly longer for the robotic assistance group (158 min vs. 118 min). In addition, the cost was almost $3000 greater despite a similar length of stay, and no difference in complications was shown. The authors concluded that this was a good training case; however, one should be cautioned by the fact that 40 cases were not sufficient for an expert team to match their conventional results [20].

These data question why the putative advantages of robotic assistance fail to translate into tangible superiority in the operating room. In addition, the recurring theme of high cost needs to be addressed by proponents before widespread adoption can be encouraged. Future investigations should focus on direct comparisons with conventional laparoscopic colorectal surgery with an emphasis beyond subjective parameters, which do not translate into superior clinical outcomes with at least equivalent resource consumption [20].

22.3 HPB Procedures

Pancreatic resection is amongst the most complex and challenging of abdominal operations. Even in highly experienced centers, open pancreatic surgery is associated with morbidity rates of 30–40 % and mortality rates of approximately 2 % [21, 22]. New, minimally invasive techniques may reduce postoperative morbidity. Therefore, in recent years, laparoscopic pancreatic surgery has been introduced as an alternative to open surgery. Laparoscopic techniques have potential benefits; they can decrease pain and blood loss, fewer complications, faster recovery, and shorter hospital length of stay (LOS) [15, 23]. Early experiences have shown that laparo-scopic pancreatic surgery is safe and feasible in selected patients, and that morbidity rates range from 16 to 40 % [24, 25]. Although a growing number of studies on laparoscopic pancreatic surgery have been published, it has not gained wide acceptance. This is probably explained by the known limitations of conventional laparoscopic surgery, such as the decreased range of motion this technique affords and the two-dimensional vision of the operative field, which make its practice difficult.

The use of a robotic system may overcome some of these shortcomings. Robot-assisted surgery provides three-dimensional vision and a magnified view of the operative field. These advantages, combined with the increased freedom of movement of surgical instruments and the elimination of tremor, lead to improved precision in operative technique and may lead to safer anastomoses compared with laparoscopic pancreatic surgery.

For highly selected patient, robotic PD is feasible with similar morbidity and mortality compared to open or purely laparoscopic approaches. Data on cost analysis are lacking, and further studies are needed to evaluate also the cost-effectiveness of the robotic approach for PD in comparison to open or laparoscopic techniques [26].

The emergence of minimally invasive surgery for liver resection procedures has thrived with the introduction of novel technologies, including flexible fiber-optic imaging systems, and hemostatic options, such as clips, staplers, and electrical or ultrasonic energy-induced hemostasis, and laparoscopic liver resection has been shown to be safe in experienced hands, with acceptable morbidity and mortality rates for both minor and major hepatic resections [27, 28]. Previous studies conducted on selected groups of patients have shown that the 5-year survival rates for patients undergoing laparoscopic HCC resection were comparable to those of patients undergoing open hepatic resection [28, 29]. The advantages of minimally invasive surgery are well known. Shorter hospital stays, decreased postoperative pain, rapid return to preoperative activity, improved cosmesis, and decreased postoperative ileus are among the benefits of the laparoscopic approach [27]. However, laparoscopic liver surgery, although it has benefitted from advances in minimally invasive surgery, is not without inherent limitations, including limited degrees of freedom for manipulation, fulcrum effect against the port, tremor amplification, awkward ergonomics, and two-dimensional imaging adaptation [4].

Robotic liver resection has emerged as a new modality in the field of minimally invasive surgery. However, the effectiveness of this approach for liver resection is not yet known. Robotic methods may have the potential to overcome certain laparoscopic disadvantages, but few studies have drawn a matched comparison of outcomes between robotic and laparoscopic liver resections. Tsung et al. published the largest series comparing robotic to laparoscopic liver resections. Patients undergoing robotic liver surgery had significantly longer operative times (median: 253 vs. 199 min) and overall room times (median: 342 vs. 262 min) compared with their laparoscopic counterparts. However, the robotic approach allowed for an increased percentage of major hepatectomies to be performed in a purely minimally invasive fashion (81 % vs. 7.1 %, $P<0.05$) [30].

Robotic and laparoscopic liver resection display similar safety and feasibility for hepatectomies. Although a greater proportion of robotic cases were completed in a totally minimally invasive manner, there were no significant benefits over laparoscopic techniques in operative outcomes [30]. The feasibility and safety of robotic surgery for HCC has been displayed in many studies, with favorable short-term outcome. However, the long-term oncologic results remain uncertain [31, 32]. In the subgroup analysis of minor liver resection, when compared with the conventional laparoscopic approach, the robotic group had similar blood loss, morbidity rate, mortality rate, and R0 resection rate. However, the robotic group had a significantly longer operative time (202.7 min vs. 133.4 min) [31].

Robotic liver resection is safe and feasible in experienced hands. It requires an expert patient-side surgeon with advanced laparoscopic skills. Wristed instruments are useful in a variety of maneuvers, such as looping Glissonian pedicles (especially on the left side of the liver) and in suturing bleeding points. Long-term oncologic

outcomes are unclear, but short-term perioperative results indicate that robotic liver resection is comparable to conventional laparoscopic liver resection [32].

In conclusion, many advanced surgical procedures benefit from a minimally invasive approach. Future assessments of the relative role of three-dimensional conventional laparoscopy versus robotic assistance are required to confirm the relative impact of the approaches on value-based surgical care. The impact of learning curve, adoption, and technical complications should be the measures used for these comparisons to ultimately define the cost efficiency of robotic-assisted laparoscopic surgery compared to conventional laparoscopy. Potential future cost savings for both hospitals and patients can be found in shorter operative times as surgeons complete their learning curves. This will also allow more procedures to be performed, which spreads the fixed costs of the robot over more patients. Also improved surgical technique coupled with shorter OR times could lead to even shorter hospital stays decreasing costs to patients and allowing for further revenue opportunities for hospitals.

Finally, as robotic technology expands its cost, just like the cost of all other technologies before it, will decrease over time with the inevitable advent of competitors in the market place. It may be this factor in the end that provides the greatest cost savings to both patients and hospitals, allowing more patients the indisputable benefits of minimally invasive surgery within an economically responsible framework.

22.4 Key Points

- The fixed (equipment and maintenance) and variable (instruments) costs for robotic surgery are higher than both conventional laparoscopic or open surgery.
- The OR costs of robotic surgery are negatively impacted by the increased length of the procedure over open surgery (though not necessarily over conventional laparoscopic surgery).
- When the total (fixed, variable, OR, and hospital stay) costs for robotic surgery and open surgery

are comparable, it is due to a considerable shortening of the length of hospital stay after the robotic surgery, resulting in total cost savings. However, these data are almost exclusively comparisons for moving from open to robotic.

- Conventional laparoscopic surgery shares the minimally invasive benefits of robotic surgery and is less expensive due to lower variable costs; however, there remain many procedures that the majority of surgeons are not able to perform laparoscopically due to the prohibitively long learning curve. This will need to be compelling data confirming that the learning curve and adoption rates for robotic assistance are superior to conventional laparoscopic surgery.

References

1. Reynolds Jr W. The first laparoscopic cholecystectomy. JSLS. 2001;5(1):89–94.
2. Bucher P, et al. Randomized clinical trial of laparoendoscopic single-site versus conventional laparoscopic cholecystectomy. Br J Surg. 2011;98(12):1695–702.
3. Idrees K, Bartlett DL. Robotic liver surgery. Surg Clin North Am. 2010;90(4):761–74.
4. Kitisin K, et al. A current update on the evolution of robotic liver surgery. Minerva Chir. 2011;66(4): 281–93.
5. Hyung WJ. Robotic surgery in gastrointestinal surgery. Korean J Gastroenterol. 2007;50(4):256–9.
6. Antoniou SA, et al. Robot-assisted laparoscopic surgery of the colon and rectum. Surg Endosc. 2012;26(1):1–11.
7. Falk V, et al. Influence of three-dimensional vision on surgical telemanipulator performance. Surg Endosc. 2001;15(11):1282–8.
8. Chen CC, Falcone T. Robotic gynecologic surgery: past, present, and future. Clin Obstet Gynecol. 2009;52(3):335–43.
9. Bolenz C, et al. Cost comparison of robotic, laparoscopic, and open radical prostatectomy for prostate cancer. Eur Urol. 2010;57(3):453–8.
10. Visco AG, Advincula AP. Robotic gynecologic surgery. Obstet Gynecol. 2008;112(6):1369–84.
11. Smith A, et al. Cost analysis of robotic versus open radical cystectomy for bladder cancer. J Urol. 2010; 183(2):505–9.
12. Satava RM. Robotics in colorectal surgery: telemonitoring and telerobotics. Surg Clin North Am. 2006; 86(4):927–36.
13. Lucas SM, Baber J, Sundaram CP. Determination of patient concerns in choosing surgery and preference for laparoendoscopic single-site surgery and assessment of satisfaction with postoperative cosmesis. J Endourol. 2012;26(6):585–91.
14. Memon S, et al. Robotic versus laparoscopic proctectomy for rectal cancer: a meta-analysis. Ann Surg Oncol. 2012;19(7):2095–101.
15. Schwenk W et al. Short term benefits for laparoscopic colorectal resection. Cochrane Database Syst Rev, 2005(3): p. CD003145.
16. Tyler JA, et al. Outcomes and costs associated with robotic colectomy in the minimally invasive era. Dis Colon Rectum. 2013;56(4):458–66.
17. Fung AK, Aly EH. Robotic colonic surgery: is it advisable to commence a new learning curve? Dis Colon Rectum. 2013;56(6):786–96.
18. Huettner F, et al. One hundred and two consecutive robotic-assisted minimally invasive colectomies—an outcome and technical update. J Gastrointest Surg. 2011;15(7):1195–204.
19. Deutsch GB, et al. Robotic vs. laparoscopic colorectal surgery: an institutional experience. Surg Endosc. 2012;26(4):956–63.
20. de Souza AL, et al. Robotic assistance in right hemicolectomy: is there a role? Dis Colon Rectum. 2010;53(7):1000–6.
21. Winter JM, et al. 1423 pancreaticoduodenectomies for pancreatic cancer: a single-institution experience. J Gastrointest Surg. 2006;10(9):1199–210. discussion 1210-1.
22. Kleeff J, et al. Distal pancreatectomy: risk factors for surgical failure in 302 consecutive cases. Ann Surg. 2007;245(4):573–82.
23. Keus F, Gooszen HG, van Laarhoven CJ. Open, small-incision, or laparoscopic cholecystectomy for patients with symptomatic cholecystolithiasis. An overview of Cochrane Hepato-Biliary Group reviews. Cochrane Database Syst Rev, 2010(1): p. CD008318.
24. Gumbs AA, et al. Laparoscopic pancreatoduodenectomy: a review of 285 published cases. Ann Surg Oncol. 2011;18(5):1335–41.
25. Gagner M, Palermo M. Laparoscopic Whipple procedure: review of the literature. J Hepatobiliary Pancreat Surg. 2009;16(6):726–30.
26. Cirocchi R, et al. A systematic review on robotic pancreaticoduodenectomy. Surg Oncol. 2013;22(4):238–46.
27. Reddy SK, Tsung A, Geller DA. Laparoscopic liver resection. World J Surg. 2011;35(7):1478–86.
28. Nguyen KT, Gamblin TC, Geller DA. World review of laparoscopic liver resection-2,804 patients. Ann Surg. 2009;250(5):831–41.
29. Tranchart H, et al. Laparoscopic resection for hepatocellular carcinoma: a matched-pair comparative study. Surg Endosc. 2010;24(5):1170–6.
30. Tsung A, et al. Robotic versus laparoscopic hepatectomy: a matched comparison. Ann Surg. 2014;259(3): 549–55.
31. Lai EC, Yang GP, Tang CN. Robot-assisted laparoscopic liver resection for hepatocellular carcinoma: short-term outcome. Am J Surg. 2013;205(6):697–702.
32. Ho CM, et al. Systematic review of robotic liver resection. Surg Endosc. 2013;27(3):732–9.

W. Conan Mustain and Bradley J. Champagne

Abstract

The use of robotic surgery has increased dramatically despite a paucity of data demonstrating clinical benefits of the technology. While the technical advantages of the da Vinci platform may facilitate a minimally invasive approach to difficult operations in confined spaces, many of the procedures for which it is being used could be accomplished more efficiently with conventional laparoscopy. Such is the case with segmental colectomy, where laparoscopic resection is quickly becoming the gold standard for benign and malignant disease. The da Vinci system may improve success rates of minimally invasive rectal resection, especially in select patients, but robotic colorectal surgery is not for everyone; not every patient and not every surgeon.

Keywords

Robotic • Colorectal • Total mesorectal excision • Cost-effective • Learning curve

23.1 Maintaining Perspective

The authors of this book have offered their collective knowledge and experience to provide the reader with a comprehensive guide to robotic colorectal surgery (RCS). While colorectal surgery may lag behind urology and gynecology in the widespread application of robotics, the very publication of this text is a testament to the growing interest in the technology. Anyone who has sat at the platform of the da Vinci Surgical System (Intuitive Surgical®, Inc., Sunnyvale, CA) can appreciate the technical advantages offered by the three-dimensional high-definition optics, stable camera platform, articulating instruments, and ergonomic interface. Surgeons with extensive experience in RCS report excellent clinical outcomes and an overwhelmingly

W.C. Mustain, M.D. • B.J. Champagne, M.D.,
F.A.C.S., F.A.S.C.R.S. (✉)
University Hospitals—Case Medical Center,
11100 Euclid Avenue, LKS-5047, Cleveland,
OH 446, USA
e-mail: William.Mustain@UHhospitals.org

© Springer International Publishing Switzerland 2015
H. Ross et al. (eds.), *Robotic Approaches to Colorectal Surgery*,
DOI 10.1007/978-3-319-09120-4_23

positive surgeon experience. There is great enthusiasm among surgeons and patients for increased access to robotic surgery.

While the technological advantages of robotic surgery may help overcome some shortcomings of conventional laparoscopy, it is important to realize that there is a relatively small number of procedures in which the "limitations" of laparoscopy are actually limiting. The benefits of the robot are best realized when working in confined spaces with limited visualization, particularly when precise movements and complex maneuvers such as suturing and knot tying are required. This explains the overwhelming application of the technology to prostatectomy, as well as its growing presence in otolaryngology and cardiac surgery, where other minimally invasive options are unavailable. In these cases, this highly sophisticated and expensive piece of medical technology may allow surgeons to offer minimally invasive procedures that would otherwise not be possible. Advocates of robotic surgery for rectal cancer suggest that total mesorectal excision (TME), particularly in a narrow male pelvis, is an example of such a procedure. On the contrary, cholecystectomy, hysterectomy, and segmental colectomy are routinely and efficiently performed laparoscopically with a high degree of success and excellent clinical outcomes. The growing application of robotics to procedures such as these calls into question the judgment of surgeons and hospital administrators alike. This situation is further complicated when "key opinion leaders" on robotic TME attempt to demonstrate advantages of the robot over routine laparoscopic colectomy. This perfunctory approach presents a credibility issue that may dampen the enthusiasm by all to adopt robotics for the difficult proctectomy, where it may truly be advantageous.

Before advocating for the expansion of RCS, we should review the facts. First, the use of the da Vinci robot has exploded across surgical specialties in recent years, largely driven by aggressive marketing. General surgery, including colorectal surgery, is one of the fastest growing segments of the robotic market. Secondly (contrary to sales pitches and marketing strategies) every aspect of robotic surgery, from the platform itself, to the service contract, to the instruments, is associated with a significant expense. As neither private nor public payers increase reimbursement for use of the robot, these costs are borne by the institution [1]. In some settings, this is countered by the ability to offer an otherwise unavailable operation, but often this is simply the price of being modern. Third, minimally invasive approaches to colorectal surgery have been utilized for over 20 years [2]. Laparoscopic colorectal surgery (LCS) has been proven to decrease length of stay, lower complication rates, and reduce hospital costs, while achieving equivalent oncologic outcomes [3–5]. The number of surgeons offering LCS is growing annually in community and teaching hospitals of all sizes [6]. Lastly, at present there are no large studies suggesting that RCS is associated with improved outcomes compared to conventional LCS. There may be a benefit of robotics in the treatment of rectal cancer, with recent studies showing lower conversion rates and similar oncologic outcomes for robotic TME compared to conventional laparoscopy [7, 8]. However, competent minimally invasive surgeons must resist the temptation of technology and the pressure from industry and administrators to use da Vinci for all colorectal resections, just because they can. We must maintain perspective.

23.1.1 Robotic Surgery is on the Rise

Sales of the da Vinci Surgical System and the prevalence of robotic surgery have increased dramatically in last decade. As of December 31, 2013 Intuitive Surgical had installed 2966 da Vinci systems in over 2000 hospitals worldwide, including 2083 units in the United States and 476 in Europe [9]. This is a more than threefold increase from the roughly 800 units installed by 2007 [10]. More striking is that 1166 of these units were sold in 2012 and 2013 alone. In the last 10 years, over 1.5 million operations worldwide have been conducted with the use of the da Vinci system [11]. In 2013, an estimated 523,000 robotic operations were performed, up 16 % compared to approximately 450,000 in 2012. This annual rate of growth was considered modest in light of the overall 155 % increase since 2009 [9, 10].

Historically, the most common applications of the robot have been in urology and gynecology. According to market share data from Intuitive Surgical, in 2011, 83 % of prostatectomies in the United States were performed robotically [11]. Since its approval for use in gynecology in 2005, da Vinci has become a commonly utilized platform for performance of benign hysterectomy. In a 6-year period, robotic hysterectomy has expanded to account for more than 25 % of the more than 600,000 hysterectomies performed annually in the United States [11, 12]. By comparison, over the same period the rate of laparoscopic hysterectomy remained stable at just over 35 %. In recent years, there has been a substantial increase in robotic use for abdominal procedures, including cholecystectomy, foregut surgery, and colorectal surgery. In 2013, general surgery overtook urology as the second most common category of da Vinci use in the United States [9].

The first robotic-assisted colectomy was described by Weber et al. in 2002 [13]. Prior to 2007 only five series of more than ten patients appeared in the literature, focused primarily on segmental colectomy [14–18]. Specific data on the current frequency of RCS are limited but a recent analysis of the Premier Hospital Database found that, for minimally invasive segmental colectomy performed between 2009 and 2011, the robotic approach was used for 548 out of 25,758 cases (2.1 %) [19]. In data from the US Nationwide Inpatient Sample, the robotic approach was used for 0.9 % of all segmental colectomies in 2010, but appears to be increasing at an exponential rate [20]. Based on the volume of publications in the literature, robotic TME for rectal cancer appears to be gaining more traction than robotic colectomy in recent years. Over 1000 robotic pelvic dissections for rectal cancer have been described in the literature, with rectal resections outpacing colon resections since 2008 [21, 22]. Clearly, robotic surgery is on the rise. The challenge is to remember that the robot is a highly sophisticated and very expensive tool, and not an exciting new toy. As such, not every operation, every surgeon, or even every hospital needs a robot.

23.1.2 The Robot Is Expensive

Perhaps the most consistent finding in the existing literature on the surgical robot is the significant increase in cost associated with its use. Turchetti et al. recently published a systematic review of the cost analysis literature on robotic vs. conventional laparoscopic surgery from 2000 to 2010 [23]. One hundred percent of the articles analyzed, covering eight different procedures from four different specialties, found the robotic approach to be significantly more expensive than conventional laparoscopy, despite most studies excluding the purchase and maintenance costs from their analyses. Regarding (RCS), Juo et al. recently reported data on segmental colectomy from the US Nationwide Inpatient Sample [20]. In a propensity score-matched cohort, robotic colectomy was associated with significantly higher per hospital day ($3407 vs. $2617) and total hospitalization cost ($14,847 vs. $11,966) than laparoscopic colectomy. Interestingly, patients treated by robotics were more likely to have private insurance and had a higher household income than patients treated by laparoscopic colorectal surgery or open colectomy.

Financial considerations of robotic surgery must include direct equipment costs, utilization costs, and revenue impact. Depending on the model and specifications, the da Vinci surgical system retails for between $1 and $2.5 million [23]. The cost of the system can be paid upfront or can be amortized over the first 3000–6000 procedures performed on the machine. In addition to the direct cost of the platform, Intuitive Surgical requires an annual service agreement ranging from $100,000 to $170,000 per year. The impact of these costs on an institution is often considered in light of the volume of robotic cases, where cost per case is calculated by dividing expenditures by number of robotic procedures performed. Lost in this equation, however, is the fact that no additional funds are collected on a per case basis when the robot is used, as Medicare and private insurers do not pay for a robot surcharge. Whether a hospital uses it for 5 cases or 500 cases, it will still pay roughly $3 million in the first 5 years to own a robot. Considering that in 2010, 131 of the hospitals in the United States with a da Vinci robot had 200 beds or fewer [24], these upfront costs may be impossible to overcome by any potential increases in market share or procedure volume.

Even if the price of purchase and maintenance of the robot is ignored, there is still a direct, measurable increase in cost per case due to consumables and utilization costs. The da Vinci system requires the use of proprietary, limited-use, disposable instruments, which are not covered under the service agreement. Intuitive Surgical reports that for 2013 instruments and accessories generated an average of $1980 in revenue per case, and over $1 billion annually [25], with future target revenue for instruments and accessories exceeding that of system and service revenue combined. Utilization costs associated with robotic surgery are difficult to calculate and variably reported, but most series report an increase in operating room times for robotic procedures compared to conventional laparoscopy owing to time spent docking and undocking the platform, as well as exchanging instruments [26–30]. Length of hospital stay has been reported to be shorter after robotic surgery compared with open surgery, but no different than conventional laparoscopy [20, 31]. Rates of postoperative complications and readmission are not significantly affected by use of the robot [18, 32–34]. The revenue impact of robot surgery must also be considered, including the effects on hospital volume, surgeon recruitment and retention, marketing, and public perception. These measures are difficult to calculate.

23.1.3 Minimally Invasive Colorectal Surgery Is Accomplished Well by Conventional Laparoscopy

LCS has been shown by multiple randomized controlled trials to be safe and effective, with improved short-term outcomes when compared to open surgery. The use of laparoscopy results in decreased pain, faster recovery, less blood loss, and improved lymph node harvest when compared to open surgery. Not surprisingly, as a result of these benefits, (LCS) is associated with fewer postoperative complications [4]. Furthermore, (LCS) is associated with shorter hospital stays and, despite higher per day costs, an overall reduction in hospital costs compared to open surgery [20]. Oncologic outcomes of laparoscopic resection for colorectal cancer have been proven to be equivalent to open surgery [35–37]. Consequently, (LCS) is now considered the gold standard for colon resection for benign and malignant disease.

After a prolonged period of adoption, met with some early resistance, the use of LCS is now steadily increasing. In the University Health System Consortium from 2008 to 2011, LCS was attempted in 42.2 % of colon resections, with a conversion rate of 15.8 %. During the study period, the rate of laparoscopic colon surgery increased, while the rate of open surgery and conversion decreased [6]. In 2010, the Nationwide Inpatient Sample reported 48.3 % of all segmental colectomies were performed laparoscopically [20]. General surgery resident experience with (LCS) has also increased dramatically in the last 10 years [38]. In a recent survey of graduating chief residents, 93 % reported feeling comfortable performing laparoscopic colectomy [39]. The American Board of Colon and Rectal Surgery and the Accreditation Council for Graduate Medical Education (ACGME) recently increased the minimum requirement for laparoscopic colorectal resections from twenty to fifty, though specific requirements for disease process and type of resection are still lacking. As current and future generations of trainees enter practice, the rate of (LCS) will continue to increase.

The learning curve for laparoscopic colectomy has been studied extensively with varying results. Most authors agree that roughly 50 cases are required for a surgeon to reach full proficiency [40–42]. Beyond this point, conversion rates and complications tend to reach a steady state, while ongoing reductions in operative time are realized with increased experience. The utilization of a hand-assist device may shorten the learning curve and permit performance of LCS in challenging and complex cases, while retaining the benefits of laparoscopy [43, 44]. Much as it did for cholecystectomy in the 1990s, laparoscopy is rapidly becoming the standard rather than the exception in segmental colectomy. In the era of value-based medicine, the use of expensive new technologies for procedures we already do well should be strongly discouraged in the absence of a proven benefit.

23.1.4 Data Showing Superiority of Robotics over Laparoscopy Are Lacking

The number and frequency of publications on RCS have increased dramatically in the last few years. The body of literature on RCS has grown from a few single-institution studies to include large meta-analyses [45–47], long-term oncologic follow-ups [8], and two, small randomized trials [48, 49]. Of more than 20 studies directly comparing robotics with LCS, only one has shown a significant reduction in complications with the use of robotics. In a series of 113 low anterior resection (56 robotic vs. 57 laparoscopic colorectal surgeries) Baik et al. [50] reported serious complications in 5.4 % of robotic vs. 19.3 % of laparoscopic resections ($P=0.025$). The authors also found that conversion to open surgery (0.0 % vs. 10.5 %, $P=0.013$) and mesorectal specimens graded as less than complete (7.1 % vs. 24.6 %, $P=0.033$) occurred less frequently in the robotic group. While this low conversion rate is impressive and may highlight the true benefit of RCS for low rectal dissections, nineteen other studies comparing RCS and laparoscopic colorectal surgery have failed to show a significant difference in conversion rates [51]. Furthermore, the serious complication rate of nearly twenty percent in the laparoscopic group is higher than expected in expert hands.

In the only prospective, randomized trial to date, Park et al. [49] examined short-term outcomes in 70 patients with right-sided colon cancer randomized to robotic and laparoscopic right colectomies. The authors reported no difference in conversion, pain scores, time to resumption of diet, length of stay, lymph node harvest, or morbidity between the two groups. Use of the robot was associated with statistically significant increases in operative time (195 min vs. 130 min, $P<0.001$) and total costs ($12,235 vs. $10,320, $P=0.013$). The authors concluded that RCS cannot be proposed as a routine approach for right colectomy.

23.2 The Right Place for the Robot

The primary advantages of the da Vinci system are realized in procedures confined to a small space where improved exposure and intricate movements are required. Most minimally invasive colorectal operations require operating in more than one region of the abdomen and typically do not require precision tasks like suturing and knot tying. For this reason, robotics offers little advantage in the minds of most advanced laparoscopists [52, 53]. The likely exception to this point may be for low rectal cancer in a male pelvis. As opposed to segmental colectomy, laparoscopic TME in a narrow male pelvis is technically challenging even to experienced laparoscopists. In the CLASICC trial, which included both colon and rectal resections, conversion rates for rectal cancer approached 35 %, with both male sex and rectal cancer identified as risk factors for conversion [54]. In the United States, a limited number of centers possess both a sufficient volume of rectal cancer and surgeons with advanced laparoscopic skills to consistently perform minimally invasive TME with low rates of conversion. The technological advantages offered by the da Vinci robotic system, especially the latest generation da Vinci Xi, may make the dissection slightly more favorable and allow completion of the dissection in difficult cases where conversion rates are highest. Any tool that improves our ability to offer a minimally invasive operation, especially in the most challenging low rectal cancers should be considered. Data to substantiate this theory of improved performance for low rectal cancer with robotic surgery is lacking but will likely be published over the next 5 years.

23.3 Is It for Everyone?

"Does the robot make sense for me?" is a difficult question asked by patients, surgeons, and hospital administrators alike. A discussion of the complex healthcare economics influencing a hospital or Accountable Care Organization's decision on whether or not to invest in a da Vinci robot is beyond the scope of this chapter. In today's climate, it is much less likely that a physician group will have to make a decision on the purchase of a robot, than on whether or not to incorporate the use of a hospital-owned robot into their practice. Surgeons with prior experience in robotics will likely be drawn to positions offering access to the da Vinci system. As organizations seek to maximize the use of their robots to offset the cost, surgeons may be encouraged or even pressured to acquire robotic training and begin using the system. With regard to (RCS), sound judgment is required to ensure that this expensive and specialized technology is utilized in a cost-effective manner, with an emphasis on quality rather than novelty. While each surgeon and circumstance is unique, we present four generalized, hypothetical surgeons who may be considering RCS, with our opinion on the appropriateness of RCS in their practices. In the sections that follow the term "colorectal surgeon" refers to a surgeon performing both colon and rectal resections, as opposed to one with specific board certification.

23.3.1 The Experienced Robotic Colorectal Surgeon

A surgeon who has had extensive experience with (RCS), who has already mastered the learning curve, will likely make meaningful use of the robot if given the opportunity. At present, a handful of surgical oncology fellowships and colorectal residencies at specialized centers offer trainees a significant exposure to robotic TME for rectal cancer. Surgeons trained in these programs will likely seek out or be recruited to institutions with easy access to the da Vinci system and are uniquely qualified to build high-volume robotic rectal cancer practices early in their careers. Based on fellowship training, these surgeons can assemble dedicated OR teams, streamline equipment pick sheets, and establish protocols to maximize efficiency. Similarly, a surgeon who has already developed a robust robotic rectal cancer practice will be able to transfer these skills to a new institution if necessary. It is practical for surgeons with this level of experience, when working in a hospital that already owns a robot, to use the technology for this specific purpose.

Though unlikely, it is possible that in centers performing a high volume of robotic TME the application of robotics to segmental colectomy may bear some consideration. If highly efficient systems are in place to streamline robotic surgery across the spectrum, it may become easier and more efficient to use the robot for colectomy than to switch to conventional laparoscopy on a case-by-case basis. Recognizing that this will result in a higher per-case cost to the institution, it may help to reinforce existing protocols and maximize efficiency of all robotic surgery across the institution. However, for the reasons already stated, we find it unlikely that an experienced and skilled laparoscopic surgeon will find any advantage in using the robot for routine colectomy.

23.3.2 The Experienced Laparoscopic Colorectal Surgeon

For experienced surgeons routinely performing both colon and rectal operations laparoscopically, the adoption of robotics should be strongly scrutinized prior to consideration. In the hands of an expert surgeon, LCS is extremely safe and highly efficient. With the refinements of modern laparoscopic instrumentation, the da Vinci system offers a few alluring features but little true advantage to proficient laparoscopic surgeons.

For these surgeons the robot may be safe and feasible, as well as fun and exciting, but it is certain to be more expensive and time-consuming than a procedure they already do quite well. Akin to the general surgeon using the robot to remove a gallbladder, we must be careful not to let the lure of a new toy drive us away from what already works.

This is not to say that experienced laparoscopists should not endeavor to familiarize themselves with the robot for its potential application to the difficult proctectomy. Virtually, all of the learning-curve data on RCS originate from surgeons with extensive LCS experience, who have an expectedly easier transition to robotic surgery than laparoscopic novices. These surgeons are familiar with the visualization and surgical anatomy of the pelvis and will likely experience an easy transition to robotic surgery for selected cases. An example is the obese male with a low rectal cancer, in whom the risk of conversion is high. Also, learning the da Vinci system may facilitate minimally invasive multivisceral resections when collaborating with urologists and gynecologists who are robotically proficient but lack advanced laparoscopic skills. However, unlike those surgeons who have chosen to make robotic TME their niche, the routine use of robotics by experts in LCS will likely result in significant increases in cost with no improvement in outcomes.

23.3.3 The Laparoscopic Colon Surgeon Doing Open Proctectomy

While the prevalence of laparoscopic colectomy is increasing dramatically, the majority of TME for rectal cancer is still done by open low anterior resection. Laparoscopic TME has been proven in multiple randomized controlled trials (RCTs) to have similar oncologic outcomes to open TME [55–57], while reducing blood loss, surgical site infections, and length of stay [58]. However, adoption of laparoscopy for rectal cancer has been slow in the United States, and the majority of TME is still performed in an open fashion. Many skilled pelvic surgeons who have adopted

and become proficient in laparoscopic colectomy, still manage rectal cancer by open TME due to the technical challenges of the operation. The confines of the narrow pelvis, the limitations of conventional laparoscopic instruments, and the lack of a capable assistant may all be factors in a surgeon's inability or unwillingness to offer laparoscopic TME. For these surgeons, the robot may provide the additional tools necessary to make the jump to minimally invasive pelvic surgery. The ability to offer a previously unavailable, minimally invasive approach to proctectomy will benefit patients in terms of postoperative pain, faster return to work, and lower perioperative complications, but may also benefit the hospital by reducing length of stay and eventually increasing volume of referrals. In this setting, the robot is a tool, which is complementary to the open and laparoscopic skills the surgeon already possesses and can help fill a specific need. We believe this scenario is one in which robotic surgery has the greatest potential to provide a meaningful benefit.

23.3.4 The Laparoscopic Colectomy Novice

Surgeons who perform exclusively open colectomy and little or no pelvic surgery may view the robot as a way to ease the transition to minimally invasive colectomy. However, unlike in the pelvis, where the challenges of tight confines, steep angles, and limited visualization can be overcome by the advantages of the robot, minimally invasive colectomy requires broad, sweeping movements in a larger, more dynamic field. In this setting the shortcomings of the robot, particularly the lack of tactile feedback and physical isolation from the bedside assistant, make it a dangerous tool in the hands of an inexperienced operator. For those surgeons with good laparoscopic skills interested in transitioning to minimally invasive colectomy, other options exist beyond the expensive and potentially hazardous leap to robotics. A number of laparoscopic colectomy "mini-fellowships" are offered around the country every year, as well as courses at many of the major surgical meetings. For those with a lower comfort level with laparoscopy, the use of a hand-assist device may provide a more comfortable bridge between open and laparoscopic colectomy. By providing greater tactile feedback, hand-assist shortens the learning curve for LCS and has been found to result in lower conversion rates as well as shorter operative times than conventional laparoscopy [59, 60]. Regardless of the specific technique, we agree with most authors that a surgeon should acquire advanced laparoscopic skills before transitioning to the robot [61].

23.4 When Is the Right Time to Learn?

Our belief is that RCS is primarily indicated for challenging rectal resections in the hands of well-trained laparoscopic surgeons with a high degree of comfort with open TME. If this is to be the place of the robot in colorectal surgery, it is worth considering who should learn to use the robot and when. Studies show a high degree of comfort with LCS among graduating general surgery residents. Certainly, there is no reason why LCS should be restricted to those with specialized postgraduate training. The widespread adoption of LCS by general surgeons will be beneficial to society as a whole as more patients will experience the benefits of this proven technique. On the contrary, RCS is a specialized technical approach for a specific subset of patients best treated by surgeons with a dedicated interest in complex pelvic surgery.

With the implementation of duty hour restrictions and the 80-h workweek, efforts must be made to maximize the operative experience in general surgery residency. The total operative volume of graduating residents has been on the decline and the comfort level with more complex procedures has suffered as a result. Many subspecialties have opted for integrated programs to allow residents to narrow their focus at an earlier point in training and optimize the resident experience. As such, we believe there is no role for training in RCS during general surgery residency. While some exposure to the technology may facilitate a resident's understanding of relevant anatomy and dissection planes, high volumes of RCS in residency will likely produce a trained bedside assistant who has less operative experience as the result of lost time.

The 1-year residency in colorectal surgery is designed to instruct fully trained general surgeons in the comprehensive, expert care of diseases of the colon and rectum. With the advent of laparoscopy, advanced endoscopic techniques, biologic therapies for IBD, high-resolution anoscopy, and other advanced technologies, the ability of training programs to successfully accomplish this goal has been tested. The core essentials of colorectal surgery (high quality TME, surgical management of IBD, and complex anorectal disease) are just as important today as they were 30 years ago, but now must be taught alongside newer treatments in fewer man-hours. Not every colorectal surgeon will become a high-volume robotic rectal cancer surgeon, but every colorectal surgeon should be an expert laparoscopist. For this reason, we feel that the mandatory incorporation of RCS into training programs for colorectal surgery should be strongly discouraged. Some training programs, many of them home to the authors of this book, perform high volumes of RCS. Trainees of these programs will benefit from the expertise of their mentors, but program directors must be attentive that other essential skills are not overlooked by overemphasis on this specific technique.

We believe the ideal time for training in RCS is after colorectal residency, once a solid foundation of high-quality pelvic surgery and LCS has been developed. At that point, surgeons who feel that the robot may improve their ability to offer minimally invasive rectal resection may seek specific training on the da Vinci platform. In a recent publication, Melich et al. [62] examined the learning curve of just such a surgeon, with fellowship training in open and laparoscopic surgery, who adopted the use of robotics for TME at the beginning of his academic career. This thorough review of Dr. Byung Soh Min's detailed personal records provides an intricate, albeit anecdotal, look into the learning curve of robotic TME for a well-trained colorectal surgeon.

In his first ten cases, robotic TME took significantly longer than laparoscopic, by nearly 2 hours. This was primarily attributable to longer extracorporeal time (port placement, docking, anastomosis, and closure) and slower splenic flexure mobilization. Inferior mesenteric artery (IMA) dissection and pelvic dissection times were only slightly longer at the outset. With increased experience, all phases of the operation became faster in both approaches, with the exception of extracorporeal time for laparoscopy. After 40 cases, operative times of robotic TME had dropped below that of laparoscopic, primarily due to a 60 % reduction in extracorporeal time. IMA dissection and splenic flexure mobilization times became similar between the techniques, becoming more efficient as case volume increased. At roughly 50 cases, the time required for pelvic dissection became significantly shorter with the robotic approach and has remained so throughout his experience. Conversion rates were low with both approaches and no significant difference in complications was observed.

Not every general surgery or colorectal residency is the same. Faculty members at various institutions have different interests and levels of expertise, which will invariably influence the experience of their trainees. As the number of surgeons trained in robotic surgery increases, exposure to RCS during training will likewise increase. However, with a limited time in which to master the ever-expanding "fundamentals" of their craft, general surgery and colorectal surgery residents must be strategically placed so as to maximize the number of procedures in which they are confident and competent. We feel that a heavy emphasis on robotics at any level of training may be sacrificing fundamentals in favor of flash. We believe that the ideal scenario is that in which a surgeon who has mastered the anatomy and the technique of open TME, who has a foundation in LCS, applies these skills to the simultaneous development of laparoscopic and robotic skills for minimally invasive proctectomy. A surgeon with this foundation can expect successful outcomes and rapid progression with both approaches and will be equipped to utilize either approach as a tool toward accomplishing the goal of providing minimally invasive cancer care.

23.5 Summary

The da Vinci surgical system is a technologically advanced surgical platform that may facilitate the minimally invasive performance of technically demanding operations in challenging anatomic locations. Despite this specialized indication, this sophisticated and costly equipment is increasingly being utilized for procedures that are routinely performed by conventional laparoscopy. In the realm of colorectal surgery, the difficulty encountered in performing laparoscopic TME for rectal cancer is a potential opportunity for improvement with the use of the surgical robot. Enthusiasm for the use of robotics across the spectrum of colorectal surgery must be tempered by a careful consideration of the current state of RCS. To put things in perspective, the use of robotic surgery is growing exponentially, driven largely by aggressive marketing on behalf of the manufacturer. The da Vinci robot is very expensive and its use adds significant costs to any operation. LCS is a safe and efficient approach to benign and malignant diseases of the colon and rectum, and current data do not support an improvement in outcomes with the use of robotic surgery. Training in RCS and application of the technology should be restricted to experienced pelvic surgeons with a fundamental grasp of laparoscopy, seeking to improve their success with minimally invasive rectal resection. The robot is not for everyone; the use of robotics for segmental colectomy and the requirement of mandatory robotic training during colorectal residency are not appropriate at this time.

23.6 Key Points

- The use of robotic surgery is increasing rapidly across multiple specialties, despite significantly higher costs and a lack of clinical evidence showing superiority to conventional laparoscopic techniques.
- Laparoscopic colorectal surgery is widely practiced and is associated with excellent clinical and oncologic outcomes. Use of the surgical robot has not been shown to improve clinical

outcomes compared to laparoscopic colorectal surgery and is associated with increased cost.

- TME for rectal cancer is a technically challenging operation in a confined location, which may benefit from the improved visualization and precision movements provided by the da Vinci surgical system.

- Use of the da Vinci robot may facilitate completion of minimally invasive surgery for rectal cancer in specialized centers, where a high-volume practice may justify the cost of the technology.

- Dedicated training in robotic colorectal surgery is best undertaken during or after colorectal fellowship by surgeons with a specific interest in minimally invasive rectal cancer surgery. Mandatory incorporation of robotic training into colorectal fellowship is not appropriate at this time.

References

1. Lotan Y. Is robotic surgery cost-effective: no. Curr Opin Urol. 2012;22(1):66–9.
2. Jacobs M, Verdeja JC, Goldstein HS. Minimally invasive colon resection (laparoscopic colectomy). Surg Laparosc Endosc. 1991;1(3):144–50.
3. Clinical Outcomes of Surgical Therapy Study G. A comparison of laparoscopically assisted and open colectomy for colon cancer. N Engl J Med. 2004;350(20): 2050–9.
4. Kennedy GD, Heise C, Rajamanickam V, Harms B, Foley EF. Laparoscopy decreases postoperative complication rates after abdominal colectomy: results from the national surgical quality improvement program. Ann Surg. 2009;249(4):596–601.
5. Fleshman J, Sargent DJ, Green E, Anvari M, Stryker SJ, Beart Jr RW, et al. Laparoscopic colectomy for cancer is not inferior to open surgery based on 5-year data from the COST Study Group trial. Ann Surg. 2007;246(4):655–62. discussion 62-4.
6. Simorov A, Shaligram A, Shostrom V, Boilesen E, Thompson J, Oleynikov D. Laparoscopic colon resection trends in utilization and rate of conversion to open procedure: a national database review of academic medical centers. Ann Surg. 2012;256(3):462–8.
7. D'Annibale A, Pernazza G, Monsellato I, Pende V, Lucandri G, Mazzocchi P, et al. Total mesorectal excision: a comparison of oncological and functional outcomes between robotic and laparoscopic surgery for rectal cancer. Surg Endosc. 2013;27(6):1887–95.
8. Park EJ, Cho MS, Baek SJ, Hur H, Min BS, Baik SH, et al. Long-term oncologic outcomes of robotic low anterior resection for rectal cancer: a comparative study with laparoscopic surgery. Ann Surg. 2015; 261(1):129–37.
9. Annual Report 2013 [press release]. Intuitive Surgical, Inc.
10. Barbash GI, Glied SA. New technology and health care costs—the case of robot-assisted surgery. N Engl J Med. 2010;363(8):701–4.
11. Available from http://www.davincisurgery.com/facts. php.
12. Dubeshter B, Angel C, Toy E, Thomas S, Glantz JC. Current Role of robotic hysterectomy. J Gynecol Surg. 2013;29(4):174–8.
13. Weber PA, Merola S, Wasielewski A, Ballantyne GH. Telerobotic-assisted laparoscopic right and sigmoid colectomies for benign disease. Dis Colon Rectum. 2002;45(12):1689–94. discussion 95-6.
14. Giulianotti PC, Coratti A, Angelini M, Sbrana F, Cecconi S, Balestracci T, et al. Robotics in general surgery: personal experience in a large community hospital. Arch Surg. 2003;138(7):777–84.
15. Anvari M, Birch DW, Bamehriz F, Gryfe R, Chapman T. Robotic-assisted laparoscopic colorectal surgery. Surg Laparosc Endosc Percutan Techniq. 2004;14(6): 311–5.
16. DeNoto G, Rubach E, Ravikumar TS. A standardized technique for robotically performed sigmoid colectomy. J Laparoendosc Adv Surg Techniq Part A. 2006; 16(6):551–6.
17. Rawlings AL, Woodland JH, Crawford DL. Telerobotic surgery for right and sigmoid colectomies: 30 consecutive cases. Surg Endosc. 2006; 20(11):1713–8.
18. D'Annibale A, Morpurgo E, Fiscon V, Trevisan P, Sovernigo G, Orsini C, et al. Robotic and laparoscopic surgery for treatment of colorectal diseases. Dis Colon Rectum. 2004;47(12):2162–8.
19. Davis BR, Yoo AC, Moore M, Gunnarsson C. Robotic-assisted versus laparoscopic colectomy: cost and clinical outcomes. JSLS. 2014;18(2):211–24.
20. Juo YY, Hyder O, Haider AH, Camp M, Lidor A, Ahuja N. Is minimally invasive colon resection better than traditional approaches?: First comprehensive national examination with propensity score matching. JAMA Surg. 2014;149(2):177–84.
21. Baek SK, Carmichael JC, Pigazzi A. Robotic surgery: colon and rectum. Cancer J. 2013;19(2):140–6.
22. Papanikolaou IG. Robotic surgery for colorectal cancer: systematic review of the literature. Surg Laparosc Endosc Percutan Techniq. 2014;24(6):478–83.
23. Turchetti G, Palla I, Pierotti F, Cuschieri A. Economic evaluation of da Vinci-assisted robotic surgery: a systematic review. Surg Endosc. 2012;26(3):598–606.
24. Carreyrou J. Surgical robot examined in injuries. Wall Street J. 2010 May 4, 2010.
25. Intuitive Surgical I. Investor Presentation Q3 2014. 2014.

26. Morino M, Beninca G, Giraudo G, Del Genio GM, Rebecchi F, Garrone C. Robot-assisted vs. laparoscopic adrenalectomy: a prospective randomized controlled trial. Surg Endosc. 2004;18(12):1742–6.

27. Heemskerk J, van Dam R, van Gemert WG, Beets GL, Greve JW, Jacobs MJ, et al. First results after introduction of the four-armed da Vinci Surgical System in fully robotic laparoscopic cholecystectomy. Digest Surg. 2005;22(6):426–31.

28. Morino M, Pellegrino L, Giaccone C, Garrone C, Rebecchi F. Randomized clinical trial of robot-assisted versus laparoscopic Nissen fundoplication. Br J Surg. 2006;93(5):553–8.

29. Rawlings AL, Woodland JH, Vegunta RK, Crawford DL. Robotic versus laparoscopic colectomy. Surg Endosc. 2007;21(10):1701–8.

30. Sarlos D, Kots L, Stevanovic N, Schaer G. Robotic hysterectomy versus conventional laparoscopic hysterectomy: outcome and cost analyses of a matched case-control study. Eur J Obstet Gynecol Reprod Biol. 2010;150(1):92–6.

31. Bolenz C, Gupta A, Hotze T, Ho R, Cadeddu JA, Roehrborn CG, et al. Cost comparison of robotic, laparoscopic, and open radical prostatectomy for prostate cancer. Eur Urol. 2010;57(3):453–8.

32. Park JS, Choi GS, Lim KH, Jang YS, Jun SH. Robotic-assisted versus laparoscopic surgery for low rectal cancer: case-matched analysis of short-term outcomes. Ann Surg Oncol. 2010;17(12):3195–202.

33. Baek SJ, Kim SH, Cho JS, Shin JW, Kim J. Robotic versus conventional laparoscopic surgery for rectal cancer: a cost analysis from a single institute in Korea. World J Surg. 2012;36(11):2722–9.

34. Helvind NM, Eriksen JR, Mogensen A, Tas B, Olsen J, Bundgaard M, et al. No differences in short-term morbidity and mortality after robot-assisted laparoscopic versus laparoscopic resection for colonic cancer: a case-control study of 263 patients. Surg Endosc. 2013;27(7):2575–80.

35. Lacy AM, Garcia-Valdecasas JC, Delgado S, Castells A, Taura P, Pique JM, et al. Laparoscopy-assisted colectomy versus open colectomy for treatment of nonmetastatic colon cancer: a randomised trial. Lancet. 2002;359(9325):2224–9.

36. Veldkamp R, Kuhry E, Hop WC, Jeekel J, Kazemier G, Bonjer HJ, et al. Laparoscopic surgery versus open surgery for colon cancer: short-term outcomes of a randomised trial. Lancet Oncol. 2005;6(7):477–84.

37. Bonjer HJ, Hop WC, Nelson H, Sargent DJ, Lacy AM, Castells A, et al. Laparoscopically assisted vs open colectomy for colon cancer: a meta-analysis. Arch Surg. 2007;142(3):298–303.

38. Alkhoury F, Martin JT, Contessa J, Zuckerman R, Nadzam G. The impact of laparoscopy on the volume of open cases in general surgery training. J Surg Educ. 2010;67(5):316–9.

39. Friedell ML, VanderMeer TJ, Cheatham ML, Fuhrman GM, Schenarts PJ, Mellinger JD, et al. Perceptions of graduating general surgery chief residents: are they confident in their training? J Am Coll Surg. 2014;218(4):695–703.

40. Li JC, Hon SS, Ng SS, Lee JF, Yiu RY, Leung KL. The learning curve for laparoscopic colectomy: experience of a surgical fellow in an university colorectal unit. Surg Endosc. 2009;23(7):1603–8.

41. Li JC, Lo AW, Hon SS, Ng SS, Lee JF, Leung KL. Institution learning curve of laparoscopic colectomy—a multi-dimensional analysis. Int J Colorectal Dis. 2012;27(4):527–33.

42. Kayano H, Okuda J, Tanaka K, Kondo K, Tanigawa N. Evaluation of the learning curve in laparoscopic low anterior resection for rectal cancer. Surg Endosc. 2011;25(9):2972–9.

43. Loungnarath R, Fleshman JW. Hand-assisted laparoscopic colectomy techniques. Semin Laparosc Surg. 2003;10(4):219–30.

44. Yang I, Boushey RP, Marcello PW. Hand-assisted laparoscopic colorectal surgery. Techniq Coloproctol. 2013;17 Suppl 1:S23–7.

45. Memon S, Heriot AG, Murphy DG, Bressel M, Lynch AC. Robotic versus laparoscopic proctectomy for rectal cancer: a meta-analysis. Ann Surg Oncol. 2012;19(7):2095–101.

46. Lin S, Jiang HG, Chen ZH, Zhou SY, Liu XS, Yu JR. Meta-analysis of robotic and laparoscopic surgery for treatment of rectal cancer. World J Gastroenterol. 2011;17(47):5214–20.

47. Yang Y, Wang F, Zhang P, Shi C, Zou Y, Qin H, et al. Robot-assisted versus conventional laparoscopic surgery for colorectal disease, focusing on rectal cancer: a meta-analysis. Ann Surg Oncol. 2012;19(12):3727–36.

48. Baik SH, Ko YT, Kang CM, Lee WJ, Kim NK, Sohn SK, et al. Robotic tumor-specific mesorectal excision of rectal cancer: short-term outcome of a pilot randomized trial. Surg Endosc. 2008;22(7):1601–8.

49. Park JS, Choi GS, Park SY, Kim HJ, Ryuk JP. Randomized clinical trial of robot-assisted versus standard laparoscopic right colectomy. Br J Surg. 2012;99(9):1219–26.

50. Baik SH, Kwon HY, Kim JS, Hur H, Sohn SK, Cho CH, et al. Robotic versus laparoscopic low anterior resection of rectal cancer: short-term outcome of a prospective comparative study. Ann Surg Oncol. 2009;16(6):1480–7.

51. Kim CW, Kim CH, Baik SH. Outcomes of robotic-assisted colorectal surgery compared with laparoscopic and open surgery: a systematic review. J Gastrointest Surg. 2014;18(4):816–30.

52. Pucci MJ, Beekley AC. Use of robotics in colon and rectal surgery. Clin Colon Rectal Surg. 2013;26(1):39–46.

53. Satava RM. Robotics in colorectal surgery: telemonitoring and telerobotics. Surg Clin North Am. 2006;86(4):927–36.

54. Thorpe H, Jayne DG, Guillou PJ, Quirke P, Copeland J, Brown JM, et al. Patient factors influencing conversion from laparoscopically assisted to open surgery for colorectal cancer. Br J Surg. 2008;95(2):199–205.

55. Laurent C, Leblanc F, Wutrich P, Scheffler M, Rullier E. Laparoscopic versus open surgery for rectal cancer: long-term oncologic results. Ann Surg. 2009;250(1): 54–61.

56. Kang SB, Park JW, Jeong SY, Nam BH, Choi HS, Kim DW, et al. Open versus laparoscopic surgery for mid or low rectal cancer after neoadjuvant chemoradiotherapy (COREAN trial): short-term outcomes of an open-label randomised controlled trial. Lancet Oncol. 2010;11(7):637–45.

57. Jayne DG, Thorpe HC, Copeland J, Quirke P, Brown JM, Guillou PJ. Five-year follow-up of the Medical Research Council CLASICC trial of laparoscopically assisted versus open surgery for colorectal cancer. Br J Surg. 2010;97(11): 1638–45.

58. Vennix S, Pelzers L, Bouvy N, Beets GL, Pierie JP, Wiggers T, et al. Laparoscopic versus open total mesorectal excision for rectal cancer. Cochrane Database Systematic Rev. 2014;4: CD005200.

59. Marcello PW, Fleshman JW, Milsom JW, Read TE, Arnell TD, Birnbaum EH, et al. Hand-assisted laparoscopic vs. laparoscopic colorectal surgery: a multicenter, prospective, randomized trial. Dis Colon Rectum. 2008;51(6):818–26.

60. Moloo H, Haggar F, Coyle D, Hutton B, Duhaime S, Mamazza J, et al. Hand assisted laparoscopic surgery versus conventional laparoscopy for colorectal surgery. Cochrane Database Syst Rev 2010(10): CD006585.

61. Bokhari MB, Patel CB, Ramos-Valadez DI, Ragupathi M, Haas EM. Learning curve for robotic-assisted laparoscopic colorectal surgery. Surg Endosc. 2011; 25(3):855–60.

62. Melich G, Hong YK, Kim J, Hur H, Baik SH, Kim NK, et al. Simultaneous development of laparoscopy and robotics provides acceptable perioperative outcomes and shows robotics to have a faster learning curve and to be overall faster in rectal cancer surgery: analysis of novice MIS surgeon learning curves. Surg Endosc. 2015;29(3):558–68.

Index

© Springer International Publishing Switzerland 2015
H. Ross et al. (eds.), *Robotic Approaches to Colorectal Surgery*,
DOI 10.1007/978-3-319-09120-4

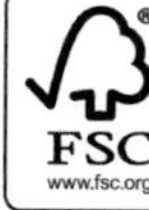

MIX
Papier aus verantwortungsvollen Quellen
Paper from responsible sources
FSC® C105338

If you have any concerns about our products,
you can contact us on
ProductSafety@springernature.com

In case Publisher is established outside the EU,
the EU authorized representative is:
Springer Nature Customer Service Center GmbH
Europaplatz 3, 69115 Heidelberg, Germany

Printed by Libri Plureos GmbH
in Hamburg, Germany